ANNUAL REVIEW
OF NURSING RESEARCH

Volume 24, 2006

Annual Review
of Nursing Research

Volume 24, 2006

Focus on Patient Safety

JOYCE J. FITZPATRICK, PhD, RN, FAAN
Series Editor

PATRICIA W. STONE, PhD, MPH, RN
PATRICIA HINTON WALKER, PhD, RN, FAAN
Volume Editors

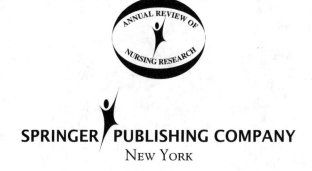

SPRINGER PUBLISHING COMPANY
NEW YORK

To purchase copies of other volumes of the *Annual Review of Nursing Research* at 10% off the list price, go to www.springerpub.com/ARNR.

Copyright © 2007 Springer Publishing Company, LLC

Springer Publishing Company, LLC
11 West 42nd Street, 15th Floor
New York, NY 10036

Acquisitions Editor: Sally J. Barhydt
Managing Editor: Mary Ann McLaughlin
Project Manager: Joanne Bowser
Cover Design: Joanne E. Honigman
Composition: Techbooks

07 08 09 10/5 4 3 2 1

ISBN-0-8261-4136-6
ISSN-0739-6686

ANNUAL REVIEW OF NURSING RESEARCH is indexed in *Cumulative Index to Nursing and Allied Health Literature* and *Index Medicus*.

Printed in the United States of America by Bang Printing

Contents

Contributors

Carol Dean Baker, RN, MSN
Assistant Professor
Georgia College & State University
Macon, Georgia

Suzanne Bakken, RN, DNSc, FAAN
The Alumni Professor of Nursing and
   Professor of Biomedical
   Informatics
Columbia University School of
   Nursing
New York, New York

Mary A. Blegen, RN, PhD, FAAN
Professor and Director
Center for Collaboration in Patient
   Safety
School of Nursing, University of
   California–San Francisco
San Francisco, California
Formerly Professor and Associate
   Dean for Research
School of Nursing
University of Colorado at Denver and
   Health Sciences
Denver, Colorado

Gaya Carlton, MS, RN
Doctoral Student
School of Nursing
University of Colorado at Denver and
   Health Sciences
Denver, Colorado

Jill Scott-Cawiezell, PhD, RN
Assistant Professor
Sinclair School of Nursing
University of Missouri-Columbia
Columbia, Missouri

Sean P. Clarke, PhD, RN, CRNP
Center for Health Outcomes and
   Policy Research
School of Nursing
University of Pennsylvania
Philadelphia, Pennsylvania

Leanne M. Currie, DNSc
Assistant Professor of Nursing
Columbia University School of
   Nursing
New York, New York

**Josephine Hegarty, PhD, MSc, BSc,
   RGN**
Senior Lecturer
School of Nursing and Midwifery
National University of Ireland
   (University College Cork)
Cork, Ireland

**Rodney W. Hicks, MSN, MPA,
   ARNP**
Research Coordinator
Center for the Advancement of
   Patient Safety
United States Pharmacopeia
Rockville, Maryland

Patricia Hinton Walker, PhD, RN, FAAN
Dean and Professor
Graduate School of Nursing
Uniformed Services University of the Health Sciences
Bethesda, Maryland

Lela Holden, MSN, RN
Colonel, United States Air Force
Chief Nurse Executive
55th Medical Group, Ehrling Bergquist Clinic
Offutt Air Force Base
Omaha, Nebraska

Karen Dorman Marek, PhD, MBA, RN, FAAN
Associate Professor
UW-Milwaukee College of Nursing
Milwaukee, Wisconsin

Geraldine McCarthy, PhD, MSN, Med, RGN
Professor of Nursing
Catherine McAuley School of Nursing and Midwifery
Brookfield Health Sciences Complex
National University of Ireland (University College Cork)
Cork, Ireland

Elizabeth Merwin, PhD, RN, FAAN
Associate Dean for Research
University of Virginia School of Nursing
Charlotte, Virginia

Dawn O'Sullivan, BSc, RGN
Research Assistant
School of Nursing and Midwifery
National University of Ireland (University College Cork)
Cork, Ireland

Ann Marie B. Peterson, RN, BS, MS, CNS
CNS Nursing Department, NIH Clinical Center
National Institutes of Health
Bethesda, Maryland
and Doctoral Student
Graduate School of Nursing
Uniformed Services University of the Health Sciences
Bethesda, Maryland

Patricia W. Stone, PhD, MPH, RN
Assistant Professor
Columbia University School of Nursing
New York, New York

Deirdre Thornlow, MN, RN
Doctoral Student
School of Nursing
University of Virginia
Charlotte, Virginia

Amy Vogelsmeier, MSN, RN, BC, GCNS
John A. Hartford Foundation
2005–2007 Building Academic Geriatric Nursing Capacity Scholar
and Doctoral Student
Sinclair School of Nursing
University of Missouri–Columbia
Columbia, Missouri

Linda J. Wanzer, MSN, RN, CNOR
Colonel, United States Army Nurse Corps
Director, Perioperative Clinical Nurse Specialist Program and Doctoral Student
Graduate School of Nursing
Uniformed Services University of the Health Sciences
Bethesda, Maryland

Preface

Patient safety is one of the most important topics in health care literature today. It also represents a rapidly developing research area for both nurse scientists and other health care researchers, and, based on the problems addressed, it is necessarily interdisciplinary in nature. In this 24th volume of the *Annual Review of Nursing Research*, the editors and contributors examine research on key aspects of patient safety.

In Chapter 1, the volume editors, Patricia W. Stone and Patricia Hinton Walker, and two co-authors, Gaya Carlton and Lela Holden, present the conceptual organization for the volume, including attention to the context of patient safety research and the terminology found in the literature. Included in this introductory chapter is discussion of the work of the Institute of Medicine (IOM) and the shaping of the patient safety research agenda by the Agency for Health-care Research and Quality (AHRQ).

The patient safety content of this volume is organized into five sections. Part I is the introduction that gives a brief history of the patient safety movement and discusses Reason's theory of human error. Part II, Patient Safety Indicators, includes three chapters, each highlighting a different nursing-sensitive patient safety indicator. Gaya Carlton and Mary A. Blegen address medication errors in Chapter 2, Leanne M. Currie reviews fall and injury prevention research in Chapter 3, and Ann Marie B. Peterson and Patricia Hinton Walker present the review of hospital-acquired infections in Chapter 4. In each of these chapters, authors briefly address the historic research on the particular topic while focusing the majority of their work on recent research.

Part III of this volume focuses on setting-specific patient safety research (e.g., hospitals, home health, and long-term care). In Chapter 5, Mary A. Blegen presents a discussion of the research related to patient safety in acute care units in hospitals, including important issues of staffing and educational preparation of providers. In Chapter 6, Linda J. Wanzer and Rodney W. Hicks focus their review on the peri-operative environment, including same-day surgery, the pre-operative holding area, the operating room (including anesthesia), and postanesthesia care units. In Chapter 7, Karen Dorman Marek and Carol Dean Baker highlight the patient safety research related to home visit programs for the elderly, including attention to patient satisfaction and quality of life. Chapter 8, authored by Jill Scott-Cawiezell and Amy Vogelsmeier, addresses the research related to patient safety in nursing homes; this chapter includes attention to issues of organizational teamwork, communication, and leadership.

Part IV includes chapters related to emerging issues in patient safety. Chapter 9, Informatics for Patient Safety, is authored by Suzanne Bakken; Sean P. Clarke looks at organizational climate and culture factors in Chapter 10. In Chapter 11, Elizabeth Merwin and Deirdre Thornlow address methodologies used in nursing research to improve patient safety, including survey research, secondary data analysis, observation, measurement, provider-focused research, and qualitative methods.

Part V of this volume includes a chapter on international nursing research. In Chapter 12, Geraldine McCarthy, Josephine Hegarty, and Dawn O'Sullivan provide an historical analysis of nursing research in Ireland. Included in this analysis are studies on clinical practice, nursing management, professional issues, and nursing education.

As in previous volumes, we are indebted to a number of contributors who have made this work possible. First, we thank the Advisory Board, who first suggested this topic for a volume more than 5 years ago; we are pleased that it has come to fruition. Second, we thank the volume editors and chapter authors in this volume for contributing their expertise to the disciplinary and interdisciplinary literature on patient safety. And finally, our deepest thanks go to our readers for nearly a quarter-century of continued support for the *Annual Review of Nursing Research* series.

Joyce J. Fitzpatrick, PhD, RN, FAAN
Series Editor

PART I

Introduction

Chapter 1

The Intersection of Patient Safety and Nursing Research

Patricia Hinton Walker, Gaya Carlton, Lela Holden, and Patricia W. Stone

ABSTRACT

The individual and collective discussions of the patient safety issue in the United States have mounted from a low roar to a deafening din in the past 10 years. In this chapter the authors (1) discuss the context of patient safety over the past decade and the federal response to the problem, (2) briefly present Reason's theory of human error, which frames much of the safety research, and (3) provide a glossary of terms.

Keywords: patient safety, nursing

The individual and collective discussions of the patient safety issue in the United States have mounted from a low roar to a deafening din in the past 10 years (Cullen, Bates, & Leape, 2000; Leape, 2005; Leape, 1994). This is fortunate because this complex issue, with its many facets, has considerable human and financial costs and, as such, can no longer be ignored. In this chapter the authors (1) discuss the context of patient safety over the past 10 years and the federal response to the problem, (2) briefly present Reason's theory of human error, which frames much of the safety research, and (3) provide a glossary of terms.

Federal organizations, including the Institute of Medicine (IOM) and the Agency for Healthcare Research and Quality (AHRQ) (Hickman, Severance, & Feldstein, 2003; Classen, Pestotnik, Evans, Lloyd, & Burke, 1997) as well as the Veterans' Administration and the Department of Defense (2006), are heavily invested in articulating the range of patient safety concerns and identifying solutions. The publications produced in recent years by the IOM in particular formulate a powerful framework from which to investigate patient safety in general and its more precise components (Institute of Medicine, 1996; Institute of Medicine, 2000; Institute of Medicine, 2001; Institute of Medicine, 2004).

The major work that captured the scope of errors and their effect on patients in the United States was the IOM's book *To Err Is Human* (2001), which included reference to the landmark research known as the Harvard Medical Practice Study. This research was the first of its kind to highlight population estimates of adverse events, both unavoidable as well as due to negligence. Researchers conducted a retrospective, random review of 30,121 records from 51 randomly selected acute care, nonpsychiatric hospitals in New York State in 1984. An adverse event was defined as an unintended injury that was caused by medical management and that resulted in measurable disability. The findings were staggering; Adverse events occurred in 3.7% of the hospitalizations, with 1.7% (13,451) resulting in death within New York hospitals in 1984. In addition, 27.6% of the adverse events were evaluated as due to negligence (Brennan & Leape, 1991). These results have been reported extensively in health care literature ever since. However, the actual numbers of deaths related to patient safety errors has been disputed and there are resulting calls for better information systems to help understand the problem more fully (Kopec, Levy, Kabir, Reinharth, & Shagas, 2005). The extrapolation of these results to the more than 33 million admissions in U.S. hospitals implies that tens of thousands die annually from medical errors, which makes it the eighth-leading cause of death, surpassing cancer or motor vehicle accidents (Institute of Medicine, 2000).

Drug-related adverse events were reported in the second part of the Harvard Medical Practice Study (Leape et al., 1991). The incidence of adverse drug events (ADEs) accounted for 19% of the total adverse events, and 18% of that number were considered related to negligence, defined as failure to meet the standard of care reasonably expected of an average physician qualified to take care of the patient. An ADE is defined as an injury resulting from medical intervention involving a drug. In addition, in recent years, the annual deaths associated with medication errors alone was estimated to be 7,391, which represented a 2.57-fold increase from 1983 to 1993 (Phillips, Christenfeld, & Glynn, 1998).

The IOM's next major publication about patient safety, *Crossing the Quality Chasm* (Institute of Medicine, 2001), again compiled the research data and offered suggestions for finding a way forward. This publication added intensity and focus to the discussion on patient safety by recommending six aims for establishing 21st century health care: safety followed by effective, patient-centered, timely, efficient, and equitable health care. The IOM also stressed that health care should be "evidence-based . . . and systems-oriented" (p. 20). Part of this publication included a comprehensive literature review that captured significant research on topics ranging from immunizations to preventable deaths. The section about ADEs was exemplified by researchers who examined 4,031 adult admissions to two tertiary care hospitals over a 6-month period in a prospective design that compared intensive care units (ICUs) and non-ICUs selected from a stratified random sample (Cullen et al., 1997). The rate of ADEs in ICUs was 19 events per 1,000 patient days, twice as high as the 10 events per 1,000 days in the non-ICUs. These data reinforced earlier research that sicker patients are more likely to experience an ADE (Avorn, 1997).

A third IOM patient safety report directly examined the critical role of nurses in relationship to patient safety (Institute of Medicine, 2004). Nursing actions, such as ongoing assessment of patients' health status, are directly related to better outcomes (Mitchell & Shortell, 1997). Nursing vigilance also defends patients against errors. A study of medication errors in two hospitals over a 6-month period found that nurses were responsible for intercepting 86% of all medication errors made by physicians, pharmacists, and others involved in providing medications for patients before the error reached the patient (Leape et al., 1995). To this end, the IOM concluded that defenses must be created in all organizational components: (1) leadership and management, (2) the workforce, (3) work processes, and (4) organizational culture. Further, there is indication that working conditions that promote patient safety also will provide a safer work environment for employees (DeJoy, Gershon, Murphy, & Wilson, 1996; McGee, 1999; Institute of Medicine, 2000; Lin, Ahern, Gershon, & Grimes, 1998; DeJoy, Searcy, Murphy, & Gershon, 2000). Because the health care workplace has been identified as a high-risk environment, this is an important consideration, and efforts to improve the health and safety of health care workers are needed (Gershon, 1985; Gershon, Vlahov, Kelen, Conrad, & Murphy, 1995; Guastello, Gershon, & Murphy, 1999). In particular, two types of occupational hazards are prevalent in health care workers: musculoskeletal injuries and needlestick injuries (Centers for Disease Control and Prevention, 2000; Stone, 2004).

These reports from the IOM and several significant large-scale descriptive studies, in the early- to mid-1990s, captured the scope and the gravity of the problem of safety. The literature from this period also captured and espoused a new way of thinking about errors using a systems framework of "no blame, no shame" (Vicente, 2003). The consensus is now strong and passionately expressed that a new paradigm is needed to reduce the tragic cost in human and financial terms of preventable medical errors. Specifically, excessive emphasis on the individual and much less emphasis on the systems components of health care is no longer adequate as a framework for conceptualizing safety and error and especially for finding solutions that work over the long term.

In 2001, the AHRQ was designated by Congress (along with other federal agencies) to provide leadership in implementing the country's research response to the 1999 IOM report on medical errors. As a result of this charge by Congress, AHRQ developed an agenda for patient safety research and has subsequently awarded $50 million in grants, contracts, and other activities for the purpose of reducing medical errors and improving patient safety. This appropriation represents the single largest investment made by the federal government in patient safety (www.ahrq.gov/qual/pscongrpt/psinisum.htm).

Leaders at AHRQ also established a Center for Quality Improvement and Safety that, as a result, has become the leader of patient safety education, dissemination of best practices, and development of standards and measures (Leape, Berwick, & Bates, 2002; Leape & Berwick, 2005). This federal agency was charged with the development of the research agenda and with $50 million in funding made available by the 107th Congress as a response to the IOM report on patient safety, awarded 94 new grants and contracts and conducted other activities to fund research as follows:

- Supporting demonstration projects to report medical errors data—24 projects at $24.7 million for
  —studying different methods of collecting data on errors
  —analyzing data already collected to identify factors that put patients at risk for medical errors
- Using computers and information technology (IT) to prevent medical errors
  —22 projects at $5.3 million for development and testing of the use of computers and IT to
  —reduce medical errors
  —improve patient safety
  —improve quality of care
- Understanding the effect of working conditions on patient safety
  —Eight projects at $3 million to examine how the following affect health care and patient safety:
  —staffing
  —fatigue

—stress
—sleep deprivation
—issues studied in aviation and manufacturing
- Developing innovative approaches to improving patient safety
  —23 projects at $8 million to research and develop
    —innovative approaches to improve patient safety
    —geographically diverse locations across nationwide
- Disseminating research results
  —Seven projects at $2.4 million to
    —educate clinicians and others about the results of patient safety research
    —seek new approaches to improve provider education
    —develop curricula, continuing education, and simulation models
    —provide other provider training strategies
- Additional patient safety research initiatives
  —Remaining $6.4 million for 10 other projects, including
    —supporting meetings of state and local officials
    —advance local patient safety initiative

In each of the succeeding fiscal years since the initial funding, AHRQ continued to devote millions of dollars of its budget to patient safety research, although since 2004 the majority of funds have been earmarked for IT implementation and research.

REASON'S APPROACH FRAMES PATIENT SAFETY RESEARCH

A cognitive psychologist has helped frame and articulate the new paradigm related to patient safety. James Reason added clarity by specifying the differences between slips and lapses and those of mistakes (Reason, 1997; Reason, 1990). The former constitute errors in execution, and the latter are errors in planning. The basic premise of Reason's approach is that humans are fallible and errors are to be expected, even within the best organizations. Errors are viewed as consequences rather than causes having their origins in "upstream" systemic factors rather than in the perversity of human nature. Such systemic factors include recurrent error traps in the workplace and organizational processes that allow error occurrence. Countermeasures are based on the assumption that although human condition cannot be changed, conditions under which humans work can. Central to the system approach is the idea that all hazardous technologies (e.g., airline industry, nuclear plants, space program) employ barriers and safeguards (i.e., system defenses) against error. When an adverse event occurs, it is important to determine how and why the defenses failed, not who blundered.

Reason illustrated system accidents using a Swiss cheese model where slices of cheese are lined up on a trajectory and represent barriers and safeguards. In an ideal world, each slice would be intact; however, in reality they have many holes continually opening, closing, and shifting location, representing opportunity for error. The presence of holes in any one slice does not usually result in a bad outcome, but when many slices momentarily line up to permit a trajectory of accident opportunity, errors may occur. Holes in the defenses arise for two reasons: active failures and latent conditions. Most adverse events involving a combination of the two. Active failures are defined as unsafe acts committed by people in direct contact with the system or patient and are in the form of slips, lapses, fumbles, mistakes, and procedural violations. Active failures have a direct and generally short-lived effect on the integrity of the defenses or barriers.

In addition, Reason (1997) articulated the difference between active and latent errors, an important distinction that is referenced by those who espouse a systems approach to safety. Active errors are those at the "sharp end" of the system and are the result of actions or violations that have a direct effect and usually in an immediate but short-lived manner. These active errors occur at the human-system interface and tend to be unique to a specific event. By contrast, latent conditions often offer compelling explanation for errors that go beyond issues related to the individual and are part of the system. Latent conditions are defined as inevitable "resident pathogens" within the system. James Reason (1997) explains:

> Latent conditions are to technological organizations what resident pathogens are to the human body. Like pathogens, latent conditions—such as poor design, gaps in supervision, undetected manufacturing defects or maintenance failures, unworkable procedures, clumsy automation, shortfalls in training, less than adequate tools and equipment—may be present for many years before they combine with local circumstances and active failures to penetrate the system's many layers of defenses . . . They arise from strategic and other top-level decisions . . . and the impact of these decisions spreads through the organization, shaping a distinctive corporate culture and creating error-producing factors within individual workplaces. (p. 10)

Errors may arise from decisions made by builders, designers, top level management, and procedural writers. So they may not themselves be mistakes, but all strategic decisions have the potential to introduce pathogens into the system. Latent conditions in turn consist of two kinds of adverse effects: error-provoking conditions within the workplace (e.g., time pressure, fatigue, understaffing, inadequate equipment, inexperience) and long-lasting holes or weaknesses in the defenses (e.g., untrustworthy alarms and indicators, design and construction deficiencies, unworkable procedures). Either of these may lie dormant for years before combining with active failures to create opportunity for error. Latent conditions can be identified and corrected before adverse events occur, as opposed to active failures, whose forms often are difficult to foresee. This understanding enables proactive management of latent conditions rather than reactive risk management (Reason, 1997).

Reason goes on to explain (1997) that latent conditions are present in all systems and often are related to resource allocation. In addition, latent conditions may lie dormant for a long time until conditions are such that the interaction with local circumstances defeats the organization's defenses and generates errors. Finally, unlike the sharp-end interface with active errors, latent conditions generally arise from the upper echelons and infrastructure of organizations.

The paradigm and mantra of systems thinking now pervade the medical and nursing (Leape & Fromson, 2006; Pape, 2003; Pape, 2001). Researchers built numerous descriptive summaries, poignant anecdotes, and analytical discussions on Reason's work to emphasize that systems failures usually precede medical errors. For example, if two drugs are packaged in an almost identical manner and are placed close to each other, a health care professional will, no doubt, eventually get confused and administer the wrong drug. Such packaging and placement are systems problems. These researchers all advanced the understanding of error in health care from 1990 to the early 2000s. There is broad recognition that errors are an inevitable component of human activities, including health care, and can be managed appropriately even if never eliminated. Learning how to manage errors more appropriately requires acknowledging that medical errors are not the result of ignorance, malice, laziness, or greed on the part of individuals or organizations. If meaningful medical cultural change is to occur, it must be based on the realization that error is a matter of "system flaws, not character flaws" (Leape, 1994, p. 1857).

In summary, the gravity of ADEs has been firmly established in the medical and nursing literature since the early 1990s, and a more sophisticated framework in terms of systems has been implanted. A basic, fundamental groundwork has been laid in the nursing research, even if the designs are not impressive in their rigor. The one study that is quasi-experimental in design is a step forward from the descriptive level of research to identify management interventions that have the potential for improving patient outcomes and safety (Pape, 2001). As always, more information is needed.

GLOSSARY OF PATIENT SAFETY TERMS

As issues related to medical errors are discussed, it is important to have a consistent vocabulary to help health care professionals categorize errors and adverse events. Categorizing and classifying errors and adverse events provides a structured way to ensure that when anyone talks about an error, he or she is not really discussing an adverse event. To help clarify the need for a structured term set related to patient safety, examine the word "error." Most leading safety experts agree that an error is an unintended act, either of omission or commission, or an act that does not achieve its intended outcome. Not all errors result in an adverse event or injury. For example, a medication may be administered late, but there may not be any negative outcomes for the patient. Therefore, it should not be classified as an ADE.

For data collection purposes and clinical improvement efforts, the categorizing of an error as an adverse event could result in inaccurate data collection. Of more concern is that improvement efforts could be focused on the wrong problem or issues. Clarity and preciseness of terminology and definitions provides a basis for understanding and comparability for clinicians and researchers.

The First Consulting Group has prepared a patient safety glossary in collaboration with the VHA Inc., to help clinicians, researchers, and others understand and use consistent vocabulary related to patient safety issues (Association of peri Operative Registered Nurses, 2006). This vocabulary was developed by patient safety experts and reflects the latest research and expert opinion on the topic and given to the contributing authors of this volume. To conserve space, we have listed only one definition for each term here. Feedback about this vocabulary can be sent to the Association of peri Operative Registered Nurses (research@aorn.org). Those comments, feedback, and suggestions will be provided to the First Consulting Group.

Accident—An event that involves damage to a defined system that disrupts the ongoing or future output of the future.

Active error—An error that occurs at the level of the frontline operator and whose effects are felt almost immediately.

Active failure—An error that is precipitated by the commission of errors and violations. These are difficult to anticipate and have an immediate adverse impact on safety by breaching, bypassing, or disabling existing defenses.

Adverse drug event (ADE)—An injury resulting from the use of a drug.

Adverse drug reaction (ADR)—A response to a drug which is noxious and unintended, and which occurs at doses normally used in man for the prophylaxis, diagnosis, or therapy of disease, or for the modification of physiological function.

Adverse event—An injury caused by medical management rather than the underlying condition of the patient.

Compliance error—Inappropriate resident behavior regarding adherence to a prescribed medication regimen.

Deteriorated drug error—Administration of a medication when the physical or chemical integrity of the dosage form has been compromised, such as expired medications, medications not properly stored, or medications requiring refrigeration that are left out at room temperature.

Dispensing error—The failure to dispense a medication upon physician order (omission error) or within a specified period of time from receipt of the medication order or reorder (time error); dispensing the incorrect drug, dose, dosage form; failure to dispense correct amount of medication; inappropriate, incorrect, or inadequate labeling of medication; incorrect or inappropriate preparation, packaging, or storage of medication prior to dispensing; dispensing of expired, improperly stored, or physically or chemically compromised medications.

Error—The failure of a planned action to be completed as intended (i.e., error of execution) or the use of a wrong plan to achieve an aim (i.e., error of planning).

Error of commission—An error that occurs as a result of an action taken. Examples include when a drug is administered at the wrong time, in the wrong dosage, or using the wrong route; surgeries performed on the wrong side of the body; and transfusion errors involving blood cross-matched for another patient.

Error of omission—An error which occurs as a result of an action not taken, for example, when a delay in performing an indicated cesarean section results in a fetal death, when a nurse omits a dose of a medication that should be administered, or when a patient suicide is associated with a lapse in carrying out frequent patient checks in a psychiatric unit. Errors of omission may or may not lead to adverse outcomes. (Also see "Omission Error.")

Extra dose error—The administration of duplicate doses to a resident or administration of one or more dosage units in addition to those that were ordered. May include administration of a medication dose after the order was discontinued (which also could be considered an "Unauthorized Drug Error").

Injury—Untoward harm occurring to a patient.

Latent error—Errors in the design, organization, training, or maintenance that lead to operator errors and whose effects typically lie dormant in the system for lengthy periods of time.

Latent failure—An error that is precipitated by a consequence of management and organizational processes and poses the greatest danger to complex systems. Latent failures cannot be foreseen but, if detected, they can be corrected before they contribute to mishaps.

Medication error—Any preventable event that may cause or lead to inappropriate medication use or patient harm, while the medication is in the control of the health care professional, patient, or consumer.

Monitoring errors—Failure to review a prescribed regimen for appropriateness, or failure to use appropriate clinical or laboratory data for adequate assessment of resident response to prescribed therapy.

Omission error—The failure to administer an ordered dose to a resident by the time the next dose is due, assuming there has been no prescribing error. Exceptions would include a resident's refusal to take the medication and failure to administer the dose because of recognized contraindications. (Also see "Error of Omission.")

Potential adverse drug event—An incident with potential for injury related to a drug.

Potential adverse event—An error of medical management that does not result in injury ("near misses").

Potential error—A mistake in prescribing, dispensing, or planned medication administration that is detected and corrected through intervention before actual medication administration.

Prescribing error—The inappropriate selection of a drug (based on indication, contraindications, known allergies, existing drug therapy, and other factors); dose; dosage form; quantity; route of administration; concentration; rate of administration; or inappropriate or inadequate instructions for use of a medication ordered by a physician or other authorized prescriber.

Preventable adverse drug event—An ADE due to an error or preventable by any means currently available.

Preventable adverse event—An adverse event attributable to an error.

Safety—Freedom from accidental injury.

Sentinel event—An unexpected occurrence involving death or serious physical or psychological injury, or the risk thereof. Serious injury specifically includes loss of limb or function. The phrase "or the risk thereof" includes any process variation for which a recurrence would carry a significant chance of a serious adverse outcome. Such events are called "sentinel" because they signal the need for immediate investigation and response.

Type A—[ADEs] that are related to a drug's pharmacological characteristics and are usually dose-dependent, predictable, and preventable.

Type B—[ADEs] that are idiosyncratic or allergic in nature and are not dose-dependent or related to a drug's pharmacological characteristics.

Unauthorized drug error—The administration of a medication to a resident for which the physician did not write an order. This category includes a dose given to the wrong resident, dose given that was not ordered, administration of the wrong drug or a discontinued drug, and doses given outside a stated set of clinical parameters or protocols.

Unpreventable adverse drug event—An adverse [drug] event that is not attributable to an error

Unpreventable adverse event—An adverse event that is not attributable to an error.

Wrong administration technique error—Use of an inappropriate procedure or improper technique in the administration of a drug. Examples of wrong technique errors include incorrect manipulation of inhalers, failure to maintain sanitary technique with medications, not wiping an injection site with alcohol, failure to use proper technique when crushing medications, failure to check nasogastric tube placement or flushing NG tube before and after administration of medication, failure to wash hands or improper hand washing technique used.

Wrong dosage form error—The administration of a medication in a dosage form different from the one that was ordered by the prescriber. This could include crushing a tablet prior to administration without an order from the prescriber.

Wrong dose error—When the resident receives an amount of medication that is greater than or less than the amount ordered by the prescriber.

Wrong drug preparation error—A medication incorrectly formulated or manipulated before administration, such as incorrect or inaccurate dilution or reconstitution, failure to shake suspensions, crushing medications that should not be crushed, mixing drugs that are physically or chemically incompatible, and inadequate product packaging.

Wrong rate error—The incorrect rate of administration of a medication to a resident. May occur with intravenous fluids or liquid enteral products.

Wrong route error—The administration of a medication to a resident by a route other than that ordered by the physician or doses administered via the correct route but at the wrong site (eg, left eye instead of right eye).

Wrong time error—The failure to administer a medication to a resident within a predefined interval from its scheduled administration time. This interval should be established by each facility and clearly stated in the facility's policies. Different intervals may be established for different drugs or drug classes, based on the therapeutic importance of dosing.

REFERENCES

Association of periOperative Registered Nurses (2006). *Glossary of Patient Safety Terms. Association of periOperative Registered Nursing.* Retrieved 10/10/2005 from www.patientsafetyfirst.org/Information_Resources/Glossary.asp

Avorn, J. (1997). Putting adverse drug events into perspective. *Journal of the American Medical Association, 277,* 341–342.

Brennan, T. A. & Leape, L. L. (1991). Adverse events, negligence in hospitalized patients: Results from the Harvard Medical Practice Study. *Perspectives in Healthcare Risk Management, 11*, 2–8.

Centers for Disease Control and Prevention (CDC). (2000). *Worker Health Chartbook, 2000.* Cincinnati, OH: NIOSH-Publications Dissemination.

Classen, D. C., Pestotnik, S. L., Evans, R. S., Lloyd, J. F., & Burke, J. P. (1997). Adverse drug events in hospitalized patients. Excess length of stay, extra costs, and attributable mortality. *Journal of the American Medical Association, 277*, 301–306.

Cullen, D. J., Bates, D. W., & Leape, L. L. (2000). Prevention of adverse drug events: A decade of progress in patient safety. *Journal of Clinical Anesthesia, 12*, 600–614.

Cullen, D. J., Sweitzer, B. J., Bates, D. W., Burdick, E., Edmondson, A., & Leape, L. L. (1997). Preventable adverse drug events in hospitalized patients: A comparative study of intensive care and general care units. *Critical Care Medicine, 25*, 1289–1297.

DeJoy, D. M., Gershon, R. R., Murphy, L. R., & Wilson, M. G. (1996). A work-systems analysis of compliance with universal precautions among health care workers. *Health Education Quarterly, 23*, 159–174.

DeJoy, D. M., Searcy, C. A., Murphy, L. R., & Gershon, R. R. (2000). Behavioral-diagnostic analysis of compliance with universal precautions among nurses. *Journal of Occupational Health Psychology, 5*, 127–141.

Gershon, R. R. (1985). Sharps handling. *Journal of Healthcare Material Management, 3*, 111–114.

Gershon, R. R., Vlahov, D., Kelen, G., Conrad, B., & Murphy, L. (1995). Review of accidents/injuries among emergency medical services workers in Baltimore, Maryland. *Prehospital and Disaster Medicine, 10*, 14–18.

Guastello, S. J., Gershon, R. R., & Murphy, L. R. (1999). Catastrophe model for the exposure to blood-borne pathogens and other accidents in health care settings. *Accidental Analysis and Prevention, 31*, 739–749.

Hickman, D., Severance, S., & Feldstein, A. (2003). *The effect of health care working conditions on patient safety.* (Rep. No. 74). Rockville, MD: Agency for Healthcare Research and Quality.

Institute of Medicine (2004). *Keeping patients safe: Transforming the work environment of nurses.* Washington, DC: National Academy Press.

Institute of Medicine (1996). *Nursing staff in hospitals and nursing homes: Is it adequate?* Washington, DC: National Academy Press.

Institute of Medicine (2000). *To err is human: Building a safer health system.* Washington, DC: National Academy Press.

Institute of Medicine (2001). *Crossing the quality chasm: A new health system for the 21st century.* Washington, DC: National Academy Press.

Kopec, D., Levy, K., Kabir, M., Reinharth, D., & Shagas, G. (2005). Development of an expert system for classification of medical errors. *Studies in Health Technology and Informatics, 114*, 110–116.

Leape, L. L. (1994). Error in medicine. *Journal of the American Medical Association, 272*, 1851–1857.

Leape, L. L. (2005). Ethical issues in patient safety. *Thoracic Surgery Clinics, 15*, 493–501.

Leape, L. L., Bates, D. W., Cullen, D. J., Cooper, J., Demonaco, H. J., Gallivan, T., et al. (1995). Systems analysis of adverse drug events. ADE Prevention Study Group 64. *Journal of the American Medical Association, 274*, 35–43.

Leape, L. L. & Berwick, D. M. (2005). Five years after *To Err Is Human:* What have we learned? *Journal of the American Medical Association, 293*, 2384–2390.

Leape, L. L., Berwick, D. M., & Bates, D. W. (2002). What practices will most improve safety? Evidence-based medicine meets patient safety. *Journal of the American Medical Association, 288*, 501–507.

Leape, L. L., Brennan, T. A., Laird, N., Lawthers, A. G., Localio, A. R., Barnes, B. A., et al. (1991). The nature of adverse events in hospitalized patients. Results of the Harvard Medical Practice Study II. *New England Journal of Medicine, 324*, 377–384.

Leape, L. L. & Fromson, J. A. (2006). Problem doctors: Is there a system-level solution? *Annals of Internal Medicine, 144*, 107–115.

Lin, M. Y., Ahern, J. E., Gershon, R. R., & Grimes, M. (1998). The use of total quality improvement techniques to determine risk factors for back injuries in hospital workers. *Clinical Performance and Quality Health Care, 6*, 23–27.

McGee, J. (1999). ANA leads effort to protect nurses and patients. *Imprint, 46*, 37–38.

Mitchell, P. H. & Shortell, S. M. (1997). Adverse outcomes and variations in organization of care delivery. *Medical Care, 35*, NS19–NS32.

Pape, T. M. (2001). Searching for the final answer: factors contributing to medication administration errors. *Journal of Continuing Education in Nursing, 32*, 152–160.

Pape, T. M. (2003). Applying airline safety practices to medication administration. *Medsurg Nursing, 12*, 77–93.

Phillips, D. P., Christenfeld, N., & Glynn, L. M. (1998). Increase in US medication-error deaths between 1983 and 1993. *Lancet, 351*, 643–644.

Reason, J. (2000). Human error: Models and management. *West Journal of Medicine, 172*, 393–396.

Reason, J. (1997). *Managing the risks of organizational accidents.* Burlington, VT: Ashgate.

Reason, J. (1990). *Human Reason.* Cambridge: Cambridge University Press.

Stone, P. W. (2004). Nurses' Working Conditions: Implications for Infectious Disease. *Emerging Infectious Diseases, 10*, 1984–1989.

U.S. Department of Defense Patient Safety Program. (2006). Retrieved 1/15/2006 from www.afip.org/PSC/

Vicente, K. J. (2003). What does it take? A case study of radical change toward patient safety, 5. *Joint Commission Journal on Quality and Patient Safety, 29*, 598–609.

PART II

Patient Safety
Indicators

Chapter 2

Medication-Related Errors: A Literature Review of Incidence and Antecedents

Gaya Carlton and Mary A. Blegen

ABSTRACT

Patient safety has become a major concern for both society and policymakers. Since nurses are intimately involved in the delivery of medications and are ultimately responsible during the medication administration phase, it is important for nursing to understand factors contributing to medication administration errors. The purpose of this chapter is to identify the incidence of these errors and the associated factors in an attempt to better understand the problem and lessen future error occurrence. Literature review revealed both active failures and latent conditions established in Reason's theory remain prevalent in current literature where active failures often display themselves in the form of incorrect drug calculations, lack of individual knowledge, and failure to follow established protocol. Latent conditions are evidenced as time pressures, fatigue, understaffing, inexperience, design deficiencies, and inadequate equipment and may lie dormant within a system until combined with active failures to create opportunity for error. Although medication error research has shifted in emphasis toward identification of system problems inherent in error occurrence, no one force emerges as a clear antecedent, reinforcing the need for further research and replication of existing studies with emphasis placed on more dependable reporting measures through which nurses are not threatened by reprisal.

Keywords: patient safety, nursing, medication-related errors

Patient safety has become a major concern for both society and policymakers. This concern has been fueled in part by news coverage of individuals injured by serious adverse events and by the publication in 1999 of the Institute of Medicine's report *To Err Is Human: Building a Safer Health System* (Agency for Healthcare Research and Quality, 2001, July). Focus on safety by the Joint Commission on Accreditation of Healthcare Organizations has also created public awareness that errors have a large and unacceptable effect on cost and public confidence (Batcheller, Burkman, Armstrong, Chappell, & Carelock, 2004). Patient injuries resulting from drug therapy are among the most common types of hospital adverse patient events (Leape et al., 1991). Because nurses are intimately involved in and ultimately responsible for the delivery of medications, they must understand the factors that contribute to medication administration errors. The purpose of this paper is to identify the incidence of these errors and the associated factors in an attempt to better understand the problem and lessen future error occurrence.

Several terms associated with drug-related errors exist in the literature, and their amplification is necessary to clearly understand current research and the discussion that follows. While adverse drug events (ADEs)—injuries resulting from medical intervention related to a drug—include both appropriate and inappropriate use of a drug (Bates et al., 1995), medication errors—including prescribing errors, monitoring errors, patient noncompliance, dispensing errors, and administration errors (Wakefield, Wakefield, Holman, & Blegen, 1996)—are considered inappropriate. Medication administration errors further narrow the term *medication errors* by circumscribing errors that occur when the patient actually received or was supposed to have received a medication. These errors are generally associated with nursing actions and include errors of both commission and omission. Errors of commission occur when medication administration violates one or more of the five rights of medication administration: right patient, right drug, right dose, right time, and right route. Also included are drugs administered to patients with known allergies. Errors of omission, on the other hand, occur when a patient does not receive a medication that was ordered (Wakefield et al., 1999).

Several studies suggest that approximately one-third to one-half of ADEs are preventable (Bates et al., 1995; Bates, Leape, & Petrycki, 1993; Classen, Pestotnik, Evans, Lloyd, & Burke, 1997). ADE rates varied from 2.4 to 6.5 per 100 admissions among hospitals conducting ADE studies (Bates et al., 1995; Classen et al., 1997) and resulted in prolonged length of stay, increased economic burden, and increased risk of death (Classen et al., 1997). More than 770,000 people are estimated to be injured or die each year in U.S. hospitals as a direct result of ADEs (Classen et al., 1997). This, consequently, results in losses well into the million dollar range for individual hospitals (Bates et al., 1997; Classen et al., 1997). Using U.S. Department of Health and Human Services mortality data (i.e., death certificates), Phillips, Christenfeld, and Glynn (1998) estimated that medication errors accounted for 7,391 deaths nationally in 1993, a 2.57-fold increase over the 1983 reporting of 2,876 deaths. By 1993, one out of every 131 outpatient deaths and one out of 854 inpatients deaths were attributed to medication errors.

Although medication errors are multidisciplinary in nature, occurring anywhere along the health care continuum from ordering a medication through administration, the majority of actual and potential medication errors have been attributed to physician ordering, with the second largest group being nurse administration (Bates et al., 1995; Cullen et al., 1997; Douglas & Larrabee, 2003; Leape et al., 1995). In particular, a medication error study conducted by Leape et al. (1995) of 11 medical surgical units in two tertiary care hospitals over a 6-month period revealed that of 334 medication errors, 39% occurred during physician ordering, 38% during nurse administration, with the remaining 23% equally divided between pharmacy dispensing errors and transcription errors. Because nurses actually administer medications, they often assume, or are assigned, responsibility for these errors even though everyone involved in the system of medication delivery and the system itself are contributors (Wakefield, Wakefield, Holman, & Blegen, 1998).

METHODOLOGY

Antecedents of medication administration errors and the incidence of error were identified by conducting a literature review specifically focusing on medication administration errors. The review was conducted by searching the following databases: Cumulative Index to Nursing and Allied Health Literature, Journals @ Ovid Full Text, and Ovid Medline. Key words used in the search process were *medication errors, medication administration errors, adverse drug events, medication administration error reporting, medication error reporting, adverse drug event reporting, incident reports,* and *adverse event reports.* Additional literature was identified by reviewing the reference lists of journal articles identified during the literature review. In addition, known authors of literature about ADEs, medication error, medication administration error, workplace error and error reporting were used as search terms.

LITERATURE REVIEW

Medication administration is often viewed as a routine and basic nursing task when in reality it "reflects a complex interaction of a large number of specific decisions and actions, often performed under less than ideal conditions" (Wakefield et al., 1996, p. 191). Because of this complexity in the medication administration process, much more potential for error exists (Wakefield et al., 1998). In addition, medication administration is a high-frequency nursing activity, raising the potential for medication-related errors as the average number of drugs administered increases (Institute of Medicine, 1999). The following review outlines incidence of medication errors and specific antecedents as identified in the literature. Reason's (1990, 2000) theory, as explained in chapter 1, was used to guide the review along with summarizing each antecedent section in context.

Incidence

Medication errors are common, costly, and may result in injury (Barker, Flynn, Pepper, Bates, & Mikeal, 2002; Bates et al., 1995; Leape et al., 1995). Barker et al. (2002) found that nearly one of every five (19%) doses administered in their study resulted in error. Wrong time comprised 43% of the errors, followed by omissions (30%), wrong dosage (17%) and other (10%). Seven percent of errors were rated potentially harmful which equated to 40 errors per day in a typical 300 patient facility. In the nurse administration stage of their study, Leape et al. (1995) found lack of drug knowledge accounted for 15% of the problem; misuse of infusion pumps/parenteral delivery systems, 13%; slips and memory lapses, 12%; faulty drug identity checking, 10%; faulty dose checking, 10%; interaction problems with other services, 10%; lack of information about the patient (such as allergies), 10%; and other 20%. Pape (2003) reported that most medication errors occur at the point of administration, and that medication administration errors rank third in the list of causes of sentinel events leading to loss of function or patient death. However, Bates et al. (1995) reported that most errors resulted during the ordering stage (49%), followed by transcription (11%), dispensing (14%), and administration (26%).

Incidence of medication error varies by stage (ordering, transcribing, dispensing, administering) depending on the individual study findings reported, as does incidence of medication administration errors by type (wrong time, wrong dosage, omission, etc.). The literature has been inconclusive as to antecedents of medication administration errors in part due to many errors being unrecognized (Barker et al., 2002) or unreported. Most medication administration reporting systems rely on individual nurses to recognize and report medication errors (Wakefield et al., 1996); however, we know from the literature that error reporting rates vary with errors being largely underreported (Blegen et al., 2004; Fuqua & Stevens, 1988; Institute of Medicine, 1999; Leape, 1996; Meurier, 2000; Wakefield et al., 1996). As a result, incidence of medication errors remains elusive and contributes to the lack of progress toward error prevention.

Factors Related to Error

Research indicates that the majority of medication errors are due to unsafe systems rather than individual incompetence (Institute of Medicine, 1999). The literature repeatedly emphasized that diligent, competent, careful health care personnel make mistakes intermittently and even more so when activity increases (Rex, Turnbull, Allen, Voorde, & Luther, 2000). Errors are due to multiple factors in a complex health care system (Reed, Blegen, & Goode, 1998), largely owing to how the work system is designed (Berwick, 1989).

Hours Worked

Leape (2004) described design characteristics prone to error inducement as those where work exceeds the capacity of the human brain or that create conditions that generate known causes of errors such as sleeplessness and fatigue. Rogers, Hwang, Scott, Aiken, and Dinges (2004), in a national survey of nurses using self-report questionnaires, found the risks of making an error were significantly increased when registered nurses (RNs) work shifts longer than 12 hours, overtime, or more than 40 hours per week. The likelihood of making an error increased with longer work hours, and was three times higher when nurses worked shifts lasting 12.5 hours or longer. Working overtime increased the odds of making at least one error, regardless of how long the shift was originally scheduled. Data suggested a trend for increasing risk with longer shifts, and significantly elevated risk for overtime following a 12-hour shift. Although this study also involved procedural, transcription, and charting errors, note that of the 199 errors and 213 near errors, more than half of the errors (58%) and near errors (56%) involved medication administration. The relationship of errors or near errors and work hours and overtime were not affected by age, type of hospital unit, or size of hospital. Moreover, the long and unpredictable hours documented in the Rogers et al. (2004) study suggest a link between poor working conditions and threats to patient safety. These factors demonstrate Reason's theory (1990, 2000), whereby fatigue and understaffing are recognized as latent conditions.

Skill Mix

Latent failures consist of two kinds of situations: those that provoke conditions within the workplace, such as time pressure, understaffing, inadequate equipment, fatigue, and inexperience; and those that create long-lasting weaknesses in the defenses, such as untrustworthy alarms, unworkable procedures, and design and construction deficiencies. Latent conditions may lie dormant within a system for many years before they are triggered, usually by combining with active failures (e.g., unsafe acts, omissions, lapses, mistakes) to create an opportunity for error

(Reason, 2000). One such latent failure, skill mix, was identified by Blegen, Goode, and Reed (1998) in a study of 42 nursing care units in one large tertiary care hospital. An inverse relationship was found to exist between hours of care delivered by RNs and unit rates of medication errors after controlling for patient acuity. The relationship was found to be curvilinear, with decreased rates of medication errors up to the RN proportion of 87.5%. In a subsequent multisite study involving 39 nursing care units in 11 hospitals, Blegen and Vaughn (1998) found similar results. A higher RN proportion (staff mix) was associated with significantly lower rates of medication administration errors; again the relationship was nonlinear. The authors suggest several hypotheses for these results: heightened vigilance by RNs as mix increases, therefore more reporting; more severely ill patients needing more complex medications, increasing opportunity for medication error; and units with higher RN proportions having less total personnel than needed for optimal patient care.

In an earlier retrospective study utilizing records review, Grillo-Peck and Risner (1995) found no significant difference in medication error rates 6 months pre- (mean of 7.17) and post- (mean of 6.83) implementation of a nursing partnership model on a neuroscience unit (38 beds) that decreased RN skill mix from 80% to 60%. The model incorporated the philosophy of primary nursing and put the RN coordinating patient care in partnership with a patient care technician (PCT). The PCT assisted the RN by providing more direct care activities, such as hygiene, monitoring vital signs and blood glucose level, and changing dressings. This allowed more time for the RN to perform higher-level activities (those only performed by the RN), such as patient assessment, patient education, planning and coordination of patient care, and collaborating with physicians. In this study, RNs were the only caregivers who administered medications. Small sample size and use of only the adult population on one nursing care unit are noted by the authors as limiting the generalizability of the findings.

Batcheller, Burkman, Armstrong, Chappell, and Carelock (2004) found the effect of implementing a patient care team model dramatically decreased medication errors on a maternity patient care unit by 77% in the 6 months following implementation. The patient care team model focused on the key role of the RN care manager, an experienced RN with knowledge of unit routine, clinical expertise, and established physician relationships. In contrast, Lengacher et al. (1997) found an increase in medication errors on a pilot unit utilizing the Partners in Patient Care (PIPC) delivery model, in which a nurse partnered with a PIPC extender. The PIPC extender assumed delegated basic nursing functions in an effort to decrease time spent by the nurse in indirect care activities and nonclinical support services. Using an error ratio (number of medication errors divided by the number of patient days), a significant increase in medication error occurred on the pilot unit as opposed to the control unit when adjusting for patient days. The sample consisted of two nursing care units at a private, not-for-profit teaching medical center. The pilot unit (a 36-bed general surgical unit) and the control unit (34-bed orthopedic unit) were randomly selected. Medication error data were obtained from incident reports over an 18-month period.

Malloch, Milton, and Jobes (1990) found medication/intravenous errors decreased by 32% on a medical unit and 51% on a surgical unit in their study of differentiated practice among RNs. RNs were categorized either as case managers or case associates, based on individual assessment of knowledge and skill base regardless of formal education. The authors did not specify how medications were administered as a result of differentiated practice. In a related retrospective study, Poster and Pelletier (1988) found a statistically significant difference between medication error rates on the nine neuropsychiatric inpatient units using primary versus functional medication administrative systems. Five units utilized a primary system, in which each nurse administered medications for his or her assigned patients during a given shift. Four units utilized a functional system, in which a medication nurse was designated during each shift. The error rate was significantly ($p \leq .0001$) higher in the units utilizing the functional system (0.18%) versus the primary system (0.09%) in spite of the fact that five times as many doses of medication were given on units utilizing the primary system. The authors note that omission was the most frequent type of error in both systems (39% in functional and 31% in primary), followed by wrong dosage (24%) in the functional system and medication given after discontinuation in the primary system (15%). Wrong dosage is the third most frequently reported error in the primary system (13%). The most frequently reported reasons for medication error in the primary system included forgot (16%), misread medication record (13%), and transcription error (11%), while the most frequently reported reasons for medication error in the functional system included misread medication card (20%) and forgot (16%). Only one nurse cited errors in computing as the reason for medication errors involving wrong dosage.

Medication errors were found to be sensitive to nurse staffing in a secondary analysis of prospective, observational data from 95 patient care units across ten adult acute care hospitals in an integrated healthcare system (Whitman, Kim, Davidson, Wolf, & Wang, 2002). A significant inverse relationship was present between worked hours per patient day and medication errors in both cardiac and noncardiac intensive care units (ICUs); however, no significant relationship was found between staffing and medication errors in intermediate care units and medical-surgical units. These findings "suggest that environments with higher acuity patients and, most likely, greater number and more complex medication regimes per patient are sensitive to staffing alterations" (Whitman et al., pp. 637–638).

In summary, research focusing on skill mix demonstrates conflicting reports: Decreased rates of medication errors were reported with increased RN skill mix (up to 87.5%), but no significant difference was noted in a subsequent study when skill mix decreased from 80% to 60%. Research on various other partnering and differentiating practice models reported above have also been inconclusive, with some reporting decreased errors while others report an increase. Researchers from one study suggested that environments with higher acuity patients and more numerous and complex medication regimes are sensitive to staffing alterations, demonstrating Reason's (2000) Swiss cheese model where opportunity for error exits in multiple layers (see chapter 1 for more about Reason's theory of human error and Swiss cheese model). As a result of conflicting studies surrounding skill mix, further research is required to determine significance between alterations in staffing patterns and medication administration error.

Patient Acuity

A special neonatal care unit study (Vincer et al., 1989) found medication errors increased with increasing levels of newborn care. The relative risk of a medication error among patients receiving ventilator care was significantly ($p < .01$) greater (48.6 per 1,000 patient days) than in those receiving nonventilator intensive care (16.8 per 1,000 patient days), intermediate care (5.6 per 1,000 patient days), or transitional care (2.3 per 1,000 patients days). During the study, 313 medication errors occurred over 23,307 patient days, with relative risk calculated at 13.4 errors per 1,000 patient days. Drug administration errors (26.8%) and failure to follow correct procedures (17.9%) topped the list of ten major groups of medication error causes. The remaining eight groups included physician's order, drug preparation, transcription, medication card, interstitial intravenous line, unknown, other, and equipment. The two most frequent types of drug administration errors were neglecting to give a medication at the scheduled time (16.6%) and failure to regulate an intravenous infusion properly (12.8%). Outdated infusion pumps were partially attributed to intravenous regulation problems. When numbers of medication errors were compared to types of errors, the majority of errors were attributed to dosage errors (32.2%) and time errors (27.2%).

Increased level of care in this study was found relative to increased incidence of medication error. This study supports the Whitman et al. (2002) study suggesting that environments with higher-acuity patients and more numerous and complex medication regimes influence medication errors. The most frequent types of medication administration errors in this study (dosage and time) suggest time pressures and use of inadequate equipment as causes, deemed by Reason (1990; 2000) as error-provoking latent conditions. Again, multiple opportunities for error are present, increasing the potential for error occurrence.

Nurse Experience and Education Level

Secondary analysis of data collected in the studies conducted by Blegen and Vaughn (1998) and Blegen, Goode, and Reed (1998) found that a relationship existed between nurse experience and medication errors (Blegen, Vaughn, & Goode, 2001). While controlling for patient acuity, staff mix, and hours of nursing care, patient care units with a higher proportion of experienced nurses had lower medication error rates. Education level was also analyzed; patient care units with more baccalaureate-prepared nurses delivered care similar in quality to those with fewer baccalaureate nurses with one exception. Only one of four effect coefficients for nursing education was significant, suggesting that units with more baccalaureate-prepared nurses have higher rates of reported error. Although educational preparation of the nurse appeared to have an insignificant effect on quality of care, nurse experience was found to be significant. Patient care units that employed a higher proportion of experienced nurses had lower medication error rates. Inexperience demonstrates another error-provoking latent condition according to Reason's (1990; 2000) system theory.

Drug Classification and Unit Type

Certain types of medications have been reported to be more commonly associated with error. Classen et al. (1997) found that morphine, digoxin, meperidine, oxycodone, acetaminophen, imipenem, cefazolin, warfarin, and vancomycin were leading drugs associated with ADEs. Bates et al. (1993) found that antibiotics and anticoagulants also were common drugs associated with error, along with antitumor drugs. However, Cullen et al. (1997) found that although a wide variety of drugs were associated with ADEs, especially in ICUs, no group of drugs caused a disproportionate share of ADEs. Certain categories of drugs were, however, more likely to be used in specific units (e.g., cardiovascular and antihypertensive drugs in ICUs).

In a study conducted on 60 consecutive ICU admissions, Girotti, Garrick, Tierney, Chesnick, and Brown (1987) found that the majority of medication administration errors were wrong time (41.2%) or omitted doses (31.4%), and 90% of all drug errors were associated with intravenous medications. The therapeutic class of drugs also revealed a significant difference in the error rates for pH and electrolyte drugs when compared with other drug classes such as antibiotics, gastrointestinal, cardiovascular, respiratory, sedatives, and analgesics. Most errors (9 of 11) in the pH and electrolyte drug class involved administration of potassium chloride. And significantly more errors occurred during day shifts (64 errors and 2,257 opportunities for error) than on night shift (38 errors and 2,324 opportunities for error). This was despite similar opportunities for error, revealing an association between the number of admissions, discharges, and deaths during day shifts and errors committed. There were no differences in the average number of patients treated during day and night shifts, and comparison of patient classification (intensity of care) revealed no significant correlation with the number and types of errors committed between the two shifts. Statistical comparison of full-time versus part-time nurses and 12-hour shifts versus 8-hour shifts also failed to identify any statistical significance. A total of 102 errors (2.2%) were discovered in the administration of medications to 35 of the 60 patients (58%) observed in the study. The authors speculate that the ICU environment, where nurse to patient ratio is normally 1:1, could have influenced the low error rate of 2.2% because the nurse has sole responsibility for medication administration to one patient as opposed to general medical and surgical units where one nurse is responsible for administering medications to several patients or perhaps an entire unit. Verbal drugs orders by physicians may also have factored into the low error rate, because nurses only accept such orders in extreme cases. In addition, ICU nurses participate in an intensive orientation that stresses safe and accurate medication administration, possibly making them more vigilant. The authors also speculate that the observation of an error in more than 50% of the study population may be accounted for in the strict definition of drug error and the high opportunity of error in comparison with the number of patients in standard units. The data collection period for this study reflected a normal period of activity in the ICU in regard to average patient type, classification, and number of admissions and discharges (or deaths).

Cullen et al. (1997) reported that the rate of preventable and potential ADEs in ICUs was 19 events per 1,000 patient days which was nearly twice the rate of non-ICUs; the medical ICU rate of 25 events per 1,000 patient days was significantly higher than the surgical ICU rate of 14 events per 1,000 patient days. However, when adjusted for number of drugs ordered since admission or used in the previous 24 hours, no difference in rates existed between ICUs and non-ICUs. Structured interviews used during this study did not confirm that serious errors were made by exhausted, fatigued, overworked, excessively stressed individuals working in complex environments with many distractions. Most interviewees were nurses working a normal shift on their home unit with fairly stable teams that enjoyed full staffing, a normal workload, and fairly effective communications. Most obtained 5 to 7 hours of sleep before the event and reported only mild work-related stress with little stress outside work. Interviews revealed that most individuals involved in ADEs perceived they were working under normal conditions and denied fatigue, stress, or distractions at the time of the error.

Also identified in this study (Cullen et al., 1997) was the similarity in error rates among stages (ordering, transcription, dispensing, administration) and the four unit types (medical ICU, surgical ICU, general medical units, general surgical units). Preventable ADEs and potential ADEs were found more likely to be severe in ICUs than non-ICUs; however, no differences in severity of ADEs were found between medical and surgical ICUs or between medical and surgical general care units. Duration of injuries was short, and few patients experienced delayed discharges as a result of ADEs. Although trends toward longer lengths of stay (LOS) and increased costs were present, results did not reach statistical significance. This finding conflicts with results found by Classen et al. (1997) and Bates et al. (1997), where LOS associated with ADEs was extended by 1.74 and 2.2 days respectively.

Medication errors were also common in pediatric impatient settings (Kaushal et al., 2001). Children pose unique challenges during the process of ordering, dispensing, administering, and monitoring medications. Weight-based dosing is necessary for virtually all pediatric drugs, requiring more calculations than for adults. Dispensing also becomes error prone because pharmacists often find it necessary to dilute stock solutions. In addition, children have more limited reserves than adults with which to buffer errors, and they have fewer communication skills with which to warn clinicians about potential errors or adverse effects they experience (Kaushal et al., 2001).

Complex environments and medication regimes coupled with increased activity (as demonstrated during day shifts) represent latent conditions of time pressures, interruptions, and distractions, again layering error potential. Limited use of verbal orders, a 1:1 nurse-patient ratio, and an orientation stressing safe and accurate medication administration are key to limiting error according to Reason's (1990, 2000) system theory. However, the conflicting nature of existing research necessitates further exploration to clarify variable relationships.

Pre-Paradigm Shift Reflecting Perceptions of Individual Responsibility

Early research (through the mid-1990s) concerning medication errors focused on individual responsibility for error with little acknowledgement of system factor involvement. Individual responsibility was reflected in the research of Fuqua and Stevens (1988) who proposed several reasons why medication errors occur. They categorize their reasons as inadequate knowledge and skill, failure to comply with policy or procedure, failures in communication, and personal experiences. Inadequate knowledge and skill reflects lack of sound knowledge of the patient's diagnosis and the purpose of the medication. Failure to comply with policy and procedure includes neglecting to check instructions, failure to check allergies and name bands, failure to monitor a patient after a medication is given, and failure to follow the five rights of medication administration (right patient, right drug, right dose, right time, and right route). Failures in communication include incorrectly reading, hearing, or documenting a medication, including transcription errors due to illegible handwriting; hazardous abbreviations; incorrect decimal points; or unclear verbal orders. Personal experiences refer to the nurse's work experience coupled with distractions, interruptions, consecutive hours worked and work schedule.

Walters (1992) surveyed nurses (N = 334, n = 238, response rate 71%) employed at a large Midwestern tertiary care institution using a 33-item questionnaire to examine RN characteristics and perceived medication error causes. She found the major perceived causes were medications received late from the pharmacy (41.6%), RN was too busy (39.1%), RN forgetfulness or oversight (35.3%), and unclear medical administration records (35.3%). (Note: These causes are not mutually exclusive and add up to more than 100%). Respondents employed more than 1 year and those with more than 1 year of nursing experience reported making significantly fewer medication errors. Fewer than one-third of the nurses perceived system problems (21.8%) or their own disorganization (12.6%) to be causes of error. A greater number of errors made by less experienced nurses along with the citing of frequent interruptions as a perceived cause of medication errors concur with the work of Fuqua and Stevens (1988).

As reported by Fuqua and Stevens (1988), inadequate knowledge and skill, failure to comply with policy or procedure, and failures in communication demonstrate active failures (Reason, 1990; Reason, 2000) and reflect the individual responsibility associated with medication error. Personal experience is the only mentioned category that suggests medication errors occur as a result of latent conditions. Walter's (1992) research reflects heavier association with latent conditions (e.g., interruptions, RN too busy, unclear medical administration records, medications received late from the pharmacy) yet also includes RN forgetfulness and oversight as active failures. Walter's research notes the beginnings of a paradigm shift away from individual responsibility toward a system approach.

Paradigm Shift Reflecting Perceptions of System Responsibility

During the past decade, medication error research has shifted in emphasis toward identification of system problems inherent in error occurrence. This shift has been gradual and remains ongoing. Although elements of individual responsibility remain, system factors are receiving increased attention. The following studies demonstrate the gradual and ongoing shift in perception from individual responsibility to system responsibility.

Surveys received from 1,384 nurses working in 24 acute care urban and rural hospitals in Iowa identified five categories of medication administration errors (in order of frequency): physician, system, pharmacy, individual, and knowledge (Wakefield, Wakefield, Holman, & Blegen, 1998). No one category emerged as the primary perceived cause of medication administration errors, again reinforcing the complexity of medication administration "involving many individuals and disciplines," being "carried out in a complex environment," and "frequently the result of several different causes" (Wakefield et al., p. 41). These scores and relative rankings of the scores were compared across hospital type (rural, urban), unit type (medical, obstetrics, intensive care, etc.), nurse education level (LPN, ADN/diploma, BSN/advanced degree) and position (staff nurse, manager). Few differences were found with the exception of position; managers were more likely to perceive individual factors as reasons for medication administration error occurrence than were staff nurses. Staff nurses ranked individual factors as fourth highest in importance (mean = 3.0), but managers ranked individual factors as second highest (mean = 3.4). Although the mean score difference were small, staff nurses were more likely to view physician, pharmacist, and system factors as reasons for medication administration errors while managers were more likely to see physician and individual factors as causes of errors. The authors state:

> Since managers may not be involved in direct patient care they only know what the individual nurse did (or did not do), and may be unaware of the nature of the patient care environment when the error occurred. The staff nurse, functioning in a busy, complex environment realizes the many demands placed on his or her time and attention. Therefore, staff nurses view external factors as impinging on their ability to pass medications correctly but may lack an understanding of their individual contribution to errors (Wakefield et al., 1998, p. 41).

The two highest-scoring reasons for medication error occurrence within the five subscales of physician, system, pharmacy, individual, and knowledge included "interrupted while administering medications" (mean = 4.34) in the system subscale and "doctor's order not legible" (mean = 4.33) in the physician subscale. A 1–6 Likert scale was used, where 6 indicates strongly agree.

A more recent study (Mayo & Duncan, 2004) found illegible physician handwriting (mean = 3.92), distractions (mean = 4.15), and nurse being tired or exhausted (mean = 4.30) as the top three causes of medication errors. This survey examined nurses' perceptions of medication errors through randomly selected nurses in multiple settings (medical-surgical, critical care, and maternal child health) practicing in 16 Southern California acute care hospitals. Work settings represented private, government, military, and health maintenance organization hospitals where nurses were represented by the United Nurses Association of California/Union of Health Care Professionals. The survey asked nurses to rank a list of medication error causes from 1 to 10, with 1 indicating the most frequent cause. Additional items on the list included confusion between two drugs with similar names (mean = 4.55), nurse miscalculation of a dose (mean = 5.20), physician prescribing the wrong dose (mean = 5.46), nurse failing to check patient name band with medication administration record (mean = 5.87), incorrect set-up or adjustment of infusion device (mean = 6.13), poor quality or damaged medication label or packaging (mean = 7.52), and nurse confused by different types and functions of infusion devices (mean = 7.74). The sample drawn from health care union nurses and the predetermined list of medication error causes may limit generalizability of study findings.

In a pediatric-focused study ($n = 284$, 227 adult care nurses, 57 pediatric nurses) conducted by Stratton, Blegen, Pepper, and Vaughn (2004), medication error rates computed from documented occurrence reports were found to be 14.8 per 1,000 patient days on pediatric units compared to 5.66 on adult units. Nurse participants were asked to select the two most important reasons medication errors occur from a list of 14 potential reasons, excluding transcription and physician handwriting errors. Response rates were similar between pediatric nurses and adult nurses, identifying distractions and interruptions (50%, 46.9% respectively) as the most likely cause followed by inadequate RN-to-patient ratios (37%, 37.2%), volumes of medication administered (35%, 31.4%), and not double-checking doses (both 28%). Similar findings were noted by RN participants ($n = 775$) asked to respond to a survey published in the September 2002 issue of *Nursing* regarding their experiences related to increased risks and causes of medication administration errors (Cohen, Robinson, & Mandrack, 2003). Distractions and interruptions during medication administration topped the list followed by inadequate staffing and inadequate RN to patient ratios, illegibly written medication orders, incorrect dosage calculations, and similar drug names and packaging. By contrast, Leape et al. (1995) found lack of information about the drug (15%), infusion pump and parenteral delivery problems (13%), and slips and memory lapses (12%) as the most common causes of error during the nurse administration phase of medication delivery as reported during interviews of those involved.

Using self-report by 393 full-time hospital staff nurses, Balas, Scott, and Rogers (2004) found that 119 (30%) of the nurses indicated making at least one error, and 127 nurses (33%) indicated making at least one near error within a 28-day data collection period. Approximately 33% of the actual medication errors were due to late administration. In written logs, nurses expressed high patient acuity and heavy workloads as reasons for untimely medication administration. One nurse reported giving a medication 90 minutes late to one patient and 40 minutes late to a second patient due to caring for an unstable third patient. Other reasons for untimely medication administration included confusion, chaos, and getting side tracked. Wrong dosage comprised 24.1% of medication errors, with interruptions and distractions during drug preparation cited as leading causes. A nurse reported being interrupted by the charge RN twice, needing to help a circulating nurse, and needing to answer a ringing telephone all while trying to calculate a pediatric dose of liquid acetaminophen. Communication among health care providers was also cited where wrong information was given to the RN concerning a blood sugar level, consequently leading to the patient receiving an incorrect dose of insulin. Of the remaining categories of medication errors, 17.2% were reported as wrong drug, 15.5% as omissions, 7.8% as wrong patient, and 1.7% as wrong route.

In summary, the studies reviewed reflect the paradigm shift toward system responsibility, and numerous causes for medication errors were cited by nurses who reinforced the complexity of the medication administration process, which involves many disciplines and individuals and is carried out in a complex environment. Most frequently cited causes were interruptions and distractions, nurse fatigue and exhaustion, RN forgetfulness and business, high acuity and heavy workloads, inadequate staffing, confusion and chaos, medications arriving late from the pharmacy, and illegible physician orders. Managers were more likely to perceive individual factors as reasons for error, while staff nurses perceive system, physician, and pharmacy factors as reasons for error. Although the majority of the above-mentioned medication error causes reflect latent conditions (with the exception of RN forgetfulness), discrepancy exists between managers and staff nurses regarding individual responsibility (active failures) versus system problems (latent conditions), suggesting the continued presence of pre-paradigm shift perceptions among those in management positions and the ongoing nature of the paradigm shift.

IMPLICATIONS

Medication administration is a complex, high-frequency nursing activity, and the potential for medication-related errors rises as the average number of administered drugs increases (Institute of Medicine, 1999). Research has linked medication administration error to increased workload, extended work hours, level of care, understaffing, inexperience, skill mix, work shift, and unit type. This poses increased threats to patient safety, yet results are inconclusive because many study findings are contradictory. Prevention of medication administration errors relies on adequate and accurate information concerning their occurrence. Using existing reports to identify incidence of medication administration error and potential causes is difficult, given the under-reporting and the questions concerning validity and reliability of the data.

Reporting systems rely on nurses to recognize and report errors; however, many errors are unrecognized, and reporting behaviors vary widely among nurses depending on their perception of what constitutes error, fear, guilt, and the burdensome nature of reporting. Incomplete records limit potential to learn from errors and to improve quality and safety of nursing care (Meurier, 2000). Research and quality improvement projects are hampered, along with loss of ability for hospitals to diagnose their systems and prevent future errors. Changing nurses' perceptions about incident reporting, coupled with an administrative shift to a systems approach to errors, would allow for greater analysis and further research toward preventable actions. As reported by Ebright, Patterson, and Render (2002), fundamental to the success of decreasing adverse events is a change in understanding of how errors occur and the relinquishment of focus on individuals as the source of the problem. Error management is based on understanding the nature and extent of the adverse event and changing the conditions that are responsible for its occurrence (Helmreich, 2000). According to Bates et al. (1995, p. 30), "Better systems should promote fewer errors and include effective mechanisms for catching those that do occur."

Although the complexity of medication administration will continue, a fuller understanding of why and how medication administration errors occur and the issues that surround reporting of such errors will further efforts to decrease error occurrence and ultimately increase patient safety. Identifying causal or contributing factors to potential medication administration error will stimulate discussion and implementation of interventions to reduce error occurrence. And identifying the critical thinking patterns nurses employ to catch potential errors or near misses will provide data important to nursing education in teaching the administration of medications. Central to understanding is a reporting system devoid of the blame and shame currently haunting nurses in spite of recent trends that shift responsibility toward systems and away from individuals. Emphasis should be placed on data collection and the importance of analyzing errors in order to diagnose system problems (Institute of Medicine, 1999). As long as fear, shame, and guilt are associated with error admission, nurses will continue to underreport.

CONCLUSION

Early literature (through the mid-1990s) reflects the individual paradigm approach (active failures), where blame was placed at the individual level when a medication administration error was made, as supported by Cobb's (1986) development of a tool to assess medication error severity upon which disciplinary action could be based. Subsequent literature reflects a more systems-based approach (latent conditions), where defects in the system are deemed culprits of error as evidenced by implementation of barriers and safeguards (technology, system redesign) in an attempt to change the conditions under which humans work (Reason, 1990; Reason, 2000).

Both active failures and latent conditions established in Reason's theory remain prevalent in current literature, where active failures often display themselves in the form of incorrect drug calculations as with weight-based dosing, lack of individual knowledge, and failure to follow established protocol. Latent conditions are evidenced as time pressures, fatigue, understaffing, inexperience, design deficiencies, and inadequate equipment and may lie dormant within a system until combined with active failures to create opportunity for error. Although medication error research has shifted in emphasis toward identification of system problems inherent in error occurrence, the shift has been gradual and remains ongoing. No one force emerges as a clear antecedent to medication administration error, reinforcing the complexity of medication administration involving many individuals, conducted in a complex environment, and frequently the result of several causes (Wakefield et al., 1998). As a result, antecedents to medication administration errors remain elusive, demonstrating many forms in many contexts and making a clear remedy unattainable at present. Further research and replication of existing studies are necessary to ascertain incidence and antecedents with emphasis placed on more dependable reporting measures in which nurses are not threatened by reprisal. Nursing focus groups could inform research concerning antecedents of medication administration errors as well as reasons why nurses do not report error. Use of focus groups may also provide new insights given the "think tank" format and brainstorming discourse. Until more accurate reporting is achieved, researchers are only speculating using limited data.

Administration and management should be surveyed to determine the perceptions of medication error regarding the paradigm shift from individual responsibility to system factors. Degree of shift may require further education regarding system factors influencing error. Implementation of technology (e.g., computerized order entry, bar coding, medication dispensing carts) should also be researched to ascertain its effect on medication error incidence along with evaluation of cost effectiveness and new antecedents resulting from technology implementation. What kind of system workarounds have evolved since technology implementation? What kinds of errors occur as a result of workarounds? Can workarounds be prevented by upgrades and patches to current technology?

Also lacking in the literature are qualitative studies elucidating the critical thinking process nurses use in discovering and preventing near miss medication administration errors. What causes nurses to question medication orders, how the medication dosage was supplied, or administration of a particular medication? Research of this type would identify themes and patterns, thereby allowing future educational opportunities that may lead to decreased medication errors.

Medication administration errors may never be totally eradicated due to the propensity for human error and system failure, but much can be improved from the current situation. With continued research examining errors and potential errors coupled with improved reporting systems, diagnosis of system frailties and dormant antecedents is possible, thereby improving health care, increasing patient safety, and lowering health care costs. Medication errors are one of the most common causes of avoidable harm to patients (Joint Commission on Accreditation of Healthcare Organizations, 1999). "If we know how to do it better and don't, we are behaving unethically. Safety is a moral issue" (Leape, 2004).

REFERENCES

Agency for Healthcare Research and Quality. (2001, July). *Making healthcare safer: A critical analysis of patient safety practices.* Retrieved May 10, 2004, from http://www.ahrq.gov/clinic/ptsafety/summary.htm

Balas, M. C., Scott, L. D., & Rogers, A. E. (2004). The prevalence and nature of errors and near errors reported by hospital staff nurses. *Applied Nursing Research, 17*(4), 224–230.

Barker, K. N., Flynn, E. A., Pepper, G. A., Bates, D. W., & Mikeal, R. L. (2002). Medication errors observed in 36 health care facilities. *Archives of Internal Medicine, 162*(16), 1897–1903.

Batcheller, J., Burkman, K., Armstrong, D., Chappell, C., & Carelock, J. L. (2004). A practice model for patient safety: The value of the experienced registered nurse. *Journal of Nursing Administration, 34*(4), 200–205.

Bates, D. W., Cullen, D. J., Laird, N., Petersen, L. A., Stephen, D., Servi, D., et al. (1995). Incidence of adverse drug events and potential adverse drug events: Implications for prevention. *Journal of the American Medical Association, 274*(1), 29–34.

Bates, D. W., Leape, L. L., & Petrycki, S. (1993). Incidence and preventability of adverse drug events in hospitalized adults. *Journal of General Internal Medicine, 8*(6), 289–294.

Bates, D. W., Spell, N., Cullen, D. J., Burdick, E., Laird, N., Petersen, L. A., et al. (1997). The cost of adverse drug events in hospitalized patients. *Journal of the American Medical Association, 277*(4), 307–311.

Berwick, D. M. (1989). Continuous improvement as an ideal in health care. *New England Journal of Medicine, 320,* 53–56.

Blegen, M. A., Goode, C. J., & Reed, L. (1998). Nurse staffing and patient outcomes. *Nursing Research, 47*(1), 43–50.

Blegen, M. A., & Vaughn, T. (1998). A multisite study of nurse staffing and patient occurrences. *Nursing Economics, 16*(4), 196–203.

Blegen, M. A., Vaughn, T. E., & Goode, C. J. (2001). Nurse experience and education: Effect on quality of care. *Journal of Nursing Administration, 31*(1), 33–39.

Blegen, M. A., Vaughn, T., Pepper, G., Vojir, C., Stratton, K., & Boyd, M. (2004). Patient and staff safety: Voluntary reporting. *American Journal of Medical Quality, 19*(2), 67–74.

Classen, D. C., Pestotnik, S. L., Evans, R. S., Lloyd, J. F., & Burke, J. P. (1997). Adverse drug events in hospitalized patients. *Journal of the American Medical Association, 277*(4), 301–306.

Cobb, M. D. (1986). Evaluation medication errors. *Journal of Nursing Administration, 16*(4), 41–44.

Cohen, H., Robinson, E. S., & Mandrack, M. (2003). Getting to the root of medication errors. *Nursing 2003, 33*(9), 36–45.

Cullen, D. J., Sweitzer, B. J., Bates, D. W., Burdick, E., Edmondson, A., & Leape, L. L. (1997). Preventable adverse drug events in hospitalized patients: A comparative study of intensive care and general care units. *Critical Care Medicine, 25*(8), 1289–1297.

Douglas, J., & Larrabee, S. (2003). Bring barcoding to the bedside: Patient safety series, part 1 of 2. *Nursing Management, 34*(5), 36–40.

Ebright, P. R., Patterson, E. S., & Render, M. L. (2002). The new look approach to patient safety: A guide for clinical nurse specialist leadership. *Clinical Nurse Specialist, 16*(5), 247–253.

Fuqua, R. A., & Stevens, K. R. (1988). What we know about medication errors: A literature review. *Journal of Nursing Quality Assurance, 3*(1), 1–17.

Girotti, M. J., Garrick, C., Tierney, M. G., Chesnick, K., & Brown, S. J. (1987). Medication administration errors in an adult intensive care unit. *Heart and Lung, 16*(4), 449–453.

Grillo-Peck, A. M., & Risner, P. B. (1995). The effect of a partnership model on quality and length of stay. *Nursing Economics, 13*(6), 367–373.

Helmreich, R. L. (2000). On error management: Lessons from aviation. *British Medical Journal, 320*(7237), 781–785.

Institute of Medicine (1999). *To err is human: Building a safer health system.* Washington, DC: National Academy Press.

Joint Commission on Accreditation of Healthcare Organizations. (1999, November 19). *High-alert medications and patient safety.* Retrieved February 11, 2005, from www.jcaho.org/about+us/news+letters/sentinel+event+alert/sea_11.htm

Kaushal, R., Bates, D. W., Landrigan, C., McKenna, K. J., Clapp, M. D., Federico, F., et al. (2001). Medication errors and adverse drug events in pediatric inpatients. *Journal of the American Medical Association, 85*(16), 2114–2120.

Leape, L. L. (1996). Out of darkness: Hospitals begin to take mistakes seriously. *Health Systems Review, 29*(6), 21–24.

Leape, L. L. (2004, April 22). *What's new in patient safety?* Lecture presented at the University of Utah Health Systems Lecture Series. Salt Lake City, UT.

Leape, L. L., Bates, D. W., Cullen, D. J., Cooper, J., Deonaco, H. J., Gallivan, T., et al. (1995). Systems Analysis of Adverse Drug Events. *Journal of the American Medical Association, 274*(1), 35–43.

Leape, L. L., Brennan, T. A., Laird, N., Lawthers, A. G., Localio, A. R., Barnes, B. A., et al. (1991). The nature of adverse events in hospitalized patients: Results of the Harvard Medical Practice Study II. *New England Journal of Medicine, 324*(6), 377–384.

Lengacher, C. A., Mabe, P. R., Heinemann, D., VanCott, M. L., Kent, K., & Swymer, S. (1997). Collaboration in research: Testing the PIPC model on clinical and nonclinical outcomes. *Nursing Connections, 10*(1), 17–30.

Malloch, K. M., Milton, D. A., & Jobes, M. O. (1990). A model for differentiated nursing practice. *Journal of Nursing Administration, 20*(2), 20–26.

Mayo, A. M., & Duncan, D. (2004). Nurse perceptions of medication errors: What we need to know for patient safety. *Journal of Nursing Care Quality, 19*(3), 209–217.

Meurier, C. E. (2000). Understanding the nature of errors in nursing: Using a model to analyze critical incident reports of errors which had resulted in an adverse or potentially adverse event. *Journal of Advanced Nursing, 32*(1), 202–207.

Pape, T. M. (2003). Applying airline safety practices to medication administration. *Medsurg Nursing, 12*(2), 77–93.

Phillips, D. P., Christenfeld, N., & Glynn, L. M. (1998). Increase in US medication-error deaths between 1983 and 1993. *Lancet, 351*, 643–644.

Poster, E. C., & Pelletier, L. (1988). Primary versus functional medication administration: Monitoring and evaluating medication error rates. *Journal of Nursing Quality Assurance, 2*(2), 68–76.

Reason, J. (1990). *Human error.* Cambridge: Cambridge University Press.

Reason, J. (2000). Human error: Models and management. *British Medical Journal, 320*(7237), 768–770.

Reed, L., Blegen, M. A., & Goode, C. S. (1998). Adverse patient occurrences as a measure of nursing care quality. *Journal of Nursing Administration, 28*(5), 62–69.

Rex, J. H., Turnbull, J. E., Allen, S. J., Voorde, K. V., & Luther, K. (2000). Systematic root cause analysis of adverse drug events in a tertiary referral hospital. *Joint Commission Journal of Quality Improvement, 26*(10), 563–575.

Rogers, A. E., Hwang, W. T., Scott, L. D., Aiken, L. H., & Dinges, D. F. (2004). The working hours of hospital staff nurses and patient safety. *Health Affairs, 23*(4), 202–212.

Stratton, K. M., Blegen, M. A., Pepper, G., & Vaughn, T. (2004). Reporting of medication errors by pediatric nurses. *Journal of Pediatric Nursing, 19*(6), 385–392.

Vincer, M. J., Murray, J. M., Yuill, A., Allen, A. C., Evans, J. R., & Stinson, D. A. (1989). Drug errors and incidents in a neonatal intensive care unit. *American Journal of Diseases of Children, 143,* 737–740.

Wakefield, B. J., Wakefield, D. S., Holman, T. U., & Blegen, M. A. (1998). Nurses' perceptions of why medication administration errors occur. *MEDSURG Nursing, 7*(1), 39–44.

Wakefield, D. S., Wakefield, B. J., Holman, T. U., & Blegen, M. A. (1996). Perceived barriers in reporting medication administration errors. *Best Practices and Benchmarking in Healthcare, 4,* 191–197.

Wakefield, D. S., Wakefield, B. J., Uden-Holman, T., Borders, T., Blegen, M., & Vaughn, T. (1999). Understanding why medication administration errors may not be reported. *American Journal of Medical Quality, 14*(2), 81–88.

Walters, J. A. (1992). Nurses' perceptions of reportable medication errors and factors that contribute to their occurrence. *Applied Nursing Research, 5*(2), 86–88.

Whitman, G. R., Kim, Y., Davidson, L. J., Wolf, G. A., & Wang, S. L. (2002). The impact of staffing on patient outcomes across specialty units. *Journal of Nursing Administration, 32*(12), 633–639.

Chapter 3

Fall and Injury Prevention

Leanne M. Currie

ABSTRACT

Falls and related injuries are increasingly being recognized as a nursing-sensitive quality indicator, and they continue to be an unsolved patient safety problem in inpatient and outpatient care areas as well as in the community at large. The purpose of this review is to summarize the current research related to fall and injury prevention. The chapter is organized presenting research in (1) the community and (2) acute and long-term care settings. For each setting, the research that addresses risk factors, risk assessment instruments, and fall and injury prevention efforts are reviewed. There is a large body of research that investigates fall and injury prevention across the care continuum. In the community setting, targeted risk evaluation in the emergency department and management of vitamin D deficiency appear to be promising preventive methods. However, further research needs to explore staffing ratios, automated methods of assessing and communicating fall risk, improved methods and timing of risk evaluation and methods by which existing and new evidence might be translated into practice.

Keywords: patient safety, nursing, falls

Falls and related injuries continue to be an unsolved problem in inpatient and out-patient care areas as well as in the community at large. Increased attention to this problem in recent years derives from the evolving health care delivery environ-ment, which includes higher patient-to-nurse staffing ratios, cutbacks stemming from managed care, and national efforts toward improving patient safety.

Excluding the pediatric population, the incidence of falls in the United States increases with age. Approximately 32% of community-dwelling individuals over the age of 65 fall each year. This is an important issue because the life expec-tancy of Americans is also increasing; Americans over the age of 65 currently rep-resent 12% of the population, which equates to approximately 35 million people. However, this proportion is expected to increase to 19.6% (or approximately 63 million people) by 2030 (Morbidity and Mortality Weekly Report, 2003). There-fore, if the trend for increased falls in community-dwelling individuals continues, we are at risk for 20 million community-dwelling individuals falling each year.

Unintentional injury is the *fifth leading cause of death* in the general popu-lation in the United States, and falls are the second most common cause of un-intentional injury across ages. In the community setting, fall-related injuries are the most common cause of death in the persons over the age of 65, resulting in 38.4 *fall-related deaths* per 100,000 individuals 65 years or older (Hausdorff, 2001; Hornbrook et al., 1994; Lauritzen, 1996; Office of Statistics and Programming, 2005). Although the underlying status of the individual who sustains a fall may contribute to the fall and subsequent injury, the trauma related to the fall itself is most often the cause of morbidity and mortality.

Sadly, fall-related death rates have gradually increased between 1999 and 2002; from 29 to 36 per 100,000 (Office of Statistics and Programming, 2005). This is likely due to the aging population, but is a growing public health issue despite local efforts at fall prevention (Morbidity and Mortality Weekly Report, 2003; National Center for Injury Prevention and Control, 2003). Investigators have found that fall-related injuries account for up to 15% of rehospitalizations in the first month postdischarge (Mahoney et al., 2000). Whether or not this is a function of hospital processes to decrease length of stay, a function of the aging population, or yet some other unrecognized factor, it is clear that falls in the community are a public health issue that should be addressed.

Because of the magnitude of the problem, fall-related death prevention is a Healthy People 2010 (HP2010) objective. The specific goal is to reduce the num-ber of deaths resulting from falls among those aged 65 or older to no more than 34.6 per 100,000 persons from the baseline of 38.4 per 100,000. This is a growing challenge as the population ages. Despite the high risk for deaths related to falls in the geriatric population, fall prevention is neither a Health Plan Employer Data and Information Set preventive indicator nor an Agency for Healthcare Research and Quality preventive quality indicator (Levine et al., 2005).

Although not a formal nursing quality indicator for ambulatory or primary care, fall and injury prevention is a known public health issue. The gerontology physician community has carried out a large body of work toward addressing this problem; however, nursing care (e.g., primary care nurse practitioners, ambulatory care nurses) can influence fall and injury prevention in these areas as well. Indeed, as the health care provider community moves toward patient-centered care, fall and fall-related injury prevention is gradually being addressed across the care continuum, invoking the potential to effectively contend with this issue and to more clearly define the role of nursing in its prevention.

FALLS ARE A PATIENT SAFETY ISSUE

Promotion of patent safety in hospitals has been a focus of attention for nursing care and hospital quality management for decades. And fall prevention has been an individual area of concern for nurses almost 50 years (Grubel, 1959; Thurston, 1957). Indeed, for hospital-based incident reporting, an unintentional fall is considered avoidable and is therefore classified as an adverse event.

Falls are the most frequently reported adverse events in the adult inpatient setting, with fall rates ranging from 1.7 to 25 falls per 1,000 patient days depending on the care area, with geropsychiatric patients having the highest risk (Halfon, Eggli, Van Melle, & Vagnair, 2001; Leape et al., 1991; Mahoney, 1998; Morgan, Mathison, Rice, & Clemmer, 1985). Extrapolated hospital fall statistics indicate that the overall risk of a patient falling in the acute care setting is approximately 1.9% to 3% of all hospitalizations (Leape et al., 1991; Mahoney, 1998; Morgan et al., 1985). In the United States, there are approximately 37 million hospitalizations each year (Healthcare Cost and Utilization Project, 2002); therefore the resultant number of falls could reach more than 1,000,000 per year.

Injuries are reported to occur in approximately 6% to 44% of inpatient falls (Hitcho et al., 2004; Lauritzen, 1996; Morse, 1997; Resnick & Junlapeeya, 2004; Rohde, Myers, & Vlahov, 1990). Serious injuries from falls, such as head injuries or fractures, occur in a lesser proportion, 2% to 8%, of falls (Hitcho et al., 2004); however, these serious injuries are estimated to occur approximately 90,000 times per year in the United States. Deaths from falls in the inpatient environment are a relatively rare occurrence, less than 1%. However, given the hospital admission rates, it is estimated that up to 11,000 fatal falls occur per year nationwide. Most of these falls are considered preventable, and the fatal injuries from preventable falls should not occur while a patient is under hospital care.

FALLS AS A NURSING-SENSITIVE
QUALITY INDICATOR

As one of the nursing quality indicators monitored by the American Nurses Association, National Database of Nursing Quality Indicators (ANA-NDNQI) and by the National Quality Forum (American Nurses Association, 1999; National Quality Forum, 2004), falls have long been associated with the quality of nursing care in the acute care setting. Participation in the ANA-NDNQI provides hospitals with the ability to view their fall and injury rates in relation to other hospitals of similar type and size. However, participation is voluntary, and as such, has not been adopted nationally.

A second national repository for care-related fall and injury reporting is the Maryland Quality Indicator Project, which provides benchmarks for the behavioral health, long-term care, and home care settings (Maryland Quality Indicator Project, 2005). As with the ANA-NDNQI, participation in this project is voluntary on the part of the care agency, but can be beneficial as it provides the ability to benchmark with similar institutions.

In the home care setting, the Centers for Medicare & Medicaid Service's Outcome and Assessment Information Set provides the reporting basis for the patients' physical functioning. Recent efforts in home care quality seeks to include falls as a quality indicator for patients who are not completely bedbound (Hirdes et al., 2004). These data will provide a better representation of the problem and also have the potential to identify patients at risk for falls and thus prevent falls and fall-related injuries.

In the nursing home setting, the long-term care minimum data set (LTCMDS) is used for reporting all aspects of care. The LTCMDS captures fall and injury histories via assessments that are performed on admission and at regular intervals during a resident's stay. In addition, residents are evaluated for balance and ability to perform activities of daily living (ADLs), with the goal to prevent falls should the patient be deficient in these areas. However, recent work by Hill-Westmoreland and Gruber-Baldini (2005) indicated that chart reviews for a group of long-term care facilities only demonstrated 75% concordance between chart abstraction and minimum data set reporting. A more recent development in the long-term care setting, the Nursing Home Quality Initiative (NHQI), promotes the collection of a list of enhanced quality indicators, including those that track declines in functional and cognitive status (Centers for Medicare & Medicaid Services, 2003, 2005). Increased and more accurate monitoring of these elements has the potential to reduce falls among nursing home residents; however, the effect of these efforts has yet to be established.

DEFINITIONS OF FALLS AND
RELATED INJURIES

Although reporting has improved in recent years, early work in this field was troubled by inconsistencies in the definitions of falls and related injuries by which the outcome variables had different meanings depending on the definition used, making it difficult to conduct large-scale reviews (Close et al., 1999; Masud & Morris, 2001). Falls may be precipitated by intrinsic or extrinsic factors. Extrinsic factors include environmental hazards, whereas intrinsic factors include physiologic processes that may precipitate a fall. Distinguishing between intrinsic or extrinsic risk factors can facilitate identification of preventive strategies. According to Tinetti, Speechley, and Ginter (1988), a fall in the nonhospitalized geriatric population is defined as "an event which results in a person coming to rest unintentionally on the ground or lower level, not as a result of a major intrinsic event (such as a stroke) or overwhelming hazard." Agostini, Baker, and Bogardus (2001) adapted this definition for the inpatient, acute, and long-term, care areas to define a fall as "unintentionally coming to rest on the ground, floor, or other lower level, but not as a result of syncope or overwhelming external force."

Other definitions are broader and include falls related to intrinsic events such as syncope or stroke. For example, Nevitt's definition of a fall is "falling all the way down to the floor or ground, or falling and hitting an object like a chair or stair" (Nevitt, Cummings, & Hudes, 1991). The ANA-NDNQI (American Nurses Association, 2005) provides an all-inclusive definition whereby a fall is:

> an unplanned descent to the floor (or extension of the floor, e.g., trash can or other equipment) with or without injury. All types of falls are included whether they result from physiological reasons or environmental reasons. (p. 26)

The International Classification of Diseases 9 Clinical Modifications (ICD-9-CM) attributes several codes to falls, all of which have broad descriptions: accidentally bumping against moving object caused by crowd with subsequent fall (E917.6); fall on or from ladders or scaffolding (E881); fall from or out of building or other structure (E882); other fall from one level to another (E884); fall on same level from slipping, tripping, or stumbling (E885); fall on same level from collision, pushing, or shoving by or with another person (E886); and other and unspecified fall (E888) (National Center for Health Statistics, 2005). In the inpatient care setting, E888 is the code that is typically used to record a fall in a medical record. However, this ICD-9-CM code is not consistently used for reporting; therefore, institutions generally rely on incident reports as the method of identifying fall events (National Center for Health Statistics, 2005).

Fall-related injuries in the community, home care, and long-term care areas are generally characterized by ICD-9-CM diagnoses for the related injured body part. However, in the acute care setting, fall-related injuries are generally categorized as none, mild, moderate, major, and injuries that result in death. These definitions are as follows: (1) *None* indicates that the patient did not sustain an injury secondary to the fall; (2) *Minor* indicates those injuries requiring a simple intervention; (3) *Moderate* indicates injuries requiring sutures or splints; (4) *Major* injuries are those that require surgery, casting, further examination (e.g., for a neurological injury); and (5) *Deaths* are those that result from injuries sustained from the fall (American Nurses Association, 1999).

According to Morse (1997), inpatient falls can be classified into three categories: accidental falls (derived from extrinsic factors, such as environmental considerations), anticipated physiologic falls (derived from intrinsic physiologic factors, such as confusion), and unanticipated physiologic falls (derived from unexpected intrinsic events, such as a new onset syncopal event or a major intrinsic event such as stroke). According to the Morse classification (1997), approximately 78% of the anticipated physiologic falls can be identified and thus prevented. However, work that identifies precursors to unexpected intrinsic events, such as screening for predictors of syncopal events (Kumar, Thomas, Mudd, Morris, & Masud, 2003; Richardson et al., 2000, 2002) might increase the proportion of anticipated physiologic falls, which could ultimately prevent more falls.

DEFINITIONS OF FALLS IN THE CONTEXT OF MEDICAL ERRORS

A fall is consistent with the definition of a medical error, which states that an error is "the failure of a planned action to be completed as intended" (i.e., error of execution) or "the use of a wrong plan to achieve an aim" (i.e., error of planning) (Committee on Data Standards for Patient Safety, 2003; Committee on Quality of Health Care in America, 1999). In this sense, the planned action might be to ensure the patient's safety, and an error in planning might be to apply an inappropriate (or ineffective) therapy to the patient's plan of care. As an *error of commission*, which is "an error that occurs as a result of an action taken," a fall might occur when a patient is given a medication that increases the risk for falling. On the other hand, a fall might be considered an *error of omission*, "an error which occurs as a result of an action not taken," when a patient is not assessed for fall risk or when an appropriate intervention is not applied. Although not all patients fall, failure to identify those at risk can predispose caregivers to errors of omission. Falls can also arise from *latent errors* where an agency does not apply appropriate standards, sufficient training, or support for the practice-based processes regarding fall and injury prevention in the care environment. This type of error has the potential to be systematically removed from most hospital situations in the United States since the Joint Commission on Accreditation of Healthcare Organizations (JCAHO) has indicated that risk assessment for falls must be carried out on all patients who are hospitalized and that a fall prevention program must be implemented and evaluated (Joint Commission on the Accreditation of Hospitals, 2005a). A fall or fall-related injury might constitute a *monitoring error* if an appropriate clinical or laboratory evaluation is not used to identify fall risk, or worse, if the patient is not monitored to identify the presence of injury after a fall. For example, if a patient sustained a head injury after a fall, but a computed tomography scan was not performed, the patient might die from a subdural hematoma, a clinically manageable condition if detected early.

Purpose

The purpose of this review is to summarize the current research related to fall and injury prevention. The chapter is organized to present research in the community and the long-term and acute care settings. For each setting, the research that addresses risk factors, risk assessment instruments and fall and injury prevention efforts are reviewed. A growing body of research related to vitamin D (including vitamin D deficiency as a risk factor for falls and vitamin D supplementation as a preventive measure) has been carried out in a various settings. Because the settings are varied, vitamin D research is presented as it relates to each area.

Methods

MedLine, Cumulative Index to Nursing and Allied Health Literature, and Cochrane databases from 1966 to November 2005 were searched for medical subject heading terms, including individual and combinations of accidental falls, patient safety, medical errors, nursing sensitive quality indicators, and fall prevention. In addition, references from relevant articles were searched. Articles related to occupational falls, sports-related falls, alcohol-related falls and abuse-related falls were excluded. Articles that reported physiologic characteristics that are suspected to preclude falls, but that did not examine falls or fall-related injuries as outcomes, were also excluded because the research is not yet mature enough to determine the effect on falls and fall-related injuries. Further, articles that were published in a foreign language were excluded.

FALLS AND RELATED INJURIES
IN THE COMMUNITY

As previously discussed, falls and related injuries are a serious public health problem in the community. Research about these phenomena were found and categorized as risk factor identification, risk assessment instruments, and prevention strategies. Each category of research is discussed below.

Risk Factors in the Community

The pivotal research of Tinetti et al. (1988) related to fall and injury prevention in community-dwelling individuals older than 65 identified the following risk factors for falling: (1) postural hypotension, (2) use of any benzodiazepine or sedative-hypnotics, (3) use of four or more prescription medications, (4) environmental hazards, and (5) muscular strength or range of motion impairments. Other researchers have identified additional patient or treatment risk factors such as (1) comorbidities, including diabetes, diabetic foot ulcer (Wallace et al., 2002), stroke (Mackintosh, Goldie, & Hill, 2005), syncope (Rubenstein & Josephson, 2002), anemia (Dharmarajan & Norkus, 2004), Alzheimer disease (Bassiony et al., 2004), and Parkinson disease (Fink, Kuskowski, Orwoll, Cauley, & Ensrud, 2005); (2) Patient characteristics, including fallophobia (also known as "fear of falling") (Watanabe, 2005; Wilson et al., 2005), gait problems (e.g., weakness and impaired sensation) (Gerdhem, Ringsberg, Akesson, & Obrant, 2005), postural hypotension, impaired ability to perform ADLs, frailty (Delbaere, Crombez, Vanderstraeten, Willems, & Cambier, 2004; Speciale, Turco, Magnifico, Bellelli, & Trabucchi, 2004), inability to comply with recommendations (Reuben et al., 1996); and (3) Other characteristics, including, recent hospitalization (Mahoney et al., 2000), nonsupporting footwear (e.g., slippers) (Sherrington & Menz, 2003), reckless wheelchair use (Gavin-Dreschnack et al., 2005), and psychotropic medication use (Joo et al., 2002; Landi et al., 2005).

A growing body of research is investigating vitamin D deficiency as a risk factor for falls, muscle weakness related to vitamin D deficiency may prove to be a predictive factor (Dhesi et al., 2002). Dukas, Schacht, Mazor, and Stahelin (2005) have identified low creatinine clearance as an independent risk factor for falls in patients with a vitamin D deficiency.

The roles of ethnicity and race in relation to falls and injury have been studied. Reyes-Ortiz has examined risk factors for Mexican-Americans and found that in the community, the risk factors are the same as their White counterparts (Reyes-Ortiz, Al Snih, Loera, Ray, & Markides, 2004). Hanlon et al. examined predictors of falls between Caucasians and African Americans and found that African Americans were less likely to fall than Whites (OR = 0.77) (Hanlon, Landerman, Fillenbaum, & Studenski, 2002).

Risk Factors for Injury

Risk factors for injury in the community are increasingly well characterized. Porthouse and her research team performed a comprehensive cohort study of almost 4,300 women older than 70 years and confirmed the following risk factors for various types of fall-related fractures: (1) fall in the past 12 months; (2) increasing age; (3) previous fracture; (4) low body weight; and (5) maternal history of hip fracture (Porthouse et al., 2004). This work also identified that smoking was not associated with fracture risk. A growing body of research is examining vitamin D deficiency as a risk factor for fracture, however results are conflicting to date (Porthouse et al., 2004; Porthouse et al., 2005) but bear further research.

Colon-Emeric and colleagues used data from a large community epidemiologic study to identify whether historical and functional information could help to predict fracture risk (Colon-Emeric, Pieper, & Artz, 2002). The researchers identified nine characteristics that were predictors of fracture, including (1) female sex, (2) age greater than 75 years, (3) White race, (4) BMI of less than 22.8 kg/m^2, (5) history of stroke, (6) cognitive impairment, (7) one or more ADL impairments, (8) one or more Rosow-Breslau impairments (e.g., unable to perform heavy work, walk a mile, or climb stairs), and (9) anti-epileptic drug use. Ohm, Mina, Howells, Blair, and Bendick (2005) recently identified that elderly community-dwelling individuals with traumatic head injuries were more likely to die based on the use of antiplatelet therapy (RR = 2.5 for those taking antiplatelet therapies; $p = 0.016$). Many of these injury risk factors are consistent with fall risk factors, which accentuates the need to effectively screen elderly community-dwelling individuals. However, the factors that preclude patients to higher injury such as antiplatelet therapy might establish the need for additional safety measures.

Risk Assessment Instruments for the Community

Tinetti (1986) developed a fall risk assessment index based on nine risk factors, including mobility, morale, mental status, distance vision, hearing, postural blood pressure, back examination, medications, and ability to perform ADLs. This instrument has been the most widely used and tested, with a reported sensitivity and specificity of 80% and 74% respectively (Perell et al., 2001). Other instruments used in the community include following with self reported sensitivities and specificities: (1) Berg Balance Test (sensitivity = 77%; specificity = 86%), (2) Elderly Fall Screening Test (sensitivity = 93%; specificity = 78%), (3) Dynamic Gait Index (sensitivity = 85%; specificity = 38%), and (4) Timed Get Up and Go test (sensitivity = 87%; specificity = 87%) (Perell et al., 2001). Aside from the Timed Get Up and Go test, which takes less than a minute, these instruments generally take 15 to 20 minutes to complete (Perell et al., 2001). Lord et al. (2005) recently evaluated the effect of an exercise-related fall prevention program, but found that the intervention was not useful in the general community who were not screened for risk. They concluded that screening to identify individuals at high risk for falls would likely be necessary for a successful fall prevention program. Further research to identify the most accurate yet easy to use risk assessment instrument would be necessary to move these efforts forward.

A potential time point for risk assessment is in the emergency department (ED). Weigand and Gerson (2001) conducted a systematic review to examine the potential benefits of assessment of fallers while in the ED. This review and a growing body of evidence suggest that targeted assessment and referral of patients admitted to the ED because of a fall is promising (Close et al., 1999; Davison, Bond, Dawson, Steen, & Kenny, 2005; Miller, Lewis, Nork, & Morley, 1996). Although no standardized instrument has yet been developed for use in this environment, the potential for the prevention of falls and related injuries in the community would be increased with the accurate identification of patients at risk for falls in the ED.

To date, a limited number of automated community-based fall assessment instruments have been described. By far the most complex and integrated is the Fall Risk Assessment and Management System (FRAMS), which was developed by the Australia Family Practice Group for use in the community by family practice physicians (Liaw et al., 2003). FRAMS includes automated recommendations after the clinician executes a thorough patient assessment. Although this system appears promising, its efficacy has not yet been reported.

Lord, Menz, and Tiedemann (2003) describes an electronic fall risk assessment instrument that provides a method to measure several risk factors, including vision, peripheral sensation, muscle force, reaction time, and postural sway. Although this instrument is thorough, it is meant for use by a physical therapist or a physician, nurse practitioner, or physician assistant for a focused fall risk assessment rather than as a triage or screening tool. The novel aspect of this instrument is the comparison of the individual's score to the normative scores for each of the assessments. This provides the clinician with an anchor and may facilitate improved screening over time.

Another electronic fall risk assessment instrument, described by Dyer, Watkins, Gould, and Rowe (1998), is an electronic checklist in a fall prevention clinic. Unfortunately, the researchers concluded that the clinic itself was more successful than the instrument in identifying risk factors for falling, underscoring the reality that the implementation of an instrument without associated policy and procedure changes may have limited effect.

Other automated instruments derive from the domain of physical therapy in which the physical assessment is captured electronically (Dyer et al., 1998) or in which computer logic is applied to the detailed evaluations inherent in fall assessment (Lord et al., 2003). The presence of these automated systems indicates that there is movement toward computerized fall risk assessment. Indeed, many clinical information systems have adapted paper-based assessment instruments for use in the acute care setting. However, the efficacy of these systems has not been reported, and their effectiveness is likely to be constrained by the limits of the original instrument, the system in which they are placed, and the design team in ensuring that the automated instrument accurately reflects the logic of the original instrument.

Prevention Strategies in the Community

To date, several reviews have been conducted to examine the evidence available to support practice in this area (Agostini et al., 2001; Chang et al., 2004; Cumming, 2002; Gillespie, Gillespie, Cumming, Lamb, & Rowe, 2000; Gillespie et al., 2001, 2003). Gillespie and colleagues (2003), via the Cochrane Collaboration, identified the need for multipronged, interdisciplinary prevention programs; more accurate risk assessment instruments; and more research related to this complex and costly problem. Cumming (2002) reviewed 21 trials and concluded that exercise programs were the most promising and reduction of antipsychotic medications should be considered. However, Cumming also concluded that none of the reviewed research studies provided a definitive prevention strategy. Chang and collaborators (2004) conducted a similar review targeted at examining interventions for older adults in the community and found that multifactorial assessments with targeted intervention reduced risk of falls by 37% and that exercise interventions reduced fall risk by 14%. Hill-Westmoreland, Soeken, and Spellbring conducted a recent meta-analysis, including a sensitivity analysis, which identified an improved effect on fall prevention in the community when individualized management was added to exercise interventions (i.e., exercise interventions were not sufficient in and of themselves; instead, care needed to be tailored for specific individuals) (Hill-Westmoreland & Gruber-Baldini, 2005).

Researchers are exploring several other individual prevention strategies including falls clinics, exercise interventions (e.g., Tai Chi), vitamin D intake, home visits for safety checks, cataract surgery, and cardiac pacing. Falls and balance clinics (Nitz & Choy, 2004) present a promising community-based solution to the problem of falls. Clinics such as these provide focused intervention planning for patients identified at risk for falling. Accurate identification of such patients in primary care settings is the key limitation to the success of such clinics. Identification of recurrent fallers in the ED via comprehensive screening and tailored interventions has been successful at reducing recurrent falls by 36% (Davison et al., 2005) and by 38% in a nurse-led intervention that provided home assessment and tailored interventions (Lightbody, Watkins, Leathley, Sharma, & Lye, 2002). These recent studies add to early work in the Prevention of Falls in the Elderly Trial, or PROFET, which found a 61% decrease in falls for patients who were identified in the ED and who received subsequent detailed risk assessment and tailored interventions (Close et al., 1999).

Exercise-related interventions are by far the most commonly studied individual community prevention strategy and most of this research indicates that exercise is beneficial for patients with some research demonstrating that exercise regimens that involve balance training, such as Tai Chi, are more effective (Li et al., 2005; Sattin, Easley, Wolf, Chen, & Kutner, 2005; Wayne et al., 2005;

Wolf, Barnhart, Ellison, & Coogler, 1997; Wolf, Barnhart et al., 2003; Wolf, Sattin et al., 2003). Robertson, Campbell, Gardner, and Devlin (2002) performed a meta-analysis of four studies that examined effects of home exercise program. They found in the pooled effect analysis both fall and injury rates decreased by 35%. Exercise in conjunction with cognitive behavioral therapy, whereby patients are taught how to increase self-awareness about risky situations, has demonstrated promising results including a longer time before first fall and decreased injuries (Reinsch, MacRae, Lachenbruch, & Tobis, 1992). Unfortunately, this work did not demonstrate an effect on fall prevention efficacy, fear of falling, or actual fall rates (Reinsch et al., 1992).

Laboratory studies indicate that calcium and vitamin D reduce bone loss (Nieves, 2005), and a growing body of work is examining the ability for vitamin D supplementation to prevent fractures in individuals who are vitamin D deficient. However, research to date has been inconclusive, and larger, more recent studies have indicated that the use of vitamin D does not reduce fracture risk in the general community (Grant et al., 2005). However, a meta-analysis performed by Bischoff-Ferrari and team (2005) revealed that larger doses of vitamin D supplementation (700–800 IU/d) reduced the risk of fracture by up to 26%, whereas smaller doses of vitamin D (400 IU/d) did not reduce fracture risk. Although these are promising results, more research is required to identify best practice recommendations related to vitamin D deficiency screening and vitamin D supplementation. Interestingly, vitamin D might be integral in preventing falls themselves (and possibly breast and colon cancers) (Bitan, Meyer, Shinar, & Smora, 2004; Mosekilde, 2005). Recently, Latham and colleagues have demonstrated that vitamin D intake is an individual predictor for fall reduction, with the primary mechanism of action being improvement in muscle strength (Latham, Anderson, Lee et al., 2003; Latham, Anderson, & Reid, 2003).

Other researchers are exploring the ability for osteoporosis prevention medications to reduce fracture risk. Research has reported that risedronate, an oral medication for osteoporosis prevention, was effective at preventing fracture in older patients who have had a stroke (Sato, Iwamoto, Kanoko & Satoh, 2005; Sato, Kanoko, Satoh & Iwamoto, 2005).

Cardiac pacing for appropriate individuals can reduce or prevent falls related to syncopal episodes (Kenny, 1999). Other related efforts include home assessment for risk factors with the implementation of safety devices such as handrails, nonslip surfaces on stairs, and removal of throw rugs (Clemson, Cumming, & Roland, 1996; Morgan, Virnig, Duque, Abdel-Moty, & Devito, 2004; Rodriguez et al., 1995; Steinberg, Cartwright, Peel, & Williams, 2000). Researchers who conducted a recent randomized controlled trial found that thin-soled shoes were found to be the best type of shoe for patients, rather than running shoes, which have sticky soles (Robbins, Gouw, & McClaran, 1992).

Summary of Community-Based Falls and Related Injury

In summary, authors of several reviews have examined the efficacy of community-based fall and injury prevention programs. These reviewers have indicated that individualized multipronged interventions are effective at reducing falls and related injuries in the community setting (Gillespie et al., 2003). However, these interventions are not in place across primary care areas, which hinders their potential efficacy, and the aging community would likely benefit from large-scale implementation of these proven preventive interventions.

FALLS AND RELATED INJURIES IN THE ACUTE AND LONG-TERM CARE SETTINGS

Fall and related injury prevention is a major focus for both acute and long-term health care organizations. In the acute care setting, the 2005 JCAHO National Patient Safety Goals include the requirement for assessment and periodic reassessment for fall risk (Joint Commission on the Accreditation of Healthcare Organizations, 2005a). Although the goal of this requirement is to ensure that all patients are screened for falls and thus seeks to reduce harm from falls, the outcome is unpredictable because fall and injury risk assessment instruments in and of themselves have shown inconsistent effects. A more promising extension of this goal into 2006 is the additional requisite of implementing and evaluating a fall prevention program (Joint Commission on the Accreditation of Healthcare Organizations, 2005b). National compliance with these goals has the potential to significantly affect the problem of falls in the acute care setting. As mentioned earlier, efforts to streamline quality of care in the long-term care environment via improved reporting have the potential to reduce falls and related injuries in these particularly vulnerable patients; however, the successful implementation of fall prevention programs will be necessary to improve the problem.

Falls have several possible consequences. Recurrent falls have been identified as contributing to increases in the length of stay (LOS) in elderly psychiatric patients (Greene et al., 2001). A fall may also lead to a poorer quality of life because of "fallophobia," a fear of future falls and a factor that may itself contribute to fall risk (Parry, Steen, Galloway, Kenny, & Bond, 2001). Injuries occur in between 6% to 44% of falls in the acute care setting (Hitcho et al., 2004; Morse, 1997; Rohde et al., 1990). In the long-term care population between 9% to 15% of falls result in injury, with approximately 4% of these falls resulting in fractures (Francis, 2001). Additionally, patients who have underlying disease states are more susceptible to injuries. For example, osteoporosis can increase risk for fracture and bleeding disorders can increase risk for internal bleeding (Rothschild, Bates, & Leape, 2000). Fall-related injuries increase resource utilization; injuries from falls lead to increased LOS and an increased chance of unplanned re-admission or of discharge to residential or nursing home care (Frels, Williams, Narayanan, & Gariballa, 2002). Further, inpatients who have incurred an injury due to a fall have approximately 60% higher total charges than those who did not fall or those who fell and did not sustain an injury (Bates, Pruess, Souney, & Platt, 1995).

Evans, Hodgkinson, Lambert, Wood, and Kowanko (1998), via the Joanna Briggs Institute, performed a systematic review of the evidence up to 1997 for fall and injury prevention in the acute care setting. They examined 200 studies related to identification of predictors, risk assessment instrument development and testing, and fall and injury prevention interventions. Of these studies, only two were randomized controlled trials; however, one was too small to identify an effect from using bed alarms (Tideiksaar, Feiner, & Maby, 1993) and one, in which bracelets were used for patient identification, proved inconclusive (Mayo, Gloutney, & Levy, 1994). Evans and colleagues (1998) summarized that the instruments evaluated were not generalizable; however, they did not adequately compare the psychometric properties of the instruments in question. Rather, they evaluated research related to the implementation of such instruments, which was relatively weak up to that time point. In addition, Evans and colleagues identified that individual interventions were not more useful than any of the fall prevention programs that might be developed at a particular institution for a specific subset of patients. Although this conclusion may have been sufficient at that time point, the research has matured and this statement may no longer be true. More recent research has seen a growing number of randomized controlled trials, which will facilitate the ability to make stronger practice recommendations for this complex and challenging problem.

Research related to falls and related injuries in the acute and long-term care settings were identified and categorized as risk factor identification, risk assessment instruments, and prevention strategies. Each category of research is discussed below.

Acute Care and Long-Term Care Risk Factors

Factors associated with patients at risk of falling in the acute care setting have been explored extensively, particularly over the past two decades (Mahoney, 1998; Morse, 1985b, 1998; Morse, Tylko, & Dixon, 1987; Oliver, Daly, Martin, & McMurdo, 2004; Passaro et al., 2000; Perell et al., 2001). Evans, Hodgkinson, Lambert, and Wood (2001) conducted a systematic review of research related to risk factor identification for falls and identified 28 risk factors, including impaired mental status, special toileting needs, impaired physical status and to some extent age and medications. Oliver and colleagues (2004) reviewed the risk factor and risk assessment literature and identified five risk factors consistent across studies, including unsteady gait, increased toileting needs, confusion, sedative-hypnotics and history of falling. Risk factors in the long-term care environment are largely the same, with the addition of inability to transfer effectively (Becker et al., 2005) and short-term memory loss (Kron, Loy, Sturm, Nikolaus, & Becker, 2003). Although *ability to transfer* and *short-term memory function* might be characterized by unsteady gait and confusion, these items are expressly captured via the LTC-MDS.

Research has consistently demonstrated that multiple factors are associated with falling in elderly and hospitalized patients and that fall risk increases as the number of factors increases (Agostini et al., 2001; Evans et al., 1998; Morse, 1985a, 1985b, 1998; Morse et al., 1987; Oliver et al., 2004; Rubenstein, Powers, & MacLean, 2001; Tinetti & Williams, 1997). Although increased age is a strong predictor of falling in the community and has been cited as a factor for both risk of falling as well as for the severity of injury from the fall in acute care (Mahoney, 1998; Rubenstein et al., 2001), it has not always been found to be a factor in the acute care population (Currie, Mellino, Cimino, & Bakken, 2004; Hendrich, Bender, & Nyhuis, 2003; Morse, 1985a). Instead, comorbidities and impaired functional status may be more important predictors of falls and subsequent injury in this setting (Morse, 1985a; Rothschild et al., 2000). Indeed, recent work by Hendrich et al. (2003) did not support the association between increasing age (after the age of 65) and increased risk of falling in the inpatient environment. Instead, they found that confusion was the most important risk factor associated with the risk of falling. Nevertheless, age must be considered when discussing injury associated with falls because with age often comes frailty. Several researchers have identified sex as a risk factor, with female sex being a risk factor in the older population. However, more recent research has indicated that male sex contributes to fall risk in the younger population (Currie et al., 2004; Groves, Lavori, & Rosenbaum, 1993; Hendrich et al., 2003), however the cause for this has not been determined.

Harwood reviewed the literature related to visual problems and falls. The review demonstrated that uncorrected visual impairment nearly doubled the risk of falling (Harwood, 2001; Harwood et al., 2005). Cardiovascular causes of falls derive predominantly from neurally mediated disorders (e.g., vasovagal syncope) and cardiac abnormalities (e.g., arrhythmias, infarction, valvular stenosis) (Carey & Potter, 2001; Eltrafi, King, Silas, Currie, & Lye, 2000). Time of day has also been implicated. Tutuarimia, de Haan, and Limburg (1993) identified a higher rate of falls during the night shift, but this is inconsistent with other research and may in fact be explained by staffing patterns. Association of falls to the lunar cycle has also been explored, but found to be not associated with fall rates (Schwendimann, Joos, Geest, & Milisen, 2005).

Vitamin D deficiency has been implicated as a risk factor for falls and fracture in the long-term care setting (Bischoff-Ferrari et al., 2004). In addition, elevated alkaline phosphatase and low serum parathyroid hormone have been identified as predictors for falls (O'Hagan & O'Connell, 2005; Sambrook et al., 2004).

There is growing evidence of an association between low staffing ratios and an increase in the incidence of falls (Dunton, Gajewski, Taunton, & Moore, 2004; Hitcho et al., 2004; McGillis Hall, Doran, & Pink, 2004; Tutuarima et al., 1993; Whitman, Lim, Davidson, Wolf, & Wang, 2002). This recent work has identified an inverse association between licensed nurse staffing ratios and fall rates (i.e., a higher proportion of nurses is associated with lower fall rates) (Dunton et al., 2004; Loan, Jennings, Brosch, DePaul, & Hildreth, 2003; Tutuarima et al., 1993; Whitman et al., 2002). In addition, a growing body of research related to *failure to rescue*, defined as being "based on the premise that although deaths in hospitals are sometimes unavoidable, many can be prevented" (Aiken, Clarke, Sloane, Sochalski, & Silber, 2002; Clarke & Aiken, 2003; Needleman, Buerhaus, Mattke, Stewart, & Zelevinsky, 2002). This research supports the inclusion of unanticipated physiologic events into the definition of falls because the patient's safety issues should be addressed at all times. Other researchers who have examined nurse staffing ratios and fall rates have suggested that fall rates decreased with a decreasing number of nurses aids rather than licensed nursing staff (Unruh, 2003). This is supported by recent work by Krauss and colleagues (2005), who have identified that of the fallers in their case-control study, 85% of those in need of assistance or supervision with ambulation fell while not being supervised.

Certain subgroups of patients have been identified to be higher risk because of the inherent characteristics of their disease process or treatment modalities. These groups of patients include those in the care areas of geriatrics, behavioral health, oncology, rehabilitation, stroke units, and areas caring for multiple sclerosis patients.

In the behavioral health setting, fall rates range from 4.5 to 25 falls per 1,000 patient days. Researchers have investigated the risk factors in the behavioral health setting and have identified the typical faller to be a female with a history of falls who is less than 65 years of age and who is experiencing anxiety and agitation and receiving a sedative, tranquilizer, or laxative (Vaughn, Young, Rice, & Stoner, 1993). Irvin (1999) explored risk factors in the psychiatric setting and found that gait or balance problems and history of falls were the primary predictors. Although many of these characteristics are consistent with patients in the acute care setting, younger age and comorbidities such as depression and psychosis are often predictors in this population (Lim, Ng, Ng, & Ng, 2001; Poster, Pelletier, & Kay, 1991; Tay et al., 2000; Tsai, Witte, Radunzel, & Keller, 1998). In addition, treatments specific to behavioral health patients are different than those in the acute care setting. For example, patients treated for late-life depression are at risk for falling in the first weeks of using a tricyclic antidepressant and should be monitored closely in the time during which they are adjusting to the new medication (Joo et al., 2002). De Carle and Kohn (2000, 2001) have described risk factors in behavioral health patients and have identified electroconvulsive therapy as a factor that may increase the risk that a patient may fall.

Patients in rehabilitation units are also at higher risk, likely because they have suffered injuries such as stroke or head injury, which preclude muscle weakness, impaired cognition, and impulsivity (Rapport et al., 1993; Salgado, Lord, Ehrlich, Janji, & Rahman, 2004). In addition, these patients are being physically challenged, which places them in higher risk situations, and thus at higher risk for falling (Teasell, McRae, Foley, & Bhardwaj, 2002). Oncology patients may be at higher risk because of the side effects of chemotherapy or fatigue.

In the pediatric inpatient setting, fall rates range from 0 to 0.8 per 1000 patient days (Graf, 2005). These rates are low compared to adult inpatient and long-term care rates. The factors that limit the number of falls in this population are unclear, but may be related to staffing ratios and/or the common practice of parents staying with pediatric inpatients.

Injury Risk Factors

In general, injury risk factors are similar across care areas. Vassallo, Vignaraja, Sharma, Briggs, and Allen (2004) examined the risk factors associated with injury in a group of inpatient fallers and found that three factors were associated with injuries related to falls: (1) history of falls; (2) confusion; and (3) unsafe gait. In addition to these, Rothschild identified physiological processes, such as increased bleeding tendencies and osteoporosis as factors that increased risk for bleeding or fracture, (Rothschild et al., 2000). The risk for medications or physiologic factors to precipitate injuries related to bleeding have been explored on a limited basis in the inpatient population. Contrary to results in the community (Ohm et al., 2005), Stein, Viramontes, and Kerrigan (1995) found that hospitalized stroke patients who are anticoagulated are not at higher risk for falls than nonanticoagulated patients.

Acute Care Risk Assessment Instruments

Many tools have been developed to identify patients at highest risk for falling in the acute care setting (Coker & Oliver, 2003; Currie et al., 2004; Hendrich et al., 2003; Hendrich, Nyhuis, Kippenbrock, & Soja, 1995; Morse, 1997; Nyberg & Gustafson, 1996; Oliver et al., 2004). Perell et al. (2001) reviewed risk assessment tools and identified six functional assessment instruments and 15 fall risk assessment instruments developed by nursing. Vasallo and colleagues concurrently examined the predictive validity in the acute care setting of four commonly used risk assessment instruments (STRATIFY, Downton, Tullamore, and Tinetti) and found that the STRATIFY instrument was the easiest to use and was the most effective of the four at predicting falls in the first week of inpatient admission (total predictive accuracy 66.6%), but it had the poorest sensitivity (68.2%) (Vassallo, Stockdale, Sharma, Briggs, & Allen, 2005).

The risk assessment instrument that is most commonly reported on is the Morse Falls Risk Assessment Tool (Morse & Morse, 1988). In 2002, O'Connell and Myers conducted psychometric testing with this tool on a group of 1,059 patients admitted to an Australian hospital. In this study, the Morse Falls Risk Assessment Tool had a sensitivity of 83% and a specificity of 29%, but a positive predictive value of only 18%. This resulted in a high false positive rate, with the tool identifying more than 70% of patients who did not fall as being at high risk for falling. This research was confounded by the fact that the interventions were applied based on the instruments' predictions; therefore, their predictive validity cannot be conclusively stated. The STRATIFY falls prediction tool also had a low positive predictive value (30%) and relatively low sensitivity (66%) and specificity (47%) (Coker & Oliver, 2003). The Heinrich Falls Risk Model I (HFRM-I) is reported to be more robust (sensitivity = 77%; specificity = 72%) than either of the others, and the Hendrich Falls Risk Model II (HFRM-II) demonstrated even more improvement (sensitivity = 74.9%; specificity = 73.9%; positive predictive value = 75%) (Hendrich et al., 2003). The inclusion of a "get up and go" test to the HFRM-II tool was the major change between versions I and version II. The get up and go test evaluates a person's ability to rise from a chair in a single movement, which is an assessment method that has been explored in earlier falls prediction research. It is surprising that the sensitivity and specificity of the tool only increases slightly with the addition of this factor, underscoring the complexity of predicting patient falls. In addition, prospective evaluation of the use of the HFRM-II instrument has yet to be reported.

Several studies have tested the predictive validity of fall risk assessment instruments in relation to the judgment of nurses. Myers and Nikoletti (2003) concluded that neither the fall risk assessment instrument nor nurses' clinical judgment acted as a reliable predictor. Eagle et al. (1999) compared the Functional Reach Test, the Morse Falls Scale, and nurses' clinical judgment in the rehabilitation and geriatric environment. This study also concluded that the two standardized assessment processes were no better at predicting falls than the clinical judgment of nurses. A limitation to both of these studies was that the evaluation occurred only at one time point close to admission, which does not account for the variability of patient status throughout a patient's hospital stay.

In the domain of rehabilitation medicine, Ruchinskas compared structured assessments including Mini-Mental State Exam, the Geriatric Depression Scale, the Functional Intervention Model, and the clinical judgment of physical and occupational therapists on admission and discharge (Ruchinskas, 2003). This study concluded that the clinical judgment of therapists had a positive predictive power of 33% and a negative predictive power of 82%. However, the more accurate predictors of falling for the patients in their sample were a history of falls and presence of a neurological diagnosis. In the residential care environment, it was found that clinical judgment can contribute to the accurate prediction of fall risk, but is not sufficient on its own as a valid predictor (Lundin-Olsson, Jensen, Nyberg, & Gustafson, 2003). Although fall prediction research has been performed for two decades, it is clear that fall prevention is a complex problem that cannot be solved by risk assessment alone, hence the dissatisfaction with available risk assessment instruments.

Long-Term Care Assessment Instruments

Lundin-Olson, Nyberg, and Gustafson (2000) developed the Mobility Interaction Fall Chart (MIF chart), which is an instrument that measures a patient's ability to walk and talk at the same time, the ability to maintain pace while carrying a glass of water, visual impairment, and difficulty concentrating. When the predictive validity of the MIF chart was evaluated, the researchers found that the chart was helpful only when used in conjunction with clinical judgment and knowledge of a patient's history of falls, thus making the use of this instrument limited on its own (Lundin-Olsson et al., 2003). The Downton instrument, originally developed in the community setting, characterizes risk by five factors: (1) increased dependency, (2) cognitive impairment, (3) increased number of physical symptoms, (4) presence of anxiety, and (5) presence of depression (Downton & Andrews, 1991). This instrument has recently been prospectively evaluated in the long-term care setting with a reported sensitivity ranging from 81% to 95% and specificity ranging from 35% to 40% (Rosendahl et al., 2003). Although the specificity is low, this instrument might provide a standardized measure by which to identify those at risk in the long-term care environment. Becker et al. (2005) have recently described an algorithm to assess fall risk in the long-term care setting whereby long-term care residents are categorized into three subgroups: (1) Residents requiring assistance to transfer, (2) Residents able to transfer with history of falls and requiring the use of restraints, and (3) Residents able to transfer and with no history of falls but with urinary incontinence and visual impairment. The researchers found that the residents with the history of falls were at highest risk for falls, which is consistent with other research in this domain, but might be useful to tailor interventions and would warrant prospective evaluation (Becker et al., 2005).

Pediatric Risk Assessment Instruments

Falls in the acute care pediatric setting are relatively rare; however, standardized assessment may be beneficial to reduce falls and injuries in this population. Graf (2005) has recently developed an instrument for acute care pediatric risk assessment. According to Graf, factors associated with pediatric falls include (1) Seizure medication (OR 4.9), (2) Orthopedic Diagnosis, (3) Not using an IV (OR 3.6), (4) Physical and occupational therapy ordered, and (5) LOS (OR 1.84 for every 5 days). This model has a sensitivity and specificity of 69% and 84% respectively, and is being prospectively evaluated by the investigator with the hopes that standardized assessment will facilitate reduction in these already low rates.

Automated Risk Assessment

Recent national patient safety efforts highlight the promise of using informatics processes to manage patient safety issues such as the management of patient falls. However, to date, most automated risk assessment techniques in the acute care setting are electronic versions of existing fall risk assessment instruments with limited use of computerized decision support (Browne, Covington, & Davila, 2004; Currie et al., 2004). Promising new work in data mining for fall prediction has demonstrated that the LTC-MDS has the potential to use existing data to generate risk models for patients in this setting. Volrathongchai (2005) has recently explored the ability to use computerized data mining techniques to identify elderly residents of long-term care facilities who were at risk for falls. Although this work has not been prospectively evaluated, the research found that the use of these data mining techniques in conjunction with nursing knowledge had the potential to identify fallers.

Acute and Long-Term Care Prevention Strategies

The goal of any fall and injury prevention effort is to decrease adverse outcomes for the patients who are most vulnerable to falling. A beneficial consequence of fall and related injury prevention programs is the potential to streamline resource use with the added potential for decreased costs associated with this problem (Moller, 2005; Panneman, Goettsch, Kramarz, & Herings, 2003; Scuffham, Chaplin, & Legood, 2003). To date however, a ubiquitous fall and injury prevention strategy has not been identified for hospitalized patients.

Several reviews have examined fall prevention strategies in the acute and long-term care settings (Agostini et al., 2001; Chang et al., 2004; Evans et al., 1998; Oliver, Hopper, & Seed, 2000). Oliver, Hopper and Seed (2000) examined 10 studies, including three randomized controlled trials and seven prospective studies with historical controls. They found that the pooled effects ratio was 1.0 (95% CI 0.60–1.68), indicating that overall the interventions were not able to prevent falls. Agostini, Baker, and Bogardus (2001) conducted a review of the literature related to fall prevention for hospitalized and institutionalized older adults. This review did not pool the results, but instead examined the literature related to the use of armbands, bed alarms, and restraints for fall prevention, all of which will be discussed individually below.

The use of physical restraints to prevent falls has been called into question because restraints limit mobility and might contribute to injuries (Evans, Wood, & Lambert, 2003; Vassallo et al., 2005). Agostini et al. (2001) examined literature related to fall prevention via restraint and side rail use as well as fall rates when restraints were removed. Six studies were evaluated finding that restraints were associated with increased injuries and restraint and side rail removal did not increase in fall rates (Agostini et al., 2001). Evans, Wood, and Lambert (2002) also examined the literature and found 16 studies that examined restraint minimization, concluding that restraint minimization programs involving effective staff education can reduce injuries and do not increase fall rates.

Several individual fall prevention interventions have been examined, including the use of armband identification bracelets, exercise regimens, post-fall assessment, bed alarms, toileting regimens, and vitamin D supplementation. Mayo et al. (1994) conducted a randomized controlled trial to examine whether armbands would help identify high-risk patients in a rehabilitation unit and thus prevent falls in the high-risk group. The researchers, however, found that high-risk patients with an armband had higher fall rates than those without the armband. Mulrow et al. (1994) examined the effects of a physical therapy exercise intervention for frail long-term care residents and found that fall rates increased in the intervention group. However, the intervention group in this study also showed an increase in general strength and a decrease in the use of assistive devices, making one wonder whether the physical therapy intervention sought to decrease the use of assistive devices in inappropriate situations in the first place. Rubenstein and colleagues examined the ability for post-fall assessment to identify underlying factors that could be remedied to prevent further falls (Rubenstein, Robbins, Josephson, Schulman, & Osterweil, 1990). Despite widespread use, only one study from 1993 has examined bed alarms (Tideiksaar et al., 1993). Tideiksaar et al. found that bed alarms were an effective method for fall prevention (Relative Risk = 0.32), but the intervention warrants further research. An associated intervention, a movement detector, has recently been developed. A promising pilot study examined the use of a movement detection patch attached to the thigh that alerts clinicians when elderly long-term care residents were moving about (Kelly, Phillips, Cain, Polissar, & Kelly, 2002). Kelly et al. found a 91% decrease in falls during the one-week testing period. Although the product developers sponsored this study, the intervention might be suitable for select patients and bears further testing.

Bakarich, McMillan, and Prosser (1997) examined the effect of a toileting regimen for elderly confused patients with mobility problems in the acute care units of a large metropolitan teaching hospital. The researchers found that there were 53% fewer falls during shifts in which the risk assessment and toileting intervention was used, but that compliance with the assessment and intervention was difficult to maintain. More recently, Klay and Marfyak (2005) found that a continence specialist in the long-term care environment reduced falls by 58%. Vitamin D has also reduced falls in elderly females in the long-term care setting by up to 49% (Bischoff et al., 2003). Further investigation of the use of vitamin D in the acute care and rehabilitation setting for fall and injury prevention is warranted.

As with community interventions, tailored, multipronged prevention strategies are shown to be more effective than individual interventions alone. Hofmann and colleagues used three concurrent interventions—staff education, an exercise program, and environmental modifications—for a frail elderly population (Hofmann, Bankes, Javed, & Selhat, 2003). The concurrent use of these interventions decreased the fall rate by 38% and decreased the fracture rate by 50%. Haines, Bennell, Osborne, and Hill (2004) also examined a multipronged intervention involving staff and patient education, an exercise programs and the use of hip protectors. Researchers found a 22% decrease in falls and a 28% decrease in injuries in the intervention group.

One of the most promising studies by Jensen and her research team investigated the effects of a comprehensive fall risk assessment and tailored intervention program in the long-term care setting (Jensen, Lundin-Olsson, Nyberg, & Gustafson, 2002). The intervention included assessment via the MIF chart, visual evaluation, medication evaluation, and delirium screening by all members of the care team (e.g., physicians, nurses, and physical and occupational therapists). This research demonstrated that the comprehensive assessment and tailored interventions reduced falls by 51% and injuries by 77% over a 34-week period. A statistically significant reduction in falls (RR 0.71) was also found by applying a tailored plan of care to adult inpatients who were deemed at high risk for a fall based on having had a previous fall (Healey, Monro, Cockram, Adams, & Heseltine, 2004). In effect, this research used history of fall as a method to triage high-risk patients, who then received a comprehensive risk assessment with targeted interventions. This research did not demonstrate a decrease in injuries; however further research using this technique will be useful. McMurdo, Millar, and Daly (2000) found a reduction in fall rates in a group of 133 nursing home residents by up to 55% with comprehensive risk assessment and balance training, but these results were not statistically significant. A larger sample size would provide a better understanding of the effect of the intervention.

Other research examining multipronged studies has found that such interventions were not effective. A recent study in long-term care facilities found a decrease in falls that was nullified when the results were controlled for LOS (Vassallo, Vignaraja, Sharma, Hallam et al., 2004). However, controlling for LOS removes the ability for LOS to be identified as a predictor, which may be the case for patients who stay longer in a hospital setting. Kerse, Butler, Robinson, and Todd

(2004) found that, in a group of nursing homes, long-term care residents who were randomized to risk assessment followed by tailored interventions showed an increase in falls (Incident Rate Ratio 1.34; p value 0.018). Semin-Goosens, van der Helm and Bossyut (2003) evaluated the effect of a guideline with semi-structured interventions and found that fall rates in high risk neurology and medical patients were not reduced. The researchers attributed the failure to resistance by nurses to changing attitudes toward falls with the statement that nurses did not find falls "troublesome enough." However, the failure was more likely due to system issues, such as ability to implement, agreement with the guideline, and training issues, which are common with guideline implementation failures (Cabana et al., 1999; Rubinson, Wu, Haponik, & Diette, 2005). In addition, the Semin-Goosens et al. guideline did not use a standardized risk assessment instrument, which might have made it difficult to identify patients at risk.

Although the results of multipronged studies are conflicting, it is important to note, that neither the studies of multipronged interventions with effective results nor those with ineffective results have controlled for staffing ratios or skill mix.

An increasing number of studies have examined the ability to prevent injury in the acute and long-term care setting. Hip protectors have been evaluated in the long-term care environment since the early 1990s. Although early work found that hip protectors were effective in reducing hip fractures in the frail or osteoporotic elderly (Lauritzen, Petersen, & Lund, 1993), more recent work indicates that compliance with using hip protectors is difficult to maintain, making recommendation for hip protector use conditional (O'Halloran et al., 2004; O'Halloran et al., 2005). Ray and colleagues (2005) examined the ability for a 2-day staff safety education plan to reduce serious fall-related injuries. This intervention was not effective, but may have been confounded by lack of compliance with the staff interventions.

Summary of Acute and Long-Term Care Falls and Related Injuries

In summary, fall prevention in the acute and long-term care settings is a complex and demanding problem with multiple patient types and risk factors to manage. Standardized risk assessment with tailored interventions appears to be the most promising method of prevention; however implementation of comprehensive interventions can be challenging. Further research toward overcoming barriers to implementation, guideline adherence, staffing ratios, and tailored interventions for newly identified risk factors such as vitamin D deficiency are warranted. In addition, research must be conducted on a larger scale to demonstrate generalizability and to be able to translate the evidence into practice.

CONCLUSION

Falls and related injuries are an important issue across the care continuum. National efforts in the community via HP2010, in the acute care setting via JCAHO-NPSG, and in the long-term care setting via the NHQI project have the potential to significantly reduce falls and related injuries. The growing number of randomized controlled trials related to fall prevention efforts is promising. However, most of these studies have been carried out in the community and long-term care environments, with randomized controlled trials evaluating fall and injury prevention measures in the acute care setting remaining relatively rare. As with other nursing-sensitive quality indicators, recent research demonstrating an association between fall rates and nurse staffing ratios needs to be more fully explored. In addition, further research needs to investigate automated methods of assessing and communicating fall risk, better methods for risk identification, and the identification of prevention measures. Indeed, with more coordinated efforts to apply the evidence to practice, the problem of falls might be managed more effectively.

REFERENCES

Agostini, J. V., Baker, D. I., & Bogardus, S. T. (2001). *Prevention of falls in hospitalized and institutionalized older people*. Rockville, MD: Agency for Healthcare Research and Quality.

Aiken, L. H., Clarke, S. P., Sloane, D. M., Sochalski, J., & Silber, J. H. (2002). Hospital nurse staffing and patient mortality, nurse burnout, and job dissatisfaction. *Journal of the American Medical Association, 288*(16), 1987–1993.

American Nurses Association. (1999). *Nursing-sensitive quality indicators for acute care settings and ANA's safety & quality initiative*. Retrieved February 9, 2003, www.nursingworld.org/readroom/fssafe99.htm

American Nurses Association. (2005). *National database for nursing quality indicators: Guidelines for data collection and submission on quarterly indicators, version 5.0*, NDNQI, 2005.

Bakarich, A., McMillan, V., & Prosser, R. (1997). The effect of a nursing intervention on the incidence of older patient falls. *Australian Journal of Advanced Nursing, 15*(1), 26–31.

Bassiony, M. M., Rosenblatt, A., Baker, A., Steinberg, M., Steele, C. D., Sheppard, J. M., et al. (2004). Falls and age in patients with Alzheimer's disease. *Journal of Nervous and Mental Disease, 192*(8), 570–572.

Bates, D. W., Pruess, K., Souney, P., & Platt, R. (1995). Serious falls in hospitalized patients: correlates and resource utilization. *American Journal of Medicine, 99*(2), 137–143.

Becker, C., Loy, S., Sander, S., Nikolaus, T., Rissmann, U., & Kron, M. (2005). An algorithm to screen long-term care residents at risk for accidental falls. *Aging Clinical and Experimental Research, 17*(3), 186–192.

Bischoff, H. A., Stahelin, H. B., Dick, W., Akos, R., Knecht, M., Salis, C., et al. (2003). Effects of vitamin D and calcium supplementation on falls: A randomized controlled trial. *Journal of Bone and Mineral Research, 18*(2), 343–351.

Bischoff-Ferrari, H. A., Dawson-Hughes, B., Willett, W. C., Staehelin, H. B., Bazemore, M. G., Zee, R. Y., et al. (2004). Effect of Vitamin D on falls: a meta-analysis. *Journal of the American Medical Association, 291*(16), 1999–2006.

Bischoff-Ferrari, H. A., Willett, W. C., Wong, J. B., Giovannucci, E., Dietrich, T., & Dawson-Hughes, B. (2005). Fracture prevention with vitamin D supplementation: A meta-analysis of randomized controlled trials. *Journal of the American Medical Association, 293*(18), 2257–2264.

Bitan, Y., Meyer, J., Shinar, D., & Smora, E. (2004). Nurses' reactions to alarms in a neonatal intensive care unit. *Cognition, Technology & Work, 6*(2), 239–246.

Browne, J. A., Covington, B. G., & Davila, Y. (2004). Using information technology to assist in redesign of a fall prevention program. *Journal of Nursing Care Quality, 19*(3), 218–225.

Cabana, M. D., Rand, C. S., Powe, N. R., Wu, A. W., Wilson, M. H., Abboud, P. A. C., et al. (1999). Why don't physicians follow clinical practice guidelines?: A framework for improvement. *Journal of the American Medical Association, 282*, 1458–1465.

Carey, B. J., & Potter, J. F. (2001). Cardiovascular causes of falls. *Age and Ageing, 30*(Suppl. 4), 19–24.

Centers for Medicare & Medicaid Services. (2003). *Minimum data set (MDS): Draft version 3.0 for nursing home resident assessment and care screening.*

Centers for Medicare & Medicaid Services. (2005). *Nursing home quality initiative overview:* Centers for Medicare & Medicaid Services.

Chang, J. T., Morton, S. C., Rubenstein, L. Z., Mojica, W. A., Maglione, M., Suttorp, M. J., et al. (2004). Interventions for the prevention of falls in older adults: Systematic review and meta-analysis of randomised clinical trials. *British Medical Journal, 328*(7441), 680.

Clarke, S. P., & Aiken, L. H. (2003). Failure to rescue: Needless deaths are prime examples of the need for more nurses at the bedside. *American Journal of Nursing, 103*(1), 42–47.

Clemson, L., Cumming, R. G., & Roland, M. (1996). Case-control study of hazards in the home and risk of falls and hip fractures. *Age and Ageing, 25*(2), 97–101.

Close, J., Ellis, M., Hooper, R., Glucksman, E., Jackson, S., & Swift, C. (1999). Prevention of falls in the elderly trial (PROFET): A randomised controlled trial. *The Lancet, 353*(9147), 93–97.

Coker, E., & Oliver, D. (2003). Evaluation of the STRATIFY falls prediction tool on a geriatric unit. *Outcomes Management for Nursing Practice, 7*(1), 8–14; quiz 15–16.

Colon-Emeric, C. S., Pieper, C. F., & Artz, M. B. (2002). Can historical and functional risk factors be used to predict fractures in community-dwelling older adults? Development and validation of a clinical tool. *Osteoporos International, 13*(12), 955–961.

Committee on Data Standards for Patient Safety. (2003). *Patient safety: Achieving a new standard for care:* Institute of Medicine.

Committee on Quality of Health Care in America. (1999). *To err is human: Building a safer health system:* National Academies Press.

Cumming, R. G. (2002). Intervention strategies and risk-factor modification for falls prevention. A review of recent intervention studies. *Clinics in Geriatric Medicine, 18*(2), 175–189.

Currie, L. M., Mellino, L. V., Cimino, J. J., & Bakken, S. (2004). Development and representation of a fall-injury risk assessment instrument in a clinical information system. *Medinfo, 11*(Pt. 1), 721–725.

Davison, J., Bond, J., Dawson, P., Steen, I. N., & Kenny, R. A. (2005). Patients with recurrent falls attending accident & emergency benefit from multifactorial intervention—a randomised controlled trial. *Age and Ageing, 34*(2), 162–168.

de Carle, A. J., & Kohn, R. (2000). Electroconvulsive therapy and falls in the elderly. *Journal of ECT, 16*(3), 252–257.

de Carle, A. J., & Kohn, R. (2001). Risk factors for falling in a psychogeriatric unit. *International Journal of Geriatric Psychiatry, 16*(8), 762–767.

Delbaere, K., Crombez, G., Vanderstraeten, G., Willems, T., & Cambier, D. (2004). Fear-related avoidance of activities, falls and physical frailty. A prospective community-based cohort study. *Age and Ageing, 33*(4), 368–373.

Dharmarajan, T. S., & Norkus, E. P. (2004). Mild anemia and the risk of falls in older adults from nursing homes and the community. *Journal of the American Medical Director Association, 5*(6), 395–400.

Dhesi, J. K., Bearne, L. M., Moniz, C., Hurley, M. V., Jackson, S. H., Swift, C. G., et al. (2002). Neuromuscular and psychomotor function in elderly subjects who fall and the relationship with vitamin D status. *Journal of Bone and Mineral Research, 17*(5), 891–897.

Downton, J. H., & Andrews, K. (1991). Prevalence, characteristics and factors associated with falls among the elderly living at home. *Aging (Milano), 3*(3), 219–228.

Dukas, L. C., Schacht, E., Mazor, Z., & Stahelin, H. B. (2005). A new significant and independent risk factor for falls in elderly men and women: A low creatinine clearance of less than 65 ml/min. *Osteoporosis International, 16*(3), 332–338.

Dunton, N., Gajewski, B., Taunton, R. L., & Moore, J. (2004). Nurse staffing and patient falls on acute care hospital units. *Nursing Outlook, 52*(1), 53–59.

Dyer, C. A., Watkins, C. L., Gould, C., & Rowe, J. (1998). Risk-factor assessment for falls: From a written checklist to the penless clinic. *Age and Ageing, 27*(5), 569–572.

Eagle, D. J., Salama, S., Whitman, D., Evans, L. A., Ho, E., & Olde, J. (1999). Comparison of three instruments in predicting accidental falls in selected inpatients in a general teaching hospital. *Journal of Gerontological Nursing, 25*(7), 40–45.

Eltrafi, A., King, D., Silas, J. H., Currie, P., & Lye, M. (2000). Role of carotid sinus syndrome and neurocardiogenic syncope in recurrent syncope and falls in patients referred to an outpatient clinic in a district general hospital. *Postgraduate Medical Journal, 76*(897), 405–408.

Evans, D., Hodgkinson, B., Lambert, L., & Wood, J. (2001). Falls risk factors in the hospital setting: A systematic review. *International Journal of Nursing Practice, 7*(1), 38–45.

Evans, D., Hodgkinson, B., Lambert, L., Wood, J., & Kowanko, I. (1998). *Falls in acute hospitals: A systematic review:* Joanna Briggs Center for Evidence Based Nursing and Midwifery.

Evans, D., Wood, J., & Lambert, L. (2002). A review of physical restraint minimization in the acute and residential care settings. *Journal of Advanced Nursing, 40*(6), 616–625.

Evans, D., Wood, J., & Lambert, L. (2003). Patient injury and physical restraint devices: A systematic review. *Journal of Advanced Nursing, 41*(3), 274–282.

Fink, H. A., Kuskowski, M. A., Orwoll, E. S., Cauley, J. A., & Ensrud, K. E. (2005). Association between Parkinson's disease and low bone density and falls in older men: The osteoporotic fractures in men study. *Journal of the American Geriatric Society, 53*(9), 1559–1564.

Francis, R. M. (2001). Falls and fractures. Age and Ageing, 30 Supplement 4, 25–28.

Frels, C., Williams, P., Narayanan, S., & Gariballa, S. E. (2002). Iatrogenic causes of falls in hospitalised elderly patients: A case-control study. Postgraduate Medical Journal, 78(922), 487–489.

Gavin-Dreschnack, D., Nelson, A., Fitzgerald, S., Harrow, J., Sanchez-Anguiano, A., Ahmed, S., et al. (2005). Wheelchair-related falls: Current evidence and directions for improved quality care. Journal of Nursing Care Quality, 20(2), 119–127.

Gerdhem, P., Ringsberg, K. A., Akesson, K., & Obrant, K. J. (2005). Clinical history and biologic age predicted falls better than objective functional tests. Journal of Clinical Epidemiologyl, 58(3), 226–232.

Gillespie, L. D., Gillespie, W. J., Cumming, R., Lamb, S. E., & Rowe, B. H. (2000). Interventions for preventing falls in the elderly. Cochrane Database of Systematic Reviews, (2), CD000340.

Gillespie, L. D., Gillespie, W. J., Robertson, M. C., Lamb, S. E., Cumming, R. G., & Rowe, B. H. (2001). Interventions for preventing falls in elderly people. Cochrane Database of Systematic Reviews (3), CD000340.

Gillespie, L. D., Gillespie, W. J., Robertson, M. C., Lamb, S. E., Cumming, R. G., & Rowe, B. H. (2003). Interventions for preventing falls in elderly people. Cochrane Database of Systematic Reviews (4), CD000340.

Graf, E. (2005). Pediatric hosptial falls: Development of a predictor model to guide pediatric clincial practice. Paper presented at the Sigma Theta Tau International: 38th Biennial Convention, Indianapolis, IN.

Grant, A. M., Avenell, A., Campbell, M. K., McDonald, A. M., MacLennan, G. S., McPherson, G. C., et al. (2005). Oral vitamin D3 and calcium for secondary prevention of low-trauma fractures in elderly people (Randomised evaluation of calcium or vitamin D, RECORD): A randomised placebo-controlled trial. The Lancet, 365(9471), 1621–1628.

Greene, E., Cunningham, C. J., Eustace, A., Kidd, N., Clare, A. W., & Lawlor, B. A. (2001). Recurrent falls are associated with increased length of stay in elderly psychiatric inpatients. International Journal of Geriatric Psychiatry, 16(10), 965–968.

Groves, J. E., Lavori, P. W., & Rosenbaum, J. F. (1993). Accidental injuries of hospitalized patients. A prospective cohort study. International Journal of Technological Assessment in Health Care, 9(1), 139–144.

Grubel, F. (1959). Fall: A principal patient incident. Hospital Management, 88, 37–38.

Haines, T. P., Bennell, K. L., Osborne, R. H., & Hill, K. D. (2004). Effectiveness of targeted falls prevention programme in subacute hospital setting: Randomised controlled trial. British Medical Journal, 328(7441), 676.

Halfon, P., Eggli, Y., Van Melle, G., & Vagnair, A. (2001). Risk of falls for hospitalized patients: A predictive model based on routinely available data. Journal of Clinical Epidemiology, 54(12), 1258–1266.

Hanlon, J. T., Landerman, L. R., Fillenbaum, G. G., & Studenski, S. (2002). Falls in African American and white community-dwelling elderly residents. Journals of Gerontology. Series A: Biological Sciences and Medical Sciences, 57(7), M473–478.

Harwood, R. H. (2001). Visual problems and falls. Age and Ageing, 30(Suppl. 4), 13–18.

Harwood, R. H., Foss, A. J., Osborn, F., Gregson, R. M., Zaman, A., & Masud, T. (2005). Falls and health status in elderly women following first eye cataract surgery: A randomised controlled trial. *British Journal of Ophthalmology*, 89(1), 53–59.

Hausdorff, J. M. (2001). Gait variability and fall risk in community-living older adults: A 1-year prospective study. *Archives of Physical Medicine and Rehabilitation*, 82(8), 1050–1056.

Healey, F., Monro, A., Cockram, A., Adams, V., & Heseltine, D. (2004). Using targeted risk factor reduction to prevent falls in older in-patients: A randomised controlled trial. *Age and Ageing*, 33(4), 390–395.

Healthcare Cost and Utilization Project. (2002). *National and regional estimates on hospital use for all patients from the HCUP Nationwide Inpatient Sample (NIS)*. Retrieved November 20, 2003, from www.ahrq.gov/HCUPnet/

Hendrich, A. L., Bender, P. S., & Nyhuis, A. (2003). Validation of the Hendrich II Fall Risk Model: A large concurrent case/control study of hospitalized patients. *Applied Nursing Research*, 16(1), 9–21.

Hendrich, A. L., Nyhuis, A., Kippenbrock, T., & Soja, M. E. (1995). Hospital falls: development of a predictive model for clinical practice. *Applied Nursing Research*, 8(3), 129–139.

Hill-Westmoreland, E. E., & Gruber-Baldini, A. L. (2005). Falls documentation in nursing homes: Agreement between the minimum data set and chart abstractions of medical and nursing documentation. *Journal of the American Geriatric Society*, 53(2), 268–273.

Hill-Westmoreland, E. E., Soeken, K., & Spellbring, A. M. (2002). A meta-analysis of fall prevention programs for the elderly: How effective are they? *Nursing Research*, 51(1), 1–8.

Hirdes, J. P., Fries, B. E., Morris, J. N., Ikegami, N., Zimmerman, D., Dalby, D. M., et al. (2004). Home care quality indicators (HCQIs) based on the MDS-HC. *The Gerontologist*, 44(5), 665–680.

Hitcho, E. B., Krauss, M. J., Birge, S., Claiborne-Dunagan, W., Fischer, I., Johnson, S., et al. (2004). Characteristics and circumstances of falls in a hospital setting: A prospective analysis. *Journal of General Internal Medicine*, 19(7), 732–739.

Hofmann, M. T., Bankes, P. F., Javed, A., & Selhat, M. (2003). Decreasing the incidence of falls in the nursing home in a cost-conscious environment: A pilot study. *Journal of the American Medical Director Association*, 4(2), 95–97.

Hornbrook, M. C., Stevens, V. J., Wingfield, D. J., Hollis, J. F., Greenlick, M. R., & Ory, M. G. (1994). Preventing falls among community-dwelling older persons: Results from a randomized trial. *Gerontologist*, 34(1), 16–23.

Irvin, D. J. (1999). Psychiatric unit fall event. *Journal of Psychosocial Nursing Mental Health Services*, 37(12), 8–16.

Jensen, J., Lundin-Olsson, L., Nyberg, L., & Gustafson, Y. (2002). Fall and injury prevention in older people living in residential care facilities. A cluster randomized trial. *Annals of Internal Medicine*, 136(10), 733–741.

Joint Commission on the Accreditation of Healthcare Organizations. (2005a). *2005 hospitals' national patient safety goals*. Retrieved February 10, 2005 from www.jcaho.org/ptaccredited+organizations/patient+safety/05+npsg/05_npsg_hap.htm

Joint Commission on the Accreditation of Healthcare Organizations. (2005b). *2006 critical access hospital and hospital national patient safety goals*. Retrieved September 26, 2005, from www.jcaho.org/accredited+organizations/patient+safety/06_npsg/06_npsg_cah_hap. htm

Joo, J. H., Lenze, E. J., Mulsant, B. H., Begley, A. E., Weber, E. M., Stack, J. A., et al. (2002). Risk factors for falls during treatment of late-life depression. *Journal of Clinical Psychiatry, 63*(10), 936–941.

Kelly, K. E., Phillips, C. L., Cain, K. C., Polissar, N. L., & Kelly, P. B. (2002). Evaluation of a nonintrusive monitor to reduce falls in nursing home patients. *Journal of the American Medical Directors Association, 3*(6), 377–382.

Kenny, R. A. (1999). SAFE PACE 2: Syncope and falls in the elderly—pacing and carotid sinus evaluation: A randomized controlled trial of cardiac pacing in older patients with falls and carotid sinus hypersensitivity. *Europace, 1*(1), 69–72.

Kerse, N., Butler, M., Robinson, E., & Todd, M. (2004). Fall prevention in residential care: A cluster, randomized, controlled trial. *Journal of the American Geriatric Society, 52*(4), 524–531.

Klay, M., & Marfyak, K. (2005). Use of a continence nurse specialist in an extended care facility. *Urologic Nursing, 25*(2), 101–102, 107–108.

Krauss, M. J., Evanoff, B., Hitcho, E. B., Ngugi, K. E., Dunagan, W. C., Fischer, I., et al. (2005). A case-control study of patient, medication, and care-related risk factors for inpatient falls. *Journal of General Internal Medicine, 20*(2), 116–122.

Kron, M., Loy, S., Sturm, E., Nikolaus, T., & Becker, C. (2003). Risk indicators for falls in institutionalized frail elderly. *American Journal of Epidemiology, 158*(7), 645–653.

Kumar, N. P., Thomas, A., Mudd, P., Morris, R. O., & Masud, T. (2003). The usefulness of carotid sinus massage in different patient groups. *Age and Ageing, 32*(6), 666–669.

Landi, F., Onder, G., Cesari, M., Barillaro, C., Russo, A., & Bernabei, R. (2005). Psychotropic medications and risk for falls among community-dwelling frail older people: An observational study. *Journals of Gerontology. Series A: Biological Sciences and Medical Sciences, 60*(5), 622–626.

Latham, N. K., Anderson, C. S., Lee, A., Bennett, D. A., Moseley, A., & Cameron, I. D. (2003). A randomized, controlled trial of quadriceps resistance exercise and vitamin D in frail older people: The Frailty Interventions Trial in Elderly Subjects (FITNESS). *Journal of the American Geriatric Society, 51*(3), 291–299.

Latham, N. K., Anderson, C. S., & Reid, I. R. (2003). Effects of vitamin D supplementation on strength, physical performance, and falls in older persons: A systematic review. *Journal of the American Geriatric Society, 51*(9), 1219–1226.

Lauritzen, J. B. (1996). Hip fractures: Incidence, risk factors, energy absorption, and prevention. *Bone, 18*(Suppl. 1), 65S–75S. Lauritzen, J. B., Petersen, M. M., & Lund, B. (1993). Effect of external hip protectors on hip fractures. *The Lancet, 341*(8836), 11–13.

Leape, L. L., Brennan, T. A., Laird, N., Lawthers, A. G., Localio, A. R., Barnes, B. A., et al. (1991). The nature of adverse events in hospitalized patients. Results of the Harvard Medical Practice Study II. *New England Journal of Medicine, 324*(6), 377–384.

Levine, R. S., Briggs, N. C., Husaini, B. A., Foster, I., Hull, P. C., Pamies, R. J., et al. (2005). HEDIS prevention performance indicators, prevention quality assessment and Healthy People 2010. *Journal of Health Care for the Poor and Underserved, 16.4*(Suppl. A), 64–82.

Li, F., Harmer, P., Fisher, K. J., McAuley, E., Chaumeton, N., Eckstrom, E., et al. (2005). Tai Chi and fall reductions in older adults: A randomized controlled trial. *Journals of Gerontology. Series A: Biological Sciences and Medical Sciences, 60*(2), 187–194.

Liaw, S. T., Sulaiman, N., Pearce, C., Sims, J., Hill, K., Grain, H., et al. (2003). Falls prevention within the Australian general practice data model: Methodology, information model, and terminology issues. *Journal of the American Medical Informatics Association, 10*(5), 425–432.

Lightbody, E., Watkins, C., Leathley, M., Sharma, A., & Lye, M. (2002). Evaluation of a nurse-led falls prevention programme versus usual care: A randomized controlled trial. *Age and Ageing, 31*(3), 203–210.

Lim, K. D., Ng, K. C., Ng, S. K., & Ng, L. L. (2001). Falls amongst institutionalized psycho-geriatric patients. *Singapore Medical Journal, 42*(10), 466–472.

Loan, L. A., Jennings, B. M., Brosch, L. R., DePaul, D., & Hildreth, P. (2003). Indicators of nursing care quality. Findings from a pilot study. *Outcomes Management, 7*(2), 51–58; quiz 59–60.

Lord, S. R., March, L. M., Cameron, I. D., Cumming, R. G., Schwarz, J., Zochling, J., et al. (2003). Differing risk factors for falls in nursing home and intermediate-care residents who can and cannot stand unaided. *Journal of the American Geriatric Society, 51*(11), 1645–1650.

Lord, S. R., Menz, H. B., & Tiedemann, A. (2003). A physiological profile approach to falls risk assessment and prevention. *Physical Therapy, 83*(3), 237–252.

Lord, S. R., Tiedemann, A., Chapman, K., Munro, B., Murray, S. M., Gerontology, M., et al. (2005). The effect of an individualized fall prevention program on fall risk and falls in older people: A randomized, controlled trial. *Journal of the American Geriatric Society, 53*(8), 1296–1304.

Lundin-Olsson, L., Jensen, J., Nyberg, L., & Gustafson, Y. (2003). Predicting falls in residential care by a risk assessment tool, staff judgment, and history of falls. *Aging Clinical and Experimental Research, 15*(1), 51–59.

Lundin-Olsson, L., Nyberg, L., & Gustafson, Y. (2000). The Mobility Interaction Fall chart. *Physiotherapy Research International, 5*(3), 190–201.

Mackintosh, S. F., Goldie, P., & Hill, K. (2005). Falls incidence and factors associated with falling in older, community-dwelling, chronic stroke survivors (>1 year after stroke) and matched controls. *Aging Clinical and Experimental Research, 17*(2), 74–81.

Mahoney, J. E. (1998). Immobility and falls. *Clinics in Geriatric Medicine, 14*(4), 699–726.

Mahoney, J. E., Palta, M., Johnson, J., Jalaluddin, M., Gray, S., Park, S., et al. (2000). Temporal association between hospitalization and rate of falls after discharge. *Archives of Internal Medicine, 160*(18), 2788–2795.

Maryland Quality Indicator Project. (2005). *Maryland Quality Indicator Project.* Retrieved May 27, 2005, from www.qiproject.org/

Masud, T., & Morris, R. O. (2001). Epidemiology of falls. *Age and Ageing, 30*(Suppl. 4), 3–7.

Mayo, N. E., Gloutney, L., & Levy, A. R. (1994). A randomized trial of identification bracelets to prevent falls among patients in a rehabilitation hospital. *Archives of Physical Medicine and Rehabilitation, 75*(12), 1302–1308.

McGillis Hall, L., Doran, D., & Pink, G. H. (2004). Nurse staffing models, nursing hours, and patient safety outcomes. *Journal of Nursing Administration, 34*(1), 41–45.

McMurdo, M. E., Millar, A. M., & Daly, F. (2000). A randomized controlled trial of fall prevention strategies in old peoples' homes. *Gerontology, 46*(2), 83–87.

Miller, D. K., Lewis, L. M., Nork, M. J., & Morley, J. E. (1996). Controlled trial of a geriatric case-finding and liaison service in an emergency department. *Journal of the American Geriatric Society, 44*(5), 513–520.

Morbidity and Mortality Weekly Report. (2003a). *Public health and aging: Nonfatal fall-related traumatic brain injury among older adults—California, 1996–1999*: Centers for Disease Control and Prevention.

Morbidity and Mortality Weekly Report. (2003b). *Public health and aging: Trends in aging—United States and worldwide*: Centers for Disease Control and Prevention.

Moller, J. (2005). Current costing models: are they suitable for allocating health resources? The example of fall injury prevention in Australia. *Accident Analysis and Prevention, 37*(1), 25–33.

Morgan, R. O., Virnig, B. A., Duque, M., Abdel-Moty, E., & Devito, C. A. (2004). Low-intensity exercise and reduction of the risk for falls among at-risk elders. *Journals of Gerontology. Series A: Biological Sciences and Medical Sciences, 59*(10), 1062–1067.

Morgan, V., Mathison, J., Rice, J., & Clemmer, D. (1985). Hospital falls: A persistent problem. *American Journal of Public Health, 75*(7), 775–777.

Morse, J. M. (1985a). Morse Fall Scale. University Park, PA: The Pennsylvania State University School of Nursing.

Morse, J. M. (1985b). A retrospective analysis of patient falls. *Revue Canadienne de Sante Publique, 76*(2), 116–118.

Morse, J. M. (1997). *Preventing Patient Falls.* Thousand Oaks, CA: Sage.

Morse, J. M. (1998). Predicting fall risk. *Canadian Journal of Nursing Research, 30*(2), 11–12.

Morse, J. M., & Morse, R. M. (1988). Calculating fall rates: Methodological concerns. *Quality Review Bulletin, 14*(12), 369–371.

Morse, J. M., Tylko, S. J., & Dixon, H. A. (1987). Characteristics of the fall-prone patient. *Gerontologist, 27*(4), 516–522.

Mosekilde, L. (2005). Vitamin D and the elderly. *Clinical Endocrinology (Oxf), 62*(3), 265–281.

Mulrow, C. D., Gerety, M. B., Kanten, D., Cornell, J. E., DeNino, L. A., Chiodo, L., et al. (1994). A randomized trial of physical rehabilitation for very frail nursing home residents. *Journal of the American Medical Association, 271*(7), 519–524.

Myers, H., & Nikoletti, S. (2003). Fall risk assessment: A prospective investigation of nurses' clinical judgement and risk assessment tools in predicting patient falls. *International Journal of Nursing Practice, 9*(3), 158–165.

National Center for Health Statistics. (2005). *International classification of diseases, ninth revision, clinical modification, sixth edition.* Retrieved December 12, 2005 from www.cdc.gov/nchs/icd9.htm

National Center for Injury Prevention and Control. (2003). *Falls and hip fractures among older adults*: Centers for Disease Control and Prevention, National Center for Injury Prevention and Control.

National Quality Forum. (2004). *Integrating behavioral healthcare performance measures throughout healthcare workshop proceedings.* Paper presented at the Integrating Behavioral Healthcare Performance Measures Throughout Healthcare Workshop, Washington, DC.

Needleman, J., Buerhaus, P., Mattke, S., Stewart, M., & Zelevinsky, K. (2002). Nurse-staffing levels and the quality of care in hospitals. *New England Journal of Medicine, 346*(22), 1715–1722.

Nevitt, M. C., Cummings, S. R., & Hudes, E. S. (1991). Risk factors for injurious falls: A prospective study. *Journal of Gerontology, 46*(5), M164–170.

Nieves, J. W. (2005). Osteoporosis: the role of micronutrients. *American Journal of Clinical Nutrition, 81*(5), 1232S–1239S.

Nitz, J. C., & Choy, N. L. (2004). The efficacy of a specific balance-strategy training programme for preventing falls among older people: A pilot randomised controlled trial. *Age and Ageing, 33*(1), 52–58.

Nyberg, L., & Gustafson, Y. (1996). Using the Downton index to predict those prone to falls in stroke rehabilitation. *Stroke, 27*(10), 1821–1824.

O'Connell, B., & Myers, H. (2002). The sensitivity and specificity of the Morse Fall Scale in an acute care setting. *Journal of Clinical Nursing, 11*(1), 134–136.

O'Hagan, C., & O'Connell, B. (2005). The relationship between patient blood pathology values and patient falls in an acute-care setting: A retrospective analysis. *International Journal of Nursing Practice, 11*(4), 161–168.

O'Halloran, P. D., Cran, G. W., Beringer, T. R., Kernohan, G., O'Neill, C., Orr, J., et al. (2004). A cluster randomised controlled trial to evaluate a policy of making hip protectors available to residents of nursing homes. *Age and Ageing, 33*(6), 582–588.

O'Halloran, P. D., Murray, L. J., Cran, G. W., Dunlop, L., Kernohan, G., & Beringer, T. R. (2005). The effect of type of hip protector and resident characteristics on adherence to use of hip protectors in nursing and residential homes—an exploratory study. *International Journal of Nursing Studies, 42*(4), 387–397.

Office of Statistics and Programming, National Center for Injury Prevention and Control, & Centers for Disease Control and Prevention. (2005). *WISQARS Injury Mortality Reports, 1999–2002.* Retrieved November 6, 2005, from http://webappa.cdc.gov/sasweb/ncipc/mortrate10_sy.html

Ohm, C., Mina, A., Howells, G., Bair, H., & Bendick, P. (2005). Effects of antiplatelet agents on outcomes for elderly patients with traumatic intracranial hemorrhage. *Journal of Trauma, 58*(3), 518–522.

Oliver, D., Daly, F., Martin, F. C., & McMurdo, M. E. (2004). Risk factors and risk assessment tools for falls in hospital in-patients: A systematic review. *Age and Ageing, 33*(2), 122–130.

Oliver, D., Hopper, A., & Seed, P. (2000). Do hospital fall prevention programs work? A systematic review. *Journal of the American Geriatric Society, 48*(12), 1679–1689.

Panneman, M. J., Goettsch, W. G., Kramarz, P., & Herings, R. M. (2003). The costs of benzodiazepine-associated hospital-treated fall Injuries in the EU: A pharmo study. *Drugs and Aging, 20*(11), 833–839.

Parry, S. W., Steen, N., Galloway, S. R., Kenny, R. A., & Bond, J. (2001). Falls and confidence related quality of life outcome measures in an older British cohort. *Postgraduate Medical Journal, 77*(904), 103–108.

Passaro, A., Volpato, S., Romagnoni, F., Manzoli, N., Zuliani, G., & Fellin, R. (2000). Benzodiazepines with different half-life and falling in a hospitalized population: The GIFA study. Gruppo Italiano di Farmacovigilanza nell'Anziano. *Journal of Clinical Epidemiology, 53*(12), 1222–1229.

Perell, K. L., Nelson, A., Goldman, R. L., Luther, S. L., Prieto-Lewis, N., & Rubenstein, L. Z. (2001). Fall risk assessment measures: An analytic review. *Journals of Gerontology. Series A: Biological Sciences and Medical Sciences, 56*(12), M761–766.

Porthouse, J., Birks, Y. F., Torgerson, D. J., Cockayne, S., Puffer, S., & Watt, I. (2004). Risk factors for fracture in a UK population: A prospective cohort study. *Quarterly Journal of Medicine, 97*(9), 569–574.

Porthouse, J., Cockayne, S., King, C., Saxon, L., Steele, E., Aspray, T., et al. (2005). Randomised controlled trial of calcium and supplementation with cholecalciferol (vitamin D3) for prevention of fractures in primary care. *British Medical Journal, 330*(7498), 1003–1009.

Poster, E. C., Pelletier, L. R., & Kay, K. (1991). A retrospective cohort study of falls in a psychiatric inpatient setting. *Hospital Community Psychiatry, 42*(7), 714–720.

Rapport, L. J., Webster, J. S., Flemming, K. L., Lindberg, J. W., Godlewski, M. C., Brees, J. E., et al. (1993). Predictors of falls among right-hemisphere stroke patients in the rehabilitation setting. *Archives of Physical Medicine and Rehabilitation, 74*(6), 621–626.

Ray, W. A., Taylor, J. A., Brown, A. K., Gideon, P., Hall, K., Arbogast, P., et al. (2005). Prevention of fall-related injuries in long-term care: A randomized controlled trial of staff education. *Archives of Internal Medicine, 165*(19), 2293–2298.

Reinsch, S., MacRae, P., Lachenbruch, P. A., & Tobis, J. S. (1992). Attempts to prevent falls and injury: A prospective community study. *Gerontologist, 32*(4), 450–456.

Resnick, B., & Junlapeeya, P. (2004). Falls in a community of older adults: Findings and implications for practice. *Applied Nursing Research, 17*(2), 81–91.

Reuben, D. B., Maly, R. C., Hirsch, S. H., Frank, J. C., Oakes, A. M., Siu, A. L., et al. (1996). Physician implementation of and patient adherence to recommendations from comprehensive geriatric assessment. *American Journal of Medicine, 100*(4), 444–451.

Reyes-Ortiz, C. A., Al Snih, S., Loera, J., Ray, L. A., & Markides, K. (2004). Risk factors for falling in older Mexican Americans. *Ethnicity and Disease, 14*(3), 417–422.

Richardson, D. A., Bexton, R., Shaw, F. E., Steen, N., Bond, J., & Kenny, R. A. (2000). Complications of carotid sinus massage—a prospective series of older patients. *Age and Ageing, 29*(5), 413–417.

Richardson, D. A., Bexton, R., Shaw, F. E., Steen, N., Bond, J., & Kenny, R. A. (2002). How reproducible is the cardioinhibitory response to carotid sinus massage in fallers? *Europace, 4*(4), 361–364.

Robbins, S., Gouw, G. J., & McClaran, J. (1992). Shoe sole thickness and hardness influence balance in older men. *Journal of the American Geriatric Society, 40*(11), 1089–1094.

Robertson, M. C., Campbell, A. J., Gardner, M. M., & Devlin, N. (2002). Preventing injuries in older people by preventing falls: A meta-analysis of individual-level data. *Journal of the American Geriatric Society, 50*(5), 905–911.

Rodriguez, J. G., Baughman, A. L., Sattin, R. W., deVito, C. A., Ragland, D. L., Bacchelli, S., et al. (1995). A standardized instrument to assess hazards for falls in the home of older persons. *Accident Analysis and Prevention, 27*(5), 625–631.

Rohde, J. M., Myers, A. H., & Vlahov, D. (1990). Variation in risk for falls by clinical department: Implications for prevention. *Infection Control and Hospital Epidemiology, 11*(10), 521–524.

Rosendahl, E., Lundin-Olsson, L., Kallin, K., Jensen, J., Gustafson, Y., & Nyberg, L. (2003). Prediction of falls among older people in residential care facilities by the Downton index. *Aging Clinical and Experimental Research, 15*(2), 142–147.

Rothschild, J. M., Bates, D. W., & Leape, L. L. (2000). Preventable medical injuries in older patients. *Archives of Internal Medicine, 160*(18), 2717–2728.

Rubenstein, L. Z., & Josephson, K. R. (2002). The epidemiology of falls and syncope. *Clinics in Geriatric Medicine, 18*(2), 141–158.

Rubenstein, L. Z., Powers, C. M., & MacLean, C. H. (2001). Quality indicators for the management and prevention of falls and mobility problems in vulnerable elders. *Annals of Internal Medicine, 135*(8 Pt 2), 686–693.

Rubenstein, L. Z., Robbins, A. S., Josephson, K. R., Schulman, B. L., & Osterweil, D. (1990). The value of assessing falls in an elderly population. A randomized clinical trial. *Annals of Internal Medicine, 113*(4), 308–316.

Rubinson, L., Wu, A. W., Haponik, E. E., & Diette, G. B. (2005). Why is it that internists do not follow guidelines for preventing intravascular catheter infections? *Infection Control and Hospital Epidemiology, 26*(6), 525–533.

Ruchinskas, R. (2003). Clinical prediction of falls in the elderly. *American Journal of Physical Medicine and Rehabilitation, 82*(4), 273–278.

Salgado, R. I., Lord, S. R., Ehrlich, F., Janji, N., & Rahman, A. (2004). Predictors of falling in elderly hospital patients. *Archives of Gerontology and Geriatrics, 38*(3), 213–219.

Sambrook, P. N., Chen, J. S., March, L. M., Cameron, I. D., Cumming, R. G., Lord, S. R., et al. (2004). Serum parathyroid hormone predicts time to fall independent of vitamin D status in a frail elderly population. *Journal of Clinical Endocrinology and Metabolism, 89*(4), 1572–1576.

Sato, Y., Iwamoto, J., Kanoko, T., & Satoh, K. (2005). Risedronate sodium therapy for prevention of hip fracture in men 65 years or older after stroke. *Archives of Internal Medicine, 165*(15), 1743–1748.

Sato, Y., Kanoko, T., Satoh, K., & Iwamoto, J. (2005). The prevention of hip fracture with risedronate and ergocalciferol plus calcium supplementation in elderly women with Alzheimer disease: A randomized controlled trial. *Archives of Internal Medicine, 165*(15), 1737–1742.

Sattin, R. W., Easley, K. A., Wolf, S. L., Chen, Y., & Kutner, M. H. (2005). Reduction in fear of falling through intense Tai Chi exercise training in older, transitionally frail adults. *Journal of the American Geriatrics Society, 53*(7), 1168–1178.

Schwendimann, R., Joos, F., Geest, S. D., & Milisen, K. (2005). Are patient falls in the hospital associated with lunar cycles? A retrospective observational study. *BMC Nursing, 4*(5).

Scuffham, P., Chaplin, S., & Legood, R. (2003). Incidence and costs of unintentional falls in older people in the United Kingdom. *Journal of Epidemiology and Community Health, 57*(9), 740–744.

Semin-Goossens, A., van der Helm, J. M., & Bossuyt, P. M. (2003). A failed model-based attempt to implement an evidence-based nursing guideline for fall prevention. *Journal of Nursing Care Quality, 18*(3), 217–225.

Sherrington, C., & Menz, H. B. (2003). An evaluation of footwear worn at the time of fall-related hip fracture. *Age and Ageing, 32*(3), 310–314.

Speciale, S., Turco, R., Magnifico, F., Bellelli, G., & Trabucchi, M. (2004). Frailty is the main predictor of falls in elderly patients undergoing rehabilitation training. *Age and Ageing, 33*(1), 84–85.

Stein, J., Viramontes, B. E., & Kerrigan, D. C. (1995). Fall-related injuries in anticoagulated stroke patients during inpatient rehabilitation. *Archives of Physical Medicine and Rehabilitation, 76*(9), 840–843.

Steinberg, M., Cartwright, C., Peel, N., & Williams, G. (2000). A sustainable programme to prevent falls and near falls in community dwelling older people: Results of a randomised trial. *Journal of Epidemiology and Community Health, 54*(3), 227–232.

Tay, S. E., Quek, C. S., Pariyasami, S., Ong, B. C., Wee, B. C., Yeo, J. L., et al. (2000). Fall incidence in a state psychiatric hospital in Singapore. *Journal of Psychosocial Nursing and Mental Health Services, 38*(9), 10–16.

Teasell, R., McRae, M., Foley, N., & Bhardwaj, A. (2002). The incidence and consequences of falls in stroke patients during inpatient rehabilitation: Factors associated with high risk. *Archives of Physical Medicine and Rehabilitation, 83*(3), 329–333.

Thurston, G. (1957). Fatal hospital falls. *British Medical Journal, 16*(51), 396–397.

Tideiksaar, R., Feiner, C. F., & Maby, J. (1993). Falls prevention: The efficacy of a bed alarm system in an acute-care setting. *Mount Sinai Journal of Medicine, 60*(6), 522–527.

Tinetti, M. E. (1986). Performance-oriented assessment of mobility problems in elderly patients. *Journal of the American Geriatric Society, 34*(2), 119–126.

Tinetti, M. E., Speechley, M., & Ginter, S. F. (1988). Risk factors for falls among elderly persons living in the community. *New England Journal of Medicine, 319*(26), 1701–1707.

Tinetti, M. E., & Williams, C. S. (1997). Falls, injuries due to falls, and the risk of admission to a nursing home. *New England Journal of Medicine, 337*(18), 1279–1284.

Tsai, Y.-F., Witte, N., Radunzel, M., & Keller, M. L. (1998). Falls in a psychiatric unit. *Applied Nursing Research, 11*(3), 115–121.

Tutuarima, J. A., de Haan, R. J., & Limburg, M. (1993). Number of nursing staff and falls: A case-control study on falls by stroke patients in acute-care settings. *Journal of Advanced Nursing, 18*(7), 1101–1105.

Unruh, L. (2003). Licensed nurse staffing and adverse events in hospitals. *Medical Care, 41*(1), 142–152.

Vassallo, M., Stockdale, R., Sharma, J. C., Briggs, R., & Allen, S. C. (2005). A comparative study of the use of four fall risk assessment tools on acute medical wards. *Journal of the American Geriatric Society, 53*(6), 1034–1038.

Vassallo, M., Vignaraja, R., Sharma, J. C., Briggs, R., & Allen, S. C. (2004). Predictors for falls among hospital inpatients with impaired mobility. *Journal of the Royal Society of Medicine, 97*(6), 266–269.

Vassallo, M., Vignaraja, R., Sharma, J. C., Hallam, H., Binns, K., Briggs, R., et al. (2004). The effect of changing practice on fall prevention in a rehabilitative hospital: The Hospital Injury Prevention Study. *Journal of the American Geriatric Society, 52*(3), 335–339.

Vassallo, M., Wilkinson, C., Stockdale, R., Malik, N., Baker, R., & Allen, S. C. (2005). Attitudes to restraint for the prevention of falls in hospital. *Gerontology, 51*(1), 66–70.

Vaughn, K., Young, B. C., Rice, F., & Stoner, M. H. (1993). A retrospective study of patient falls in a psychiatric hospital. *Journal of Psychosocial Nursing and Mental Health Services, 31*(9), 37–42.

Volrathongchai, K. (2005). *Predicting falls among the elderly residing in long-term care facilities using knowledge discovery in databases*. Unpublished Dissertation, University of Madison, Madison, WI.

Wallace, C., Reiber, G. E., LeMaster, J., Smith, D. G., Sullivan, K., Hayes, S., et al. (2002). Incidence of falls, risk factors for falls, and fall-related fractures in individuals with diabetes and a prior foot ulcer. *Diabetes Care, 25*(11), 1983–1986.

Watanabe, Y. (2005). Fear of falling among stroke survivors after discharge from inpatient rehabilitation. *International Journal of Rehabilitation Research, 28*(2), 149–152.

Wayne, P. M., Scarborough, D. M., Krebs, D. E., Parker, S. W., Wolf, S. L., Asmundson, L., et al. (2005). Tai Chi for vestibulopathic balance dysfunction: A case study. *Alternative Therapies in Health and Medicine, 11*(2), 60–66.

Weigand, J. V., & Gerson, L. W. (2001). Preventive care in the emergency department: Should emergency departments institute a falls prevention program for elder patients? A systematic review. *Academic Emergency Medicine,* 8(8), 823–826.

Whitman, G. R., Kim, Y., Davidson, L. J., Wolf, G. A., & Wang, S. L. (2002). The impact of staffing on patient outcomes across specialty units. *Journal of Nursing Administration, 32*(12), 633–639.

Wilson, M. M., Miller, D. K., Andresen, E. M., Malmstrom, T. K., Miller, J. P., & Wolinsky, F. D. (2005). Fear of falling and related activity restriction among middle-aged African Americans. *Journals of Gerontology. Series A: Biological Sciences and Medical Sciences,* 60(3), 355–360.

Wolf, S. L., Barnhart, H. X., Ellison, G. L., & Coogler, C. E. (1997). The effect of Tai Chi Quan and computerized balance training on postural stability in older subjects. Atlanta FICSIT Group. Frailty and Injuries: Cooperative Studies on Intervention Techniques. *Physical Therapy, 77*(4), 371–381; discussion 382–374.

Wolf, S. L., Barnhart, H. X., Kutner, N. G., McNeely, E., Coogler, C., & Xu, T. (2003). Selected as the best paper in the 1990s: Reducing frailty and falls in older persons: An investigation of Tai Chi and computerized balance training. *Journal of the American Geriatric Society, 51*(12), 1794–1803.

Wolf, S. L., Sattin, R. W., Kutner, M., O'Grady, M., Greenspan, A. I., & Gregor, R. J. (2003). Intense Tai Chi exercise training and fall occurrences in older, transitionally frail adults: A randomized, controlled trial. *Journal of the American Geriatric Society, 51*(12), 1693–1701.

Chapter 4

Hospital-Acquired Infections as Patient Safety Indicators

Ann Marie B. Peterson and Patricia Hinton Walker

ABSTRACT

Transmission of infection in the hospital has been identified as a patient safety problem adversely affecting patients, visitors, and health care workers. Prevention of infection should not be limited to the hospital epidemiology staff but also must involve the entire multidisciplinary team, including nurses. This chapter reviews the literature related to patient safety of nursing-authored studies of infection control in the hospital. The review indicated that there were key areas of research interest including drug resistance; hand hygiene products, procedures, and surveillance; preoperative skin preparations; health care worker transmission of infection; common procedures associated with an increased risk of transmission; and organizational issues.

Keywords: infections, patient safety, nursing

In the past 20 years, the overall incidence of health care–associated infections has increased 36% (Institute of Medicine, 2000). Infections acquired in acute care hospitals continue to be a leading cause of death in the United States (Wenzel & Edmond, 2001). Annually, more than 500,000 of the nearly 2 million patients stricken with these infections are patients in intensive care units (ICUs), and most of these infections are associated with the presence of an invasive device (such as a vascular access line, ventilator, or indwelling urinary catheter). Nearly 90,000 of these patients are estimated to die (Centers for Disease Control and Prevention, 1992). As a result of the persistent nature of this insidious problem, an objective of Healthy People 2010 is to reduce health care–associated infections in ICUs by 10% (objective 14–20) (United States Department of Health and Human Services, 2000). The total hospital-related financial burden of health care–associated infections in the United States was estimated to exceed $4.5 billion in 1992 (using the Consumer Price Inflator, this converts to $6.5 billion in 2004 dollars) (Centers for Disease Control and Prevention, 1992). However, this estimate is based on infection rates measured in the Study on the Efficacy of Nosocomial Infection Control, which was conducted in the mid-1970s, and current expenditures are likely to be higher (Haley et al., 1985).

Risk of health care–associated infections is not limited to patients (Stone, 2004). All health care workers face a wide range of hazards on the job, including blood and body fluid exposure. Nursing personnel experience these hazards most frequently (Centers for Disease Control and Prevention, 2000).

Emerging infectious diseases, including multidrug-resistant organisms and outbreaks of recognized contagious illnesses, have highlighted yet other concerns about the safety of patients and health care workers. For example, much of the worldwide Severe Acute Respiratory Syndrome (SARS) outbreak was hospital-based, and health care workers made up a large proportion of cases, accounting for 37%–63% of suspected SARS cases in highly affected countries (Varia et al., 2003).

There have been a number of studies published investigating the effectiveness of specific interventions designed and implemented by infection control and occupational health professionals to prevent health care–associated infections. Some of this evidence has been synthesized in guidelines developed by the Centers for Disease Control and Prevention (CDC) (Tablan, Anderson, Besser, Bridges, & Hajjeh, 2004; Boyce & Pittet, 2002; O'Grady et al., 2002; Garner, 1996; Wong, 2000). The purpose of this review is to synthesize the nursing research conducted in the United States over the past 10 years.

METHODOLOGY FOR REVIEWING THE RESEARCH

There has been a great deal of research conducted related to infections and infection control. Consequently, this review was limited to (1) nursing research examining health care–associated infections; (2) nursing research examining infection control in inpatient, convalescent, or rehabilitation hospitals; (3) publications written in the English language; (4) studies published during the past 10 years' research; (5) studies conducted in the United States; and (6) publications in which a nurse is listed as first or second author.

Most of the studies related to the infection control aspect of patient safety were found in medical and hospital epidemiology journals. In these journals, the nurse researcher was often listed as the second or a subsequent author; however, the author's credentials did not always reflect an affiliation with nursing. In some publications, the authors list academic credentials (such as PhD) but not the clinical credentials (i.e., registered nurse). Consequently, it is possible that some publications were missed.

A computerized search of studies was conducted using search engines for Cumulative Index of Nursing and Allied Health literature (CINAHL) and Medline for the years 1995 to 2005. Search elements included the English language, review articles, nursing research, patients, health personnel, infection control, and communicable diseases. A hand search of journals was also conducted.

Studies were evaluated for research design, study variables, findings, statistical significance, and relevance to nursing. There are a variety of ways that the research could be organized to address this broad topic. For the purposes of this publication, the authors grouped the research as into sections as follows: (1) infection transmission: vascular access devices, (2) infection transmission: blood-borne, (3) infection transmission: urinary tract and skin, (4) equipment and products associated with transmission of infection, (5) studies related to resistant organisms, (6) infection control and surveillance studies, and (7) organizational factors that enhance compliance and efficacy. The last group highlights the importance of compliance of health care workers and factors that must be addressed to change organizational behaviors. For each topic, the relevant studies are discussed and tables are provided following the narrative sections to highlight the studies by author, year, setting, and type of study, sample size, unit of analysis, focus of study, and findings.

Infection Transmission: Acquired Through Vascular Access Devices

Central venous catheter (CVC) complications and the concomitant risk related to transmission of blood-borne infections were the focus of another study (Lange, et al., 1997). In this research, catheter-related colonization, infections, and sepsis were tracked by investigators along with exit site infections. Interventions to reduce CVC complications were instituted with a corresponding decrease in infection. CVC-associated bloodstream infection was also studied by Fridkin, Pear, Williamson, Galgiani, and Jarvis (1996) during an outbreak of infections in an

ICU. This study highlighted the association between CVC infections, the use of total parenteral nutrition, and decreased nurse staffing. However, as acknowledged by the authors, a lack of device-day data was a limitation of this study (Fridkin, et al., 1996, p. 156). Robert and colleagues (2000) also studied the relationship between nurse staffing and CVC blood stream infections. They found a relationship between increased CVC infections and the assignment of float nurses to patients. Curchoe and others conducted a study in which they found a decreased bloodstream infection rate by altering the process and supplies for CVC dressing changes (Curchoe, Powers, & El-Daher, 2002).

Larson and colleagues (2005) conducted a study in a neonatal unit. Predictors of bloodstream infection included catheter and noncatheter variables along with cultures of skin flora from the hands of nurses. In this intervention study of two patient care units, it was determined that nurses with clean hands were not generally thought to have caused the transmission of gram-negative bacilli organisms in the unit. Factors recommended to be studied further as potential sources of infection were feeding procedures and complications related to the use of parenteral nutrition (Larson et al., 2005). Table 4.1 summarizes studies of infections acquired through vascular access devices.

Infection Transmission: Blood-Borne

Researchers who have contributed to the body of knowledge in preventing blood-borne infections are highlighted first. Beekmann and colleagues (2001) evaluated educational programs, policies, and procedures related to blood-borne infections and exposures in 153 hospitals using a questionnaire. From results of this study, the authors identified that improvements were needed in education and performance evaluation for physicians and additional organizational supports. Recommendations included increased use of protective devices to prevent needle-sticks and improved availability of postexposure care for staff sustaining accidental exposure to blood and body fluids (Beekmann et al., 2001). Beekmann also described challenges to epidemiology staff as they manage escalating numbers of patients with immune deficiencies, such as those using central venous access devices (Beekmann et al., p. 77).

Another category of blood-borne infections research is related to the prevention of blood and body fluid exposures. Sohn and associates evaluated the actual incidence of injuries compared to the reporting of injuries by health care workers (Sohn, Eagan, & Sepkowitz, 2004). This study demonstrated a decrease in the reported cases of sharps injuries after the hospital introduced safer products and provided education to staff. However, a survey of staff revealed a mismatch between the actual number of injuries and reports of injury to the institution (Sohn et al., 2004).

TABLE 4.1 Studies Conducted by Nurse Scientists Examining Infections Acquired Through Vascular Access Devices

Study	Setting	Type of study	Sample size	Unit of analysis	Focus of study	Findings
Fridkin et al., 1996	Hospital	Case control and cohort	692/1,068	Patients	CVC BSIs	Nurse staffing and increased use of total parenteral nutrition may have increased the incidence of BSIs
Lange et al., 1997	Hospital	Prospective observational	268	Patients	CVC complications in children	Changing practices for cleaning, dressing, accessing, and education decreased complications
Robert et al., 2000	Hospital	Case control	127	Patients	CVC BSIs and staffing	Staffing mix (use of float pool staff) and ratio of nurses to patients may influence the rate of BSIs
Curchoe, Powers, & El-Daher, 2002	Hospital	Prospective	Not stated	Patient infection rates	CVC and BSIs	Infections decreased with use of alcohol swab sticks & increase frequency of CVC dressing changes
Larson et al., 2005	Hospital	Interventional	2,935	Neonates	Gram-negative bacilli BSIs	BSIs in neonates require not only good hand hygiene but also consideration of other strategies in neonatal units

Note: BSI = blood stream infection; CVC = central venous catheter

Hepatitis C (HCV) is a blood-borne infection that is transmitted in a variety of ways. A cohort study by de Oliveira and others (2005) demonstrated findings highly suggestive of transmission of HCV related to a nursing procedure. Using a shared saline container between patients, nurses withdrew flush solution with syringes, accessed the vascular access device of the patient, and then returned to the flush container with the same syringe. This study incorporated virus genotyping procedures. Nursing procedures were later modified to prevent the potential for further transmissions. However, the implications for nursing go beyond this one procedure. Many nursing activities have the potential to cause transmission of infection due to a lack of understanding by nurses of the risks of cross-contamination.

Tuboku-Metzger and others sought to define the opinions of patients concerning the human immunodeficiency virus (HIV), Hepatitis B (HBV), and HCV related to the status of their health care worker caregivers (Tuboku-Metzger, Chiarello, Sinkowitz-Cochran, Casano-Dickerson, & Cardo, 2005). In this qualitative study designed to assess attitudes of the public, questionnaires were mailed to a sample of 3,000 individuals. More than 2,353 subjects returned completed questionnaires. Respondents gave their perceptions on the need for dentists and doctors to disclose viral status to their patients for the infections of HIV, HBV, and HCV (Tuboku-Metzger et al., 2005). Nurses need to be aware that the rights of health care workers to privacy are in direct opposition to the expectations of the public as described in this study. Table 4.2 summarizes studies examining blood-borne infections.

Infection Transmission: Urinary Tract and Skin

Urinary catheters also contribute to the transmission of infection, and this aspect of care has been studied for years as a significant infection risk for patients. Two strategies that have traditionally been implemented to reduce this type of nosocomial infection include (1) reducing the time catheterized to the minimum and (2) incorporating into practice various catheter care regimens, such as routine washing of the external section of the catheter and perineal area with soap and water. Rupp et al. (2004) examined the incidence of urinary tract infections (UTIs) in a prospective manner after the hospital initiated use of silver-coated urinary catheters. The researchers of this 2-year study of 10 patient care areas within the hospital analyzed costs, resistance to the effects of silver treatment, and rates of catheter-associated UTIs. With reduced health care resources, it is even more important that nurse researchers address cost implications to both the patient and the institution.

Skin flora is another important area related to transmission of infection. In the surgical setting, the goal has been to reduce the level of skin flora, not only at the time of surgery but ideally for some time beyond the operation. These goals

TABLE 4.2 Studies Conducted by Nurse Scientists Examining Blood-Borne Infections HIV, HBV, and HCV

Study	Setting	Type of study	Sample size	Unit of analysis	Focus of study	Findings
Beekmann et al., 2001	Hospitals	Survey	153	Hospitals	Programs for sharp safety	Education, compliance, evaluation, protected products, staffing, post-exposure events, and care were studied.
Sohn, Eagan, & Sepkowitz, 2004	Hospital	Survey	1,132/821	Staff	Sharp injuries before and after introduction of safer devices	Sharp injuries decreased after introduction of safer devices although HCW reporting did not match actual injury rate
de Oliveira et al., 2005	Clinic	Cohort	494	Patients	Hepatitis outbreak	Contamination of saline flush bags used between patients
Tuboku-Metzger et al, 2005	Homes	Qualitative	2,353	Participants	Public attitudes about hepatitis	2,353 responders varied in opinions about needed disclosure of viral status and perception of risk transmission

Note: HIV = human immunodeficiency virus; HBV = hepatitis B virus; HCV = hepatitis C virus; HCW = health care worker were aimed at reducing the risk of both operative and postoperative infections. One in vivo nonformal study was identified with 26 volunteers to test the difference between the common hospital practices using the antiseptic, povidone iodine as a preoperative body wash compared to an alcohol-based system (Seal & Paul-Cheadle, 2004). Although the sample was divided into two groups, randomization was not described for assigning subjects into the groups. For a 2-week period, subjects were restricted from contact with medicated skin or hair products or other known sources of products believed to have an effect on skin flora. Hair was removed from the skin test sites and, after 48 or more hours, skin areas were sampled for colony counts (colony-forming units). Using either of the two interventions, skin was prepared and then sampled for up to 72 hours for colony counts to determine antimicrobial efficacy. The investigators explored a system approach that combined a bath with an antiseptic given 24 hours before surgery along with an approved skin preparation at the time of the operation. Success was marked by keeping skin flora levels low for 72 hours and decreasing rates of infection (Seal & Paul-Cheadle, 2004, pp. 57–62). Table 4.3 summarizes studies conducted by nurses examining infections of the urinary tract and skin.

Equipment and Products Associated with Transmission of Infection

Medical equipment has been associated with transmission of infection as described by two research teams (Brooks et al., 1998; Milam, Hall, Pringle, & Buchanan, 2001). In the first study, the goal was to reduce the incidence of Vancomycin Resistant Enterococcus (VRE) after an outbreak (Brooks et al., 1998). A number of interventions were used such as education of staff, increased cleaning of the environment, and switching from oral and rectal temperature taking to measurement of temperature with tympanic thermometers. A 48% decrease of VRE was accomplished with these measures (Brooks et al., 1998).

Health care equipment itself can serve as a fomite, as was shown in a study of cloth covers for stethoscopes used by health care workers in a hospital in Florida (Milam et al., 2001). In this investigation, all but two of the stethoscope covers were found to contain bacteria or fungus organisms. A survey used in the study revealed that the covers were washed by staff "infrequently or never" (Milam et al., 2001). The mean frequency for washing the covers was 3.7 months. The motivation for this study began with a causal observation of a practice issue, cloth-covered stethoscopes, and the idea was followed-up with an investigation of the issue (Milam et al., 2001). Implications for nurses are that noting clinical practice issues such as unwashed stethoscope covers can count in the efforts for reduction of infection transmission. Table 4.4 summarizes studies by nurses associated with equipment and products.

TABLE 4.3 Studies Conducted by Nurses Examining Infections of the Urinary Tract and Skin

Study	Setting	Type of study	Sample size	Unit of analysis	Focus of study	Findings
Rupp et al., 2004	Hospital	Prospective non-randomized surveillance	600	Patients (rate of catheter-associated UTIs per 1000 patient days)	UTIs and silver coated urinary catheters, cost, and resistant organisms	Use of silver coated catheters reduced UTIs, costs, and incidence of resistant isolates
Seal & Paul-Cheadle, 2004	Clinic	In vivo study	26	Patient cultures	Removing skin flora with ethanol versus iodine based products	Reduction of skin flora occurred and lasted for 72 hours

Note: UTI = urinary tract infection

TABLE 4.4 Studies Conducted by Nurses Examining Infections Associated with Equipment and Products

Study	Setting	Type of study	Sample size	Unit of analysis	Focus of study	Findings
Brooks et al., 1998	Hospital	Intervention study	Not stated	Patients	Stopping an NI outbreak	Using tympanic thermometers helped to reduce infections
Milam et al., 2001	Hospital	Surveillance	22	Cultures of stethoscope covers	Fabric covers on stethoscopes	90%, or 18 of 22, of the fabric stethoscope covers were positive for bacteria or yeast

Note: NI = nosocomial infection

Studies Involving Resistant Organisms

Although neither contamination nor colonization necessarily predict infection, many authors have investigated occurrences of resistant organism infections in hospitals (Boyce, Havill, Kohan, Dumigan, & Ligi, 2004; Trick et al., 2002; Fry et al., 2005; Saiman et al., 2003; Stone et al., 2003). These investigators identified the increasing incidence of resistant organisms and linked these events to factors such as health care worker noncompliance with personal protective equipment, hand hygiene, and inadequate monitoring and treatment for resistant organisms.

In a 2004 review of publications in the area of Methicillin-resistant *staphylococcus aureus* organisms (MRSA) Boyce and fellow researchers (2004) stressed the importance of combining standard hand hygiene precautions with other measures. Other measures were routine isolation precautions including use of personal protective equipment and institution of active surveillance by culturing the nares of those patients thought likely to become infected with resistant organisms. The authors remarked about the increased costs and manpower needed for performing active surveillance or screening surveillance (Boyce et al., 2004, pp. 398–399).

In a cross-sectional evaluation study conducted by Trick et al. (2002), researchers examined VRE organisms on five floors of a rehabilitation hospital. Variables examined included rectal cultures from 74 patients and 319 cultures of specific environmental surfaces. The study found a greater incidence of VRE between incontinent versus continent patients and more positive cultures from the floors and common areas nearest the VRE positive patients. Examples of VRE-positive environmental surfaces included shower seats, the tops of counters, and commodes found in the room (Trick et al., 2002, p. 901). Other positive areas were the blood pressure cuffs, bedside blood glucose meters, bed and rail surfaces, handrails on the rehabilitation unit, washer and dryer handles, and mats (Trick et al., 2002, p. 901). Hand hygiene practices at the time of the 1999 study were soap and water for VRE-negative or unknown patients and 2% chlorhexidine gluconate for known positive patients. The VRE status was known for nine of the 13 VRE-positive patients. Methods to determine VRE status included communication from a transferring institution, clinical testing, and performing occasional surveys. Although this approach is commonly used to determine VRE status, only some of the positive patients benefited from contact isolation precautions, which contributed to transmission of organisms.

In another study by Fry et al. (2005), use of additional precautions for adult patients such as not sharing food and cigarettes, was instituted along with greater use of preventive vaccines for pneumonia and the influenza.

Saiman led a group in an investigation of neonatal patients, incorporating standard isolation precautions, along with four additional measures: (1) assigning specific nurses to the isolated infants, (2) treating the nares of infants with

Mupirocin, (3) washing babies weighing over 1500 grams with hexachlorophene, (4) protecting the eyes of infants with gauze during suction procedures, and (5) transferring some noninfected infants to other newborn ICUs (Saiman et al., 2003, pp. 317–321).

Stone and others conducted a retrospective cost analysis from the hospital perspective. In this study, the investigators examined the attributable costs and length of stay (LOS) related to extended-spectrum beta lactamase–producing *Klebsiella pneumoniae*. The investigators conservatively estimated that an outbreak of this multidrug-resistant organism in a neonatal ICU cost the hospital $146,331 and increased neonate LOS by 48.5 days (95% confidence interval 1.7 to 95.2) (Stone et al., p. 2003).

Studies like these have relevance for nursing practice. Because environmental surface contamination with these patients is not only likely to occur in the room but also on any environmental surface touched by the patient, attention to cleaning is critical. Routine disinfection of surfaces with quaternary ammonium disinfectant was used in the rehabilitation facility along with standard contact isolation precautions such as gowning, gloving, and hand hygiene with antiseptics.

Despite all the precautions taken, transmission of organisms to environmental surfaces occurred, causing potential risks to other patients and staff. Table 4.5 summarizes the research related to the resistance of organisms. In the future, research in this area may need a multidisciplinary approach including groups from medicine, nursing, respiratory therapy, nutrition, phlebotomy, and housekeeping. Because the costs and efforts of caring for patients with resistant organisms have been high, prevention of transmission of these infections should be a significant motivation for all health care workers, including nurses.

Infection Control and Surveillance Studies

Investigators have studied the incidence of infections by using surveillance techniques in order to identify both community- and hospital-acquired sources. Additionally, some researchers have assessed the effectiveness of interventions (Weinstein et al., 1999; Stover et al., 2001; Lai, Baker, & Fontecchio, 2003). In one investigation, surveillance surveys for infection from a 10-year period were combined with review of the chart and a nurse-completed risk assessment for patients. Risk for infection was increased with the use of medical devices. The investigators found that although overall infection rates did not change over time, bloodstream infections increased (Weinstein et al., 1999).

The transmission or prevalence of tuberculosis (TB) has also been studied as an infection control/surveillance approach (Stroud et al., 1995; Sepkowitz, Fella, Rivera, Villa, & DeHovitz, 1995; Christie et al., 1998). Stroud and colleagues (1995) focused on the assessment of the CDC recommendations for infection

TABLE 4.5 Resistant Infections and Infection Control Measures

Study	Setting	Type of study	Sample size	Unit of analysis	Focus of study	Findings
Trick et al., 2002	Rehabilitation hospital	Cross-sectional	74	Patient cultures	Assess contaminated hospital environmental areas for gastrointestinal VRE	Areas most contaminated with gastrointestinal VRE were: patient rooms, especially floors, but not frequent in work common areas
Saiman et al., 2003	Hospital	Surveillance	13/235	Neonates cultures and staff	Newborn ICU MRSA	Outbreak of 13 infants with MRSA HCW with MRSA
Stone et al., 2003	Hospital	Retrospective cost analysis	8	Infants cultured and costs	Neonatal intensive care nursery	An outbreak of a NI in a neonatal intensive care unit was retrospectively assessed for costs and length of stay
Boyce et al., 2004	Hospital	Literature review and surveillance cultures	442	Patients with positive surveillance cultures	Infection control measures and resistant precautions	Increase of methicillin-resistant staphylococcus aureus. Review of infections and the relationship of possible causative variables
Fry et al., 2005	Long-term care facility	Longitudinal cross-sectional	384	Patients with MDRSP	Multi-drug-resistant streptococcus pneumonia	Training for infection control prevented further cases

Note: VRE = vancomycin-resistant enterococci; MRSA = methicillin-resistant *staphylococcus aureus*; MDRSP = multidrug resistant streptococcus pneumoniae; HCW = health care worker; NI = nosocomial infection control compared to the incidence of TB in both patients and health care workers. This research supported that the CDC guidelines need to be adhered to in order to prevent transmission of TB in patients (Stroud et al., 1995). Sepkokwitz and associates (1995) found a 40% prevalence of positive tests for TB using the purified protein derivative test with staff working in a New York hospital. These results reflected a complex picture that included foreign-born nurses, some of who had received Bacillus Calmette-Guerin vaccination. In the third study, led by Christie et al. (1998), the researchers found no transmission of TB from patients to health care workers. This group examined the cost benefit ratio for TB measures when considering a community with a low incidence of TB.

Stover led a study utilizing a survey to analyze the nosocomial infection rates in 50 U.S. hospitals for children. Forty-three hospitals returned the questionnaire. The types of infections assessed were those associated with CVCs, ventilators, and urinary catheters. In the process of the study, it was determined that there was variability between facilities for infection surveillance, an identified area for future research (Stover et al., 2001, pp. 152–157).

Infections associated with ventilators were studied by several research teams (Babcock et al., 2003; Lai et al., 2003). One group used surveillance rates to document ventilator-associated pneumonia prior to and after clinical care interventions (Lai et al., 2003). The interventions consisted of elevating the head of the bed, changing to sterile water and one way enteral valves, and changing the equipment for in line suction catheters (Lai et al., 2003, pp. 859–863). The ICU managers and staff monitored patient days on the ventilator. This study demonstrated that changing nursing and respiratory therapy interventions resulted in a significant decrease in the rate of pneumonia for the ventilator patients (Lai et al., 2003, p. 859). Another study used a retrospective cohort design to record the causes of ventilator-associated pneumonia and found variance of infectious causative agents between the hospitals surveyed (Babcock et al., 2003). In these studies, summarized in Table 4.6, nurses played an important role not only in obtaining data but in understanding the role of risk factors and infection for nursing care of patients.

Organizational Factors that Enhance Compliance and Efficacy

Researchers have repeatedly demonstrated problems with health care workers' compliance to policies and procedures for infection control. Health care workers were not the only group identified as responsible for fostering conditions for ideal infection control. The institution itself has an obligation to provide the necessary systems required for patient safety in the area of infection control. Examples of these systems issues include staff education, appropriate types of products such as hand antiseptics, adequate sink availability for hand washing, and sufficient amounts and types of environmental disinfectants. The hospital must

TABLE 4.6 Infection Control and Surveillance Studies

Study	Setting	Type of study	Sample size	Unit of analysis	Focus of study	Findings
Sepkowitz et al., 1995	Hospital	Prospective	313	Staff	Prevalence of tuberculin positive staff	Staff had a 40% prevalence of a + PPD test
Stroud et al., 1995	Hospital	Retrospective cohort	38	Patients	Compliance to CDC guidelines for isolation	Adherence to guidelines reduced patient transmission
Christie et al., 1998	Hospital	Descriptive	2,275–4,356	Staff from 1986–1994	Evaluation of risk of TB for patients and staff	Communities with a low rates of TB consider cost implications of CDC guidelines
Weinstein et al., 1999	Hospital	Prevalence study (survey)	5,545	Patients with nosocomial infections	NI rate	NI rates stable overall
Stover et al., 2001	Hospital	Prevalence study (survey)	43	Participants	Nosocomial infection (NI) rate	NI and surveillance varied between facilities
Lai et al., 2003	Hospital	Surveillance and intervention	562	Patients	Ventilator-associated pneumonia	Infection rates decreased
Babcock et al., 2003	Hospital	Retrospective cohort	878	Patients with ventilator-associated pneumonia and culture results	Ventilator-associated pneumonia	Causes of infection vary between institutions

Note: TB = tuberculosis; PPD = purified protein derivative test; NI = nosocomial infections; CDC = Centers for Disease Control and Prevention ensure adequate amounts and appropriate types of personal protective equipment such as gloves, gowns, procedure masks, National Institute of Safety and Hygiene–approved respirators, sealing goggles, splash goggles, and isolation linen carts and liners. Also timely evaluation of staff performance and sufficient staffing of personnel are critical. However, current staffing shortages throughout the country have made this a difficult challenge for hospitals.

Health care organizations have an even more difficult challenge beyond the acquisition and maintenance of supplies, equipment, and human resources. The literature has shown that one of the most difficult tests for organizations has been the changing of long-term patterns of behavior, habits, the milieu, the culture, and the climate of the institution itself. The next studies highlighted in this publication demonstrate how researchers approach this organizational change and compliance.

Intervention studies in infection control at the organizational level have often resulted in behavior change of staff over the short term. Maintaining improved behaviors over the long term has been more difficult. Research has demonstrated that behavioral changes have not been long lasting unless key groups have participated in every step of the process for the change (Larson, Early, Cloonan, Sugrue, & Parides, 2000, pp. 14–22). In a study of organizational changes relative to isolation control practices conducted by Larson and associates (2000), success was demonstrated using a framework developed by Schein in 1985. The strategy incorporated participation of the administrative leadership staff in a change process using a five-point approach. In this study, the managers and their designees were intricately enmeshed in the study process at the worker level. The study results were impressive for the rates of nosocomial infections decreased in the intervention group, and behaviors were changed. Staff increased their frequency of hand hygiene, and the effect persisted over a 6-month time frame (Larson et al., 2000, pp. 14–22).

Larson used another approach to evaluate the reasons why physicians and nurses have such poor compliance to hand hygiene, a proven strategy to reduce infections (Larson, 2004, pp. 48–51). In this study, Larson adapted a survey that queried medical and nursing staff for possible beliefs about hand hygiene, especially perceived barriers. Some of the issues addressed in the survey included "awareness and agreement of guidelines, expectations of outcomes when hand hygiene was used, preferences of patients, and organizational factors such as support" (Larson, 2004, p. 50). Larson administered the survey and recommended that more work be completed on the survey tool.

In a study conducted by McKinley and colleagues (2005), the researchers used a variety of methods to attempt to change the behavior of nurses in hand hygiene. Posters, focus groups, questionnaires, and direct observation of practice were all utilized for the issue of hand hygiene. An improvement rate increase of 37% was accomplished over a year-long study. An important finding was that eliciting suggestions from the participants in the study and then implementing many of the ideas helped the patient care unit to achieve improvement (McKinley et al., 2005, pp. 368–373).

Prevention of infection in institutions has been demonstrated as a vital part of a patient safety program. For example, the influenza vaccine has been demonstrated to be an effective strategy to prevent spread of the flu in health care workers and patients and was the subject of several studies (Martinello, Jones, & Topal, 2003; Adal et al., 1996). One research team investigated reasons given by staff for not receiving the flu vaccine (Martinello et al., 2003). The investigators compared the results of a survey and knowledge test administered to both medical and nursing staff. The findings indicated a lower compliance to vaccination of nurses compared to physicians. Nurses were less knowledgeable about the vaccine compared to the physicians (Martinello et al., 2003, pp. 845–847).

Table 4.7 summaries studies related to organizational-level research conducted. Future research could be targeted to building knowledge and increasing vaccination rates of health care workers, especially nurses. Success in this area should improve the health of nurses and patients for the prevention of flu and its complications.

Other organizational-level studies are designed to assess compliance to infection control practices and efficacy of established infection control guidelines. In a review of the literature between 1984–1994, Larson and Kretzer (1995) found that health care workers were generally knowledgeable that hand hygiene has been demonstrated to be effective in decreasing transmission of infection. Despite this knowledge, they noted that compliance to hand hygiene recommendations has been low in the health care setting (pp. 88–106).

Larson also led a study in which neonatal nurses were asked to self-report hand hygiene performance using a log (Larson, Aiello, & Cimiotti, 2004). In this study, nurses were observed for the amount of time that they wore gloves and the number of times they performed hand hygiene. This was a difficult yet innovative approach to establish whether hand hygiene guidelines were being adhered to with a vulnerable patient population, premature newborns.

In another study, two types of soap dispensers were compared. Compliance improved with a hands-free dispenser compared to the standard manual dispensers for hand hygiene antiseptics. (Larson, Albrecht, & O'Keefe, 2005). The same group also conducted research designed to compare hand hygiene with antiseptic wash versus an alcohol-based antiseptic product while monitoring infections in neonatal patients and the amount of bacteria on the hands of staff. They found no differences between the products and the variables mentioned (Larson et al., 2005). Switching from the topic of hand hygiene to issues surrounding isolation and infection, the next two studies addressed some common problems found in acute care hospitals: infection outbreaks and prevention of infection with vaccinations.

Tokars and colleagues (2001) assessed the performance of staff related to isolation precautions for TB. Two hospitals were evaluated for compliance to

TABLE 4.7 Organizational Factors That Impact Hospital-Acquired Infection

Study	Setting	Type of study	Sample size	Unit of analysis	Focus of study	Findings
Adal et al., 1996	Hospital	Retrospective	171	Staff	Increasing flu vaccination in staff	Using a mobile cart to increase availability of the vaccine to staff increased vaccination
Larson, et al., 2000	Hospital	Quasi-experimental	92/860, 567/236, 989	Counting devices, electronic recordings, and patient days	Nosocomial infections Hand hygiene frequency Persistent changes in organization behaviors	Intervention group: decrease of nosocomial infection and an increase of persistent hand hygiene frequency Decrease in rates of VRE was significant
Martinello et al., 2003	Hospital	Cross-sectional study/survey	212	Participants	Knowledge of influenza vaccine	Nurses have misconceptions about the vaccine
Larson, 2004	Hospital	Survey of barriers for hand hygiene	21	Clinician results from survey tool	Attitudes of doctors and nurses	Tool (survey) scored highly for reliability and stability More testing recommended
McKinley et al., 2005	Hospital	Intervention qualitative stepwise design	38	Participant results from the survey	Poster use to improve hand hygiene practices	Focus groups, posters, questionnaire, motivators, and direct observation used to change staff behavior

Note: VRE = vancomycin-resistant enterococci

the CDC guidelines for the care of patients with active Mycobacterium TB in a study conducted from 1995–1997. The spark for the investigation was an outbreak of TB in the late 1980s and early 1990s. In this study, hospital personnel were observed for compliance in wearing personal protective equipment such as the National Institute of Occupational Health and Safety 1995–approved respirators (particulate). Patients were also observed for compliance to isolation precautions. Charts were reviewed for relevant information including genetic typing of organisms, testing, and time of isolation initiation. The records of skin testing of staff were also evaluated, and the amounts of negative pressures were monitored in the isolation rooms. The investigators found that although no transmission of TB occurred, multiple problems were identified, including delays in ordering laboratory sputum testing, a time lag in the initiation of isolation, partial noncompliance for use of respirators, and observations that patients left the isolation rooms without following isolation precautions (Tokars et al., 2001, pp. 449–455).

Several hospitals were re-surveyed to evaluate compliance to CDC guidelines for TB isolation (Manangan, Collaxo, Tokars, Paul, & Jarvis, 1999). Marked improvement occurred from the first survey to the last evaluation. For example, in 1991, a surgical mask was used by 55% of the staff when taking care of TB patients (Manangan et al., 1999, p. 337). By 1996, 94% wore the appropriate N-95 respirator recommended by CDC (Manangan et al., 1999, p. 337).

A 2001 high incidence of pneumococcal pneumonia was the impetus for a case control study of a nursing home (Tan, Ostrawski, & Bresnitz, 2003). One issue identified in this study was a lack of vaccination of elderly patients with the pneumococcal vaccine. This was the case despite state regulations that required vaccination of hospitalized patients age 65 years and older. Other problems included documentation deficiencies and resistance of residents and families to get the vaccination due to costs and a lack of knowledge of the benefits of vaccination (Tan et al., 2003, pp. 848–852). Table 4.8 provides a summary of studies designed to evaluate compliance and efficacy to infection control policies.

There are implications for nurses from these studies. Nurses have improved practice in the area of TB management by taking the lead in supporting compliance with respiratory isolation precautions. Patient monitoring and education are just two of the potential elements of an improvement plan that would benefit patients at risk for the flu, at risk for pneumococcal pneumonia, or in isolation for TB. However, more nursing research is needed to support the importance of the interventions that support patient safety in the area of infection control.

CONCLUSION

Nursing research in the area of patient safety relative to infection control has been varied, vital, and impressive. However, many of the studies presented did

TABLE 4.8 Studies Designed to Evaluate Compliance and Efficacy to Infection Control Policies

Study	Setting	Type of study	Sample size	Unit of analysis	Focus of study	Findings
Larson & Kretzer, 1995	Hospital	Review of literature for research studies	Sample sizes varied by study	Multiple variables analyzed including behaviors, attitudes, and self reports	Hand hygiene and barrier precautions	Problems identified and improvement recommended
Manangan et al., 1999	Hospital	Survey	53	Hospitals	Implementation of TB guidelines	Hospitals in areas surveyed improved in compliance to CDC guidelines for TB
Tokars et al., 2001	Hospital	Prospective observational	364	Patient cultures	Implementation Efficacy Compliance for TB practices	Multiple problems identified
Tan et al., 2003	Nursing home	Case control	9	Patient cultures, imaging studies, and vaccination records	Pneumococcal Pneumonia	Noncompliance with immunization guidelines
Larson, Aiello, & Cimiotti, 2004	Hospital	Observational & survey	119	Nurse direct observations and self report of hand washing	Hand hygiene observation and self-report	Some differences were found between observed versus self-report of hand hygiene
Larson, Albrecht, & O'Keefe, 2005	Hospital	Observational	5,568	Nurses observed for hand hygiene and measurements by electronic counters	Hand hygiene	Dispenser types affected compliance
Larson et al., 2005	Hospital	Clinical trial crossover design	119/2,932	Nurses/neonatal infections	Hand hygiene versus infection	No difference between alcohol based and antiseptic hand hygiene and infection rates or skin flora of staff.

Note: TB = tuberculosis; CDC = Centers for Disease Control and Prevention not employ an experimental design because these types of studies are difficult to conduct in the field of infection control. Some studies reported in the chapter were conducted using rigorous scientific methods. Others used informal methodology without concern for statistical power and experimental design. Although all studies cited in this publication are important, the studies that used more formal scientific approaches are more likely to generate evidence for greater applicability to other hospitals or patient groups.

The future of nursing science will depend not only on the ideas and abilities of seasoned researchers but also on the observations of clinicians at the bedside. Clinicians at the bedside are more likely to discern concerns worthy of investigation than those apart from the clinical setting. As the nursing profession continues to generate an increase in the number of nurse scientists conducting quality research, it is hoped that more research evidence will be generated to support patient safety in infection control.

Valuable nursing research in infection control will also depend on collaboration with a multidisciplinary team, including hospital departments such as microbiology, medicine, epidemiology, hospital administration, nursing, housekeeping, pharmacy, phlebotomy, respiratory therapy, materials management, and others. Research in infection control will need to incorporate a multifaceted approach integrating variables such as staff behavior models, surveys of staffs, education, infection surveillance, role modeling of behaviors, and administrative support and leadership. However, often the researchers include multiple interventions at once and, therefore, it is next to impossible to tell what facet of the intervention is actually providing the strongest effect.

Historically, health care providers and administrators were forced to use unproven strategies to fight infectious diseases like the plague and TB. Death and morbidity were rampant due to infections and inadequate countermeasures. Currently, we have some of the same infectious diseases, such as TB and newer ones, like resistant infections. However, today we have the advantages of technology and evidence-based practice studies. Future patient safety research designed to manage hospital-acquired infections will not only save lives but also improve the wellbeing of patients, staff, and visitors.

Acknowledgement is given to Susan M. Pilch, PhD, MLS, librarian at the National Institutes of Health Library, for support with the review of the literature.

REFERENCES

Adal, K. A., Flowers, R. H., Anglim, A. M., Hayden, F. G., Titus, M. G., Coyner, B. J., et al. (1996). Prevention of nosocomial influenza. *Infection Control and Hospital Epidemiology*, *17*(10), 641–648.

Babcock, H. M., Zack, J. E., Garrison, T., Trovillion, E., Kollef, M. H., & Fraser, V. (2003) Ventilator-associated pneumonia in a multi-hospital system: Differences in microbiology by location. *Infection Control and Hospital Epidemiology*, *24*, 853–858.

Beekmann, S. E., Vaughn, T. E., McCoy, K. D., Ferguson, K. J., Torner, J. C., Woolson, R. F., et al. (2001). Hospital bloodborne pathogens programs: Program characteristics and blood and body fluid exposure rates. *Infection Control and Hospital Epidemiology*, 22(2), 73–82.

Boyce, J., Havill, N., Kohan, C., Dumigan, D., & Ligi, C. (2004). Do infection control measures work for methicillin-resistant staphylococcus aureus? *Infection Control and Hospital Epidemiology*, 25, 395–401.

Boyce, J. M. & Pittet, D. (2002). Guideline for Hand Hygiene in Health-Care Settings: Recommendations of the Healthcare Infection Control Practices Advisory Committee and the HICPAC/SHEA/APIC/IDSA Hand Hygiene Task Force. *Infection Control & Hospital Epidemiology*, 23, S3–40.

Brooks, S., Khan, A., Stoica, D., Griffifth, J., Friedeman, L., Mukherji, F., et al. (1998). Reduction in Vancomycin-resistant Enterococcus and Clostridium Difficile infections following change to tympanic thermometers. *Infection Control and Hospital Epidemiology*, 19(5), 333–336.

CDC (1992, October 23). Public health focus: surveillance, prevention, and control of nosocomial infections. *Morbidity & Mortality Weekly Report*, 41, 783–787.

Center for Disease Control and Prevention (2000). *Worker Health Chartbook, 2000*. Cincinnati, OH: NIOSH-Publications Dissemination, U.S. Department of Health and Human Services, Public Health Service.

Christie, C. D., Constantinou, P., Marx, M. L., Willke, M. J., Marot, K., Mendez, F. L., et al. (1998). Low risk for tuberculosis in a regional pediatric hospital: Nine-year study of community rates and the mandatory employee tuberculin skin-test program. *Infection Control and Hospital Epidemiology*, 19(3), 168–174.

Curchoe, R. M., Powers, J., & El-Daher, N. (2002). Weekly transparent dressing changes linked to increased bacteremia rates. *Infection Control and Hospital Epidemiology*, 23(12), 730–732.

De Oliveira, A. M., White, K. L., Leschinsky, D. P., Beecham, B. D., Vogt, T. M., Moolenaar, et al. (2005). An outbreak of hepatitis C virus infections among outpatients at a hematology/oncology clinic. *Annals of Internal Medicine*, 142(11), 898–902.

Fridkin, S. K., Pear, S. M., Williamson, T. H., Galgiani, J. N., & Jarvis, W. R. (1996). The role of understaffing in central venous catheter-associated bloodstream infections. *Infection Control and Hospital Epidemiology*, 17(3), 150–158.

Fry, A., Udeagu, C., Soriano-Gabarro, M., Fridkin, S., Musinski, D., LaClaire, L., et al. (2005). Persistence of fluoroquinolone-resistant, multidrug-resistant streptococcus pneumonia in a long-term-care facility: Efforts to reduce intrafacility transmission. *Infection Control and Hospital Epidemiology*, 26, 239–247.

Garner, J. S. (1996). Guideline for isolation precautions in hospitals. Part I. Evolution of isolation practices, Hospital Infection Control Practices Advisory Committee [see comments]. *American Journal of Infection Control*, 24, 24–31.

Haley, R. W., Morgan, W. M., Culver, D. H., White, J. W., Emori, T. G., Mosser, J., et al. (1985, June 13). Update from the SENIC project. Hospital infection control: Recent progress and opportunities under prospective payment. *American Journal of Infection Control*, 97–108.

Institute of Medicine (2000). *To Err Is Human: Building a Safer Health System*. Washington DC: National Academy Press.

Lai, K. K., Baker, S. P., & Fontecchio, S. A. (2003). Impact of a program of intensive surveillance and interventions targeting ventilated patients in the reduction of ventilator-associated pneumonia and its cost-effectiveness. *Infection Control and Hospital Epidemiology, 24*(11), 859–863.

Lange, B. J., Weiman, M., Feuer, E. J., Jakobowski, D., Bilodeau, J., Stallings, V. A., et al. (1997). Impact of changes in catheter management on infectious complications among children with central venous catheters. *Infection Control and Hospital Epidemiology, 18*(5), 326–332.

Larson, E. L., Cimiotti, J. P., Haas, J., Nesin, M., Allen, A., Della-Latta, P., et al. (2005). Gram-negative bacilli associated with catheter-associated and non-catheters-associated bloodstream infections and hand carriage by healthcare workers in neonatal intensive care units. *Pediatric Critical Care Medicine, 6*(4), 457–461.

Larson, E. L., Albrecht, S., O'Keefe, M. (2005) Hand hygiene behavior in a pediatric emergency department and a pediatric intensive care unit: Comparison of use of 2 dispenser systems. *American Journal of Critical Care, 14*(4), 304–312.

Larson, E. L., Cimiotti, J., Haas, J., Parides, M., Nesin, M., Della-Latta, P., et al. (2005). Effect of antiseptic handwashing vs. alcohol sanitizer on health care-associated infections in neonatal intensive care units. *Archives of Pediatrics & Adolescent Medicine, 159*(4), 377–383.

Larson, E. (2004). A tool to assess barriers to adherence to hand hygiene guideline. *American Journal of Infection Control, 32*(1), 48–51.

Larson, E. L., Aiello, A. E., & Cimiotti, J. P. (2004). Assessing nurses' hand hygiene practices by direct observation or self-report. *Journal of Nursing Measurement, 12*(1), 77–85.

Larson, E. (2001). Hygiene of the Skin: When is clean too clean? *Emerging Infectious Diseases, 7*(2), 225–230.

Larson, E., Early, E., Cloonan, P., Sugrue, S., & Parides, M. (2000). An organizational climate intervention associated with increased handwashing and decreased nosocomial infections. *Behavioral Medicine, 26,* 14–22.

Larson, E. & Kretzer, E. K. (1995). Compliance with handwashing and barrier precautions. *Journal of Hospital Infection, 30*(suppl.), 88–106

Manangan, L. P., Collaxo, E. R., Tokars, J., Paul, S., & Jarvis, W. R. (1999). Trends in compliance with the guidelines for preventing the transmission of mycobacterium tuberculosis among New Jersey hospitals, 1989 to 1996. *Infection Control and Hospital Epidemiology, 20*(5), 337–340.

Martinello, R. A., Jones, L., & Topal, J. E. (2003). Correlation between Healthcare workers' knowledge of influenza vaccine and vaccine receipt. *Infection Control and Hospital Epidemiology, 24*(11), 845–848.

McKinley, R., Gillespie, W., Krauss, J., Harrison, S., Medeiros, R., Hawkins, M., et al. (2005). Focus group data as a tool in assessing effectiveness of a hand hygiene campaign. *American Journal of Infection control, 33*(6), 368–373.

Milam, M., Hall, M., Pringle, T., & Buchanan, K. (2001). Bacterial contamination of fabric stethoscope covers: The velveteen rabbit of health care? *Infection Control Hospital Epidemiology, 22,* 653–655.

O'Grady, N. P., Alexander, M., Dellinger, E. P., Gerberding, J. L., Heard, S. O., Maki, D. G. et al. (2002). Guidelines for the prevention of intravascular catheter-related infections. Centers for Disease Control and Prevention. *Morbidity and Mortality Weekly Report Recommendations and Reports, 51*, 1–29.

Robert, J., Fridkin, S. K., Blumberg, H. M., Anderson, B., White, N., Ray, S., et al. (2000). The influence of the composition of the nursing staff on primary bloodstream infection rates in a surgical intensive care unit. *Infection Control and Hospital Epidemiology, 21*(1), 12–17.

Rupp, M., Fitzgerald, T., Marion, N., Helget, V., Puumala, S., Anderson, J., et al. (2004). Effect of silver-coated urinary catheters: Efficacy, cost-effectiveness, and antimicrobial resistance. *American Journal of Infection Control, 32*, 445–450.

Saiman, L., Cronquist, A., Fann, Wu, F., Zhou, J., Rubenstein, D., et al. (2003). An outbreak of methicillin-resistant staphylococcus aureus in a neonatal intensive care unit. *Infection Control and Hospital Epidemiology, 24*, 317–321.

Seal, L. & Paul-Cheadle, D. (2004). A systems approach to preoperative surgical patient skin preparation. *American Journal of Infection Control, 32*, 57–62.

Sepkowitz, K. A., Fella, P., Rivera, P., Villa, N., & DeHovitz, J. (1995). Prevalence of PPD positivity among new employees at a hospital in New York City. *Infection Control and Hospital Epidemiology, 16*(6), 344–347.

Sohn, S., Eagan, J., & Sepkowitz, K. A. (2004). Safety-engineered device implementation: Does it introduce bias in percutaneous injury reporting? *Infection Control and Hospital Epidemiology, 25*(7), 543–547.

Stone, P. W. (2004). Nurses' Working Conditions: Implications for Infectious Disease. *Emerging Infectious Diseases, 10*, 1984–1989.

Stone, P. W., Gupta, A., Loughrey, M., la-Latta, P., Cimiotti, J., Larson, E., et al. (2003). Attributable costs and length of stay of an extended-spectrum beta-lactamase-producing Klebsiella pneumoniae outbreak in a neonatal intensive care unit. *Infection Control & Hospital Epidemiology, 24*, 601–606.

Stover, B., Shulman, S., Bratcher, D., Brady, M., Levine, G., & Jarvis, W. (2001). Nosocomial infection rates in US children's hospitals neonatal and pediatric intensive care units. *American Journal of Infection Control, 29*, 152–157.

Stroud, L. A., Tokars, J. I., Grieco, M. H., Crawford, J. T., Culver, D. H., Edlin, B. R., et al. (1995). Evaluation of infection control measures in preventing the nosocomial transmission of multi-drug-resistant mycobacterium tuberculosis in a New York City hospital. *Infection Control and Hospital Epidemiology, 16*(3), 141–147.

Tablan, O. C., Anderson, L. J., Besser, R., Bridges, C., & Hajjeh, R. (2004). Guidelines for preventing health-care–associated pneumonia, 2003: Recommendations of CDC and the Healthcare Infection Control Practices Advisory Committee. *Morbidity and Mortality Weekly Report Recommendations and Reports, 53*, 1–36.

Tan, C. G., Ostrawski, S., & Bresnitz, E. A. (2003). A preventable outbreak of pneumoccal pneumonia among unvaccinated nursing home residents in New Jersey during 2001. *Infection Control and Hospital Epidemiology, 24*(11), 848–852.

Tokars, J., McKinley, G., Otten, J., Woodley, C., Sordillo, E., Caldwell, J., Liss, C., Gilligan, M., Diem, L., Onorato, I., & Jarvis, W. (2001). Use and efficacy of tuberculosis infection control practices at hospitals with previous outbreaks of multi-drug resistant tuberculosis. *Infection Control and Hospital Epidemiology, 22*, 449–445.

Trick, W., Temple, R., Chen, D., Wright, B., Solomon, S., & Peterson, L. (2002). Patient colonization and environmental contamination by vancomycin-resistant enterococci in a rehabilitation facility. *Archives Physical Medicine & Rehabilitation*, 83, 899–902.

Tuboku-Metzger, J., Chiarello, L., Sinkowitz-Cochran, R., Casano-Dickerson, A., & Cardo, D. (2005). Public attitudes and opinions toward physicians and dentists infected with bloodborne viruses: Results of a national survey. *American Journal of Infection Control*, 33, 229–303.

United States Department of Health and Human Services. (2000). *Healthy people 2010/ U.S. Department of Health and Human Services*. (Conference edition ed.) Washington, DC: U.S. Department of Health and Human Services.

Varia, M., Wilson, S., Sarwal, S., McGeer, A., Gournis, E., Galanis, E., et al. (2003). Investigation of a nosocomial outbreak of severe acute respiratory syndrome (SARS) in Toronto, Canada. *Canadian Medical Association Journal*, 169, 285–292.

Weinstein, J., Mazon, D., Pantelick, E., Reagon-Cirincione, P., Dembry, L. & Hierholzer, W. (1999). A decade of prevalence surveys in a tertiary-care center: trends in nosocomial infection rates, device utilization, and patient acuity. *Infection Control and Hospital Epidemiology*, 20, 543–548.

Wenzel, R. P. & Edmond, M. B. (2001). The impact of hospital-acquired bloodstream infections. 21. *Emerging Infectious Diseases*, 7, 174–177.

Wong, E. (2000). Guideline for Prevention of Catheter-associated Urinary Tract Infections. Centers for Disease Control and Prevention [Data file].

PART III

Setting-Specific Patient Safety Research

Chapter 5

Patient Safety in Hospital Acute Care Units

Mary A. Blegen

ABSTRACT

The most visible threats to patient safety associated with nursing care occur on hospital inpatient units. Patient safety research is a new phenomenon, but it builds on the knowledge provided by quality-of-care research done previously. The purpose of this chapter is to describe the current state of the science in the area of nurse staffing and patient safety. The results of research studies published since the last round of reviews (1996–2005) are described by level of analysis, measures of nurse staffing and patient outcomes. Although research linking nurse staffing to the quality of patient care has increased markedly since 1996, the results of recent research projects do not yet provide a thorough and consistent foundation for producing solutions to the crisis in hospital nursing care. The inconsistencies are largely due to differing units of analysis (hospital, patient, care unit), variability in measures of nurse staffing, the variety of quality indicators chosen, the difficulty finding accurate measures of these indicators, and the difficulty creating risk-adjustment strategies for the indicators most sensitive to nursing care. Nursing administration and policy most urgently need research conducted with standardized data collected at the patient care unit level.

Keywords: patient safety, nursing, staffing

The most visible threats to patient safety associated with nursing care occur on hospital inpatient units. Although errors in the operating room grab more headlines, the bulk of health care–associated complications, injuries, and adverse occurrences happen in the course of routine patient care. The interdisciplinary team and the organizational system supporting its work provide the care and surveillance to facilitate patient comfort, protect from harm, and promote recovery. That the care and surveillance fall short of the high quality expected and allow too many adverse outcomes has been made clear over the past decade.

Patient safety research is a new phenomenon, but it builds on the knowledge provided by quality of care research done previously. A central issue in quality of care, and now patient safety research, is the effect of nurse staffing—the number and mix of nursing care providers and the way in which these services are organized (Aikin, 2005; Wachter, 2005). These concerns are the most recent manifestation of issues addressed by nursing research for 50 years. In 1960, Safford and Schlotfeldt reported that the results of their field experiment supported the hypothesis: "quality of nursing care could decrease as nurses' responsibilities were increased through the assignment of additional patients" (p. 152). Aydelotte and Tener (1960) did not find an increase in patient welfare, in general, when the number of professional nurses increased, although they did find a small decrease in patient complaints. Abdellah and Levine (1958) found that patient satisfaction was higher when professional registered nurse (RN) hours were higher; but, when the total nursing hours (RNs, licensed practical nurses [LPNs], and nursing assistants [NAs]) were higher, satisfaction was lower.

Two studies examined the effects of changing from team nursing to an all RN staffing model in hospitals. The first study compared the quality and cost of primary nursing and team nursing. Quality was maintained and cost decreased with primary nursing (Hinshaw, Scofield & Atwood, 1981). Eight medical units in one hospital participated in a comparison of team and primary nursing (Gardner, 1991). Gardner found higher observed quality on primary units than on team units and lower cost, but no differences in patient perceptions of care.

Research examining the effects of different models of patient care delivery continued through the 1990s. Using existing data from staffing intensity measures and patient records, two studies found that short staffing was related to poor outcomes and higher actual costs (Behner, Fogg, Frankenbach, & Robertson, 1990; Flood & Diers, 1988). A pair of studies conducted in California (Bostrom & Zimmerman, 1993; Neidlinger, Bostrom, Stricker, Hild, & Zhang, 1993) evaluated restructuring by adding nursing assistants. Patient satisfaction increased slightly in one hospital and decreased in the other. And quality of care declined slightly in each study. One study noted a decline in key documentation indicators, and the other noted an increase in adverse occurrence rates after the restructuring. In another study of two hospitals in California, Seago (1999) found that the introduction of a patient-focused care model did not bring about significant change and may have increased costs. Lengacher and colleagues described the outcomes of the Partners in Patient Care model on two randomly selected units over 18 months (6 months before to 12 months after implementation). Patient satisfaction was higher on the experimental unit before the restructuring change and declined over time. However, patient satisfaction on the control unit was lower before the restructuring and rose during the period of the study. Quality of care, as indicated by adverse events, was also lower on the experimental unit (Lengacher et al., 1996; Lengacher et al., 1997).

The restructuring and reorganization of hospitals, in response to the burgeoning cost of hospital care in the 1990s, led to declines in the hours of care provided by nurses. This was coupled with decreasing patient lengths of stay (LOS). Patients were discharged earlier than in the previous pattern, leaving only the sickest and most dependent patients in hospital beds. As the numbers of RNs and the hours they worked were constrained, the effect was an increase in inpatients' need for care with fewer RNs available to provide the care. In response to the concerns that these changes triggered, several scholars conducted reviews of the literature, published before 1997, addressing these issues (Bernreuter & Cardona, 1997; Hall, 1997; Huston, 1996; Krapohl & Larson, 1996; Prescott, 1993; Verran, 1996). These reviews concluded that the effects of nursing care delivery changes on staff and organizational outcomes have been studied; but the effects on client outcomes have not been studied sufficiently, and the effects on cost are equivocal. Further, they concluded that the models change quickly, with little evaluation of a new model before even newer models are implemented.

Concerns, widely expressed by nurses, patients, and other health providers, led to formation of the Institute of Medicine's (IOM's) Committee on the Adequacy of Nurse Staffing. This committee concluded that there was insufficient evidence linking nurse staffing and patient outcomes and that research in these areas was badly needed (Wunderlich, Sloan & Davis, 1996).

In response to the IOM report, the Agency for Health Care Policy and Research, the Division of Nursing of the Health Resources and Services Administration, and the National Institute of Nursing Research published a research agenda addressing *Nurse Staffing and Quality of Care in Health Care Organizations*. This agenda stated that "Research pertaining to nurse staffing and quality in hospitals is a high priority" and identified several key questions. These questions addressed many issues: relationships between the organization and delivery of nursing care and patient outcomes, unique skills and mix of RNs and other nursing and ancillary staff, and appropriate use of resources in an era when resources are limited. Research addressing these issues increased greatly following the IOM report and the prioritization of nurse staffing research. Although the term "patient safety" was not used in this work, the indicators used to measure quality and patient outcomes included those we now consider safety indicators: medication errors, patient falls, skin breakdown, and nosocomial infections (e.g., urinary tract, respiratory, bloodstream). Additionally, some of the research conducted in response to this call generated other nursing-sensitive patient safety indicators such as failure to rescue.

The purpose of this paper is to describe the current state of the science in the area of nurse staffing and patient safety. The results of research studies published since the last round of reviews (1996–2005) are described by level of analysis, measures of nurse staffing, and patient outcomes. The inconsistencies in this body of knowledge are noted, and implications for future research are discussed.

THE RESEARCH

The review presented in this chapter covers first the research that examined the effect of nurse staffing at the hospital level. Following that section are the review of studies done at the patient care unit level, a critique of nurse staffing measures, and a review focusing on the various quality and safety indicators.

National Data Sets and Multihospital Studies

Many of the hospital-level studies used national data sets from the Health Care Financing Administration (now the Centers for Medicare & Medicaid Services), Agency for Healthcare Research and Quality (AHRQ), and American Hospital Association (AHA). In one of the first studies linking mortality rates to nursing care, Aiken, Smith, and Lake (1994) found a negative and statistically significant relationship between nursing care intensity and patient mortality rates.

The American Nurses Association (ANA) used data from the uniform hospital discharge data set and from mandated state reports, which included costs for nursing personnel, to test the newly developed ANA Nursing Report Card (ANA, 1997; Lichtig, Knauf, Milholland, 1999). For this study, data from 502 hospitals in two states (CA, NY) in two time periods (1992 and 1994) were collected. Nursing Intensity Weights (NIW) were calculated using the state of New York's methods; adverse occurrences were identified from DRG/ICD-9 coding; total nursing hours per NIW and the percent hours provided by RNs were calculated. The statistically significant net effect of total hours of care per NIW was that higher hours of care was associated with lower length of stay and lower pressure ulcer rates. The statistically significant net effect of RN percent was that higher skill mix was associated with shorter length of stay, and lower rates of pressure ulcers, pneumonia, postoperative infection, and urinary tract infections.

Two studies of nurse staffing on patient care quality, published within the last three years, received extensive national attention (Aiken, Clarke, Sloane, Sochalski, & Silbur, 2002; Aiken, Clark, Cheung, Sloane, & Silbur, 2003; Needleman, Buerhaus, Mattke, Stewart, & Zelevinsky, 2002). The adverse outcomes that declined with higher levels of RN staffing included mortality rates, failure to rescue from complications, urinary tract infections, length of stay, pneumonia, gastrointestinal bleeding, and patient shock and arrests. These studies, using large hospital level data sets, made important contributions to understanding the effect of nursing care. Measurement choices in both studies reflect the current lack of precise indicators of the level or "dose" of this important structural variable.

Needleman and colleagues (2002) used state level data from mandatory reports of hospitals' costs and outcomes. Hours of care from each of the three types of nursing care providers (RN, LPNs, CNAs) were calculated as totals for each hospital and standardized using patient days (inpatient days with an adjustment for outpatient visits). The nursing care hours were further adjusted to reflect the differences in patient need (using DRGs) for different hospitals. Results showed that the impact of increased hours of care and of a greater proportion of care hours provided by RNs on patient outcomes was beneficial. However, it is difficult to translate the specific hours or proportions for all nurses employed in the hospital as a whole to recommendations for staffing patient care units with direct care RNs.

In the Aiken et al., study (2002; 2003), nurse staffing data came from a questionnaire survey of all nurses licensed in the state. A 50% random sample of nurses was drawn from licensure lists, response rates were good at approximately 50%. Nurse respondents indicated the hospital in which they worked, and hospitals were included in the study if at least 10 nurses from the hospital had responded to the survey. Nurse respondents who provided patient care on inpatient units were asked to indicate the number of patients assigned to them during the last shift they worked and the average number of patients was then assigned to the hospital as the patient to nurse ratio for that hospital. Likewise, the education level of the nurses who responded to the survey was used as the nurse education level for that hospital in subsequent analyses of mortality and "failure to rescue" rates for the hospital. Analyses showed that probability of patient mortality increased 6% with each additional patient a nurse was assigned to care for and decreased 5% for each 10% increase in the proportion of RNs with baccalaureate degrees.

In a partial replication of the Aikin study, Estabrooks Midodzi, Cummings, Ricker, and Giovannetti (2005) used a survey questionnaire to measure staffing in 49 hospitals in Alberta, Canada. They analyzed the effect of hospital level staffing, as indicated by nurse respondents to the survey, on the 30 day mortality rates of medical patients. Both RN staff mix and RN education were associated with decreased mortality rates after controlling for patient risks. These results support hypotheses held for years that more nurses and a higher level of nurse education have beneficial impacts on the quality of patient care. Tourangeau, Giovannetti, Tu and Wood (2002) used nurse staffing and patient discharge data from the province of Ontario. They also found that increased nurse RN staffing levels were associated with lower adjusted mortality rates.

Staffing data from the AHA have been extensively used to measure nurse staffing (Kovner & Gergen, 1998; Kovner, Jones, Zhan, Gergen & Basu, 2002; Person et al., 2004). In these studies, the nurse staffing data available included only the licensed nurses employed as a total for the entire hospital. These data combine the direct care RNs and those in administrative, management, education, and support roles.

Kovner and colleagues (1998, 2002) used data from the AHA survey and from the AHRQ Healthcare Cost and Utilization Project Nationwide Inpatient Sample. The study, reported in 1998, used data from 506 hospitals in 10 states to determine the frequency of nine postsurgical outcomes (adverse events) based on ICD-9-CM codes. Of these nine codes, four were sensitive to differences in nurse staffing. Higher nurse staffing levels were related to fewer instances of thrombosis, UTIs, and pneumonia after surgery; staffing levels were not related to the nurse-sensitive adverse events of pneumonia and venous thrombosis after invasive vascular procedures. Staffing was measured with RN and LPN hours per adjusted patient day (adjusted for outpatient visits). Co-linearity between RN hours per adjusted patient day and non-RN hours per adjusted patient day did not permit the separation of these effects. In the second study, RN full-time equivalent employees (FTEs) were associated only with reduced incidence of pneumonia.

RN and LPN staffing levels (AHA data) were grouped in quartiles by Person and colleagues (2004); and mortality rates following acute myocardial infarction were determined for hospitals in each quartile. Mortality rates (from 1994–1995 Cooperative Cardiovascular Project data) declined as RN staffing increased, and increased as LPN staffing increased. In these studies, nurse staffing included all nurses employed as administrators and other non-patient-care roles, nurses caring for patients in ambulatory and short-stay areas, and in specialized care areas such as operating and recovery units. Unlicensed assistant care hours were not included in the AHA data set.

Using only nursing care hours provided by licensed nurses omits an important factor from the analyses. Although most studies conclude that RN care has the greatest effect on quality, hospital units providing nonintensive care may staff with up to 50% non-licensed NAs. Omitting these care providers from analyses overlooks a major factor in contemporary hospital care.

Unruh (2003) used data from the state of Pennsylvania to determine the number of nurses employed. These data included RNs, LPNs, and NAs, but again included nursing personnel in all roles in the hospital. State-level discharge data were used to measure patient outcomes. The number of licensed nurses (RNs and LPNs), controlling for patient days, was associated with reduced incidence of atelectasis, decubiti, patient falls, and UTIs. Higher proportions of LPNs were associated with a reduced incidence of decubiti and pneumonia but with increased falls. Cho, Ketefian, Barkauskas, and Smith (2003) obtained unit-level direct care nursing hours for their study. The total hours of care from inpatient units for all nursing care providers were summed to the hospital level to determine the effect of nursing care on patient outcomes. RN hours of care and RN proportion of hours were also calculated. The total hours of care per patient day was associated with increased incidence of decubiti, and RN hours and RN proportion were associated with decreased pneumonia rates. No direct effect of nurse staffing was found on other patient outcomes, costs, and LOS.

Although the studies that used hospital-level staffing standardized the nursing care hours by patient load, the data available for standardizing varied from study to study. Cho et al. (2003) obtained only inpatient hours and adjusted for inpatient days only. Other studies obtained all nursing care FTEs or hours and adjusted for outpatient visits and inpatient days (Kovner et al., 2002; Needleman, 2002; Unruh, 2003). Two of these studies also adjusted for patient acuity or need for care (Needleman, 2002; Unruh, 2003). Adjusting for these different measures of patient load may produce quite different values for the nursing care variable.

These multi-institutional studies provide valuable information; however, there are several weaknesses in this group of studies. First, as Jones (1993) pointed out, it is difficult to find standardized data that reflect outcomes specifically affected by nursing care. Many studies reported only mortality rates at the level of the hospital. These data are available from large national data sets and have been useful in studies of hospital care. Mortality, however, is not the best indicator of the quality of nursing care. Other adverse outcomes may be more sensitive than mortality rates to nursing care; although nursing care is only one of the many factors leading to most of the other adverse outcomes. Until nursing develops standardized databases of its own, we must use existing data and attempt to find indicators that are sensitive to nursing care.

Second, nurse staffing data included all RNs employed in all positions in the hospital whether or not they provided direct patient care. The ratio of RNs to average patient census was used by Aiken, Smith, and Lake (1994). The total nursing care hours per adjusted patient day was used by two studies (ANA, 1997; Kovner & Gergen, 1998); and RN percent was used by one (ANA, 1997). Two studies used questionnaire survey data to determine average nurse to patient ratios (Aikin, et al., 2002; Estrabrook, et al., 2005). Several studies used state or province data to determine nursing hours (Needleman et al., 2002; Tourangeau et al., 2002).

Third, hospital was the level of analysis for most of these studies. Data used in these studies came from large databases with patient discharge data and nurse staffing data at the hospital level. Although these studies have been valuable, they have necessarily aggregated differing types of patients with differing levels of illness. Adjustments for patient severity were made at the level of the hospital (case-mix adjustments); but these cannot reflect severity of patients on separate patient care units. The effect of nurse staffing, however, is most direct at the patient care unit level.

As noted in Table 5.1 the hospital-level studies using mortality as an outcome were split in regard to finding a statistically significant effect for nurse staffing: Four statistically significant and two not significant. The studies focusing on other adverse outcomes found both significant and positive effects for nurse staffing and nonsignificant and negative effects for nurse staffing. Thus, these multisite studies do provide support for the idea that greater use of professional nurses in direct care improves patient outcomes; but this support is not entirely consistent. Lang, Hodge, Olson, Romano, and Kravitz (2004) reviewed 43 hospital-level studies published between 1980 and 2003. Of the 19 outcomes in one or more of these studies, pneumonia was most often found to be linked to nursing care (61% of studies found statistically significant results), 57% of the results linked nursing hours to mortality rates, and 50% of the results for nosocomial infections were linked to nurse staffing. In other words, 43% of the time the relationship between mortality rates and nurse staffing was not significant, and half of the time the relationship between nurse staffing and nosocomial infections was not significant. Blegen (2004) reviewed 11 studies at the hospital level published between 1997 and 2004 and found similar results. The proportion of results showing a statistically significant relationship between nurse staffing and a particular outcome was 77% for pneumonia, 75% for failure to rescue, 66% for UTIs, 57% for mortality, and 50% for patient falls and injuries. Both reviews concluded that the research evidence from hospital-level studies is inconsistent.

Patient Care Unit–Level Studies

Studies of data collected directly from hospitals have been able to derive nurse staffing variables reflecting only direct care providers at the patient care unit level (see summary in Table 5.2). The largest proportion of these studies used both total hours per patient day and RN staff mix (Blegen, Goode & Reed, 1998; Blegen & Vaughn, 1998; Sovie & Jawad, 2001); although one used only day shift nursing care hours and RN mix (Potter, Barr, McSweeney & Sledge, 2003). Several used only the RN staff mix to indicate nurse staffing (Hall, et al., 2003; Mark, Salyer, & Wan, 2003). Although these studies used more precise measures of nurse staffing, the outcome measures chosen have been uniquely defined for each study. Mark et al. (2003) and Sovie and Jawad (2001) used prospective data collection and carefully defined measures of adverse outcomes and calculated these rates at the unit level. Blegen, Goode & Reede (1998), Blegen & Vaughn (1998), and Potter et al. (2003) used existing data collected for quality assurance and calculated the ratios of adverse outcomes at the unit level. Patient perceptions of care and the outcomes of care provided the outcome measures in some cases (Hall et al., 2003; Mark et al., 2003; Potter et al., 2003; Sovie and Jawad, 2001). Studies collecting these data directly must, of necessity, be smaller studies. Unit-level analyses

TABLE 5.1 Hospital-Level Studies of Nurse Staffing and Selected Patient Outcomes

	Surgical patients							Medical patients				
	Kovner 1998	Kovner 2002	Needleman	Aiken 1994	Aiken 2002/2003	Cho	Estabrook	Needleman	Person	Unruh	ANA 1 1997	ANA 2 2000
Mortality rate	ns/r	ns/r	0	+	+	ns/r	+	0	+	ns/r	ns/r	ns/r
Failure to rescue	ns/r	ns/r	+	ns/r	+	ns/r	ns/r	+	ns/r	ns/r	ns/r	ns/r
Length of stay	ns/r	+	0	ns/r	ns/r	ns/r	ns/r	+	ns/r	ns/r	+	+
Pneumonia	+	ns/r	0	ns/r	ns/r	+	ns/r	+	ns/r	+	+	+
Pulmonary compromise/atelectasis	+	0	0	ns/r	ns/r	ns/r	ns/r	0	ns/r	+	ns/r	ns/r
Urinary tract infections	+	0	+	ns/r	ns/r	0	ns/r	+	ns/r	+	+	+
Skin breakdown	ns/r	ns/r	0	ns/r	ns/r	−	ns/r	0	ns/r	+	+	0
Deep vein thrombosis	+	0	0	ns/r	ns/r	ns/r	ns/r	0	ns/r	ns/r	ns/r	ns/r
Infections	ns/r	ns/r	0	ns/r	ns/r	0	ns/r	0	ns/r	0	+	+
Falls (injury)	ns/r	ns/r	ns/r	ns/r	ns/r	0	ns/r	ns/r	ns/r	+	ns/r	ns/r
Gastrointestinal bleed	ns/r	ns/r	0	ns/r	ns/r	ns/r	ns/r	+	ns/r	ns/r	ns/r	ns/r
Shock arrest	ns/r	ns/r	0	ns/r	ns/r	ns/r	ns/r	+	ns/r	ns/r	ns/r	ns/r

(Note: some studies included multiple indicators of nurse staffing; this summary is not able to reflect all of the complexity in the research reports)

+ = better nurse staffing improved outcome   0 = better nurse staffing had no effect

− = better nurse staffing detrimental effect   ns/r = not studied or reported

TABLE 5.2 Patient Care Unit Level Studies of Nurse Staffing and Selected Patient Outcomes

	Blegen 1	Blegen 2	Sovie — Medical units	Sovie — Surgical units	Hall (2003)	Hall (2004)	Mark	Potter	Dunton	Maryland ICUs — Amaravadi esophagectomy	Maryland ICUs — Dang AAA	Maryland ICUs — Pronovost AAA	Maryland ICUs — Dimick hepatectomy
Mortality rate	+	ns/r	ns/r	ns/r	ns/r	ns/r	ns/r	ns/r	ns/r	0	0	+	0
Complications	ns/r	ns/r	ns/r	ns/r	ns/r	ns/r	ns/r	ns/r	ns/r	+	+	0	+
Length of stay	ns/r	ns/r	ns/r	ns/r	ns/r	ns/r	0	ns/r	ns/r	+	ns/r	+	0
Medication errors	+	+	ns/r	ns/r	ns/r	+	0	0	ns/r	ns/r	ns/r	ns/r	ns/r
Patient falls	0	+	+	+	ns/r	0	0	+	+	+	+	ns/r	ns/r
Ventilator days	ns/r	ns/r	ns/r	ns/r	ns/r	ns/r	ns/r	ns/r	ns/r	+	+	ns/r	ns/r
Pneumonia	0	ns/r	ns/r	ns/r	ns/r	ns/r	ns/r	ns/r	ns/r	ns/r	ns/r	ns/r	0
Urinary tract infections	0	ns/r	+	0	ns/r	0	ns/r	ns/r	ns/r	+	ns/r	ns/r	ns/r
Skin breakdown	+	ns/r	0	+	ns/r	ns/r	ns/r	ns/r	ns/r	ns/r	ns/r	ns/r	ns/r
Infections	0	ns/r	ns/r	ns/r	ns/r	+	ns/r	ns/r	ns/r	+	ns/r	ns/r	0
Patient satisfaction	+	ns/r	+	+	+	ns/r	+	+	ns/r	ns/r	ns/r	ns/r	ns/r
Pain/Symptoms	ns/r	ns/r	ns/r	ns/r	0	ns/r	ns/r	+	ns/r	ns/r	ns/r	ns/r	ns/r
Functional status/self-care ability	ns/r	ns/r	ns/r	ns/r	+	ns/r	ns/r	+	ns/r	ns/r	nsr	ns/r	ns/r

(Note: some studies included multiple indicators of nurse staffing; this summary is not able to reflect all of the complexity in the research reports)
+ = better nurse staffing improved outcome   0 = better nurse staffing had no effect
– = better nurse staffing detrimental effect   ns/r = not studied or reported

were done with the numbers of units ranging between 32 and 124. Given these approaches to outcomes, the different indicators of staffing, and the smaller samples, it is not surprising that the results are inconsistent.

One set of research reports describing the effects of physician and nursing care on the outcomes of patients in surgical intensive care units (SICUs) used patient discharge data from all hospitals contributing to a state-level data set in Maryland. It measured nurse staffing with a survey completed by managers of SICUs in the state (Amaravadi, Dimick, Pronovost, & Lipsett, 2000; Dang, Johantgen, Pronovost, Jenckes, & Bass, 2002; Dimick, Swobody, Pronovost, & Lipsett, 2001; Pronovost et al., 1999). These researchers asked the SICU managers to indicate the usual number of patients assigned to each nurse during the day shift and during the night shift. The reports of patient:nurse ratios and other characteristics of the units were requested in 1996 and were used to predict the outcomes of patients with specific diagnoses for the previous 3 years (1994–1996). Patients on ICUs where 1–2 patients were typically assigned to each nurse had better outcomes than patients on units with a patient to nurse ratio of 3 or more. Although these studies captured direct patient care nurse staffing and systematically controlled for other factors effecting patient outcomes, the fact that nurse staffing was measured at a different time than the patient outcomes must be kept in mind while interpreting the results.

A review of 12 unit-level studies focusing on the effects of nurse staffing and published between 1997 and 2004 (Blegen, 2004) reported that the results of unit-level studies were inconsistent. Of the outcomes analyzed across these studies, only a portion of the relationships with nurse staffing were statistically significantly. Studies measuring patient perceptions of quality were positively related to nurse staffing at a statistically significant level 87% of the time. Indicators of complications were inversely related with higher nurse staffing only 75% of the time. The relationships between nurse staffing levels and other specific outcome indicators were significant 66% of the time for skin breakdown and patient falls and 50% of the time for nosocomial infections. The rest of the outcome indicators showed a beneficial relationship with nurse staffing at the patient care unit–level less than half of the time.

Taken as a whole, the results of the patient care unit studies are difficult to generalize and apply in practice. Most of these studies used only a few units from a few hospitals. The results from these small sample studies were not often statistically significant; and when they were, they were inconsistent from one study to the next. Quality of care indicators in these patient care unit studies were quite diverse. Adverse occurrence rates were the most often used indicators, and patient satisfaction was frequently used but measured differently in each study.

The strengths of these studies were that they recognized that staffing decisions are made at the level of the patient care unit and nursing care can be linked with multiple outcome indicators. Overall, these studies have shown more promise in describing the effect of nurse staffing on patient outcomes than those done at the hospital level. For the most part, however, these studies were done in a small number of hospitals, and when examining the relationship between staffing and quality of care, results are still ambiguous.

Patient care unit–level studies will become more prevalent as the National Database of Nursing Quality Indicators and the California Nursing Outcomes project build their databases. These will be joined by standardized databases created by nurse researchers in the Veterans Health Administration and military hospitals. These data sets will provide opportunity for more study and more rigorous study than has been possible in the past.

Measuring Nurse Staffing

It is crucial to the continued development of knowledge in this area that the measures of nurse staffing be at least clarified and at best standardized. The most informative method of measuring the amount of nursing care provided on inpatient care units is the hours of care provided divided by the number of patients being cared for. Known as hours per patient day (hppd), this approach is a more precise measure than nurse to patient ratio (Budreau, Balakrishnan, Titler, & Hafner, 1999). Precision is increased by capturing the hours within all categories of providers (i.e, RNs, LPNs, unlicensed assistants), the care needs of the patients (illness severity), and the volatility or turbulence in the care needs (patient turnover during the shift). Not one of these three factors, which allow precision in measurement, is included in any of the data sets generally available to researchers for analysis.

Other characteristics of the nurses and their work, as well as the hours of nursing care, also need to be considered. For example, the use of overtime hours is likely to affect the care on the unit. Overtime may lead to fatigue and errors, or less diligence in duties such as skin care (Institute of Medicine, 2003; Rogers, Hwang, Scott, Aiken, & Dinges, 2004). The competence of the RN is central to his or her ability to provide surveillance and early intervention to prevent or minimize adverse outcomes. However, there is little research addressing this topic. RN education and experience levels have been linked to the quality of care. Although difficult to show empirically, baccalaureate-prepared nurses are assumed to have stronger critical thinking skills and communication skills that are better than those of nurses prepared in other programs (Goode et al., 2001). Previous studies (Blegen, Vaughn & Goode, 2001; Tourangeau et al., 2002) found that RNs with greater average experience working on patient care units had a beneficial effect on patient outcomes; but the proportion of RNs with baccalaureate degrees did not. Aiken and colleagues (2003) reported that after controlling for hospital characteristics, patient characteristics, and other indicators of nurse staffing, a 10% increase in the proportion of RNs in the hospital with baccalaureate degrees was associated with a 5% decrease in 30-day mortality and in mortality after developing a complications. Estabrook and colleagues (2005) replicated these findings in Canada.

Patient Outcomes Related to Nurse Staffing

Studies of the effect of nurse staffing have used patient outcomes data from three general sources depending on the level of analysis. Patient-specific data have come from large databases derived from discharge summaries. These data are either analyzed at the individual patient level or aggregated to produce hospital-level rates or proportions of complications or adverse occurrences. Patient care unit–level data obtained directly from hospitals have used rates of adverse occurrences usually standardized per patient day of care. The third source of data has been the patients themselves, usually from surveys during hospitalization or surveys of recently discharged patients. Patient surveys have typically measured satisfaction with aspects of care, functional status, or health-related quality of life.

Historically, the quality of health care was measured with indicators of providers' activity. Health care quality measurement, in general, has been moving to patient outcomes instead (Hegyvary, 1991; Maas, Johnson & Moorhead, 1996). Determining that patient care outcomes are a direct result of an isolated nursing activity or medical activity is a difficult task, given the highly complex health care system. Although the trend in outcomes measurement is toward measures that relate to positive aspects of health, sources of positive outcome measures continue to be limited. The outcome-related measures of quality described in the literature more often include adverse occurrences than positive measures of quality (DesHarnais, McMahon, Wroblewski, & Hogan, 1990). The direct availability of adverse occurrence data from hospital administrative records continues to make these measures the easiest to access. Patient satisfaction and patient perceptions of quality are positive aspects that have been used as outcome indicators by hospitals. However, the sensitivity of these measures to detect actual differences in nursing care, as opposed to customer services activities, has been questioned (Bostrom, Tisnado, Zimmerman, & Lazar, 1994; Pierce, 1997). In addition, patient satisfaction and perception data are obtained with a wide variety of tools and are not often comparable across organizations.

Safety Indicators

In the past few years, national expert panels sponsored by AHRQ (2002) and the National Quality Forum (NQF) (2004), among others, have made recommendations to the health care community for standardized indicators of patient care quality and patient safety in relation to specific groups of consumers and specific groups of providers. As these indicators are collected in a standardized way across health care facilities, more precise and rigorous research will be possible. The nursing-sensitive quality indicators recommended by the NQF included seven patient outcomes: failure to rescue, pressure ulcers, patient falls, patient restraints, UTIs, central line infections, and ventilator-associated pneumonia. The hospital patient safety indicators recommended by AHRQ (2002) included complication of anesthesia, death in low-mortality DRGs, and decubitus ulcer; failure to rescue; foreign body left in; iatrogenic pneumothorax; infection due to medical care; postoperative hemorrhage, hip fracture, physiologic and metabolic derangements, pulmonary embolism or deep vein thrombosis, respiratory failure, sepsis, and wound dehiscence; technical difficulty; and transfusion reaction.

Medication Safety

Given the concern about medication safety, remarkably few studies have related medication administration errors to nurse staffing levels. Indicators of medication errors are central to most hospitals' quality improvement and risk management programs. Although many medication administration errors have no identified adverse consequences, they still reflect the potential for poor outcomes and have been used as indicators of the quality of nursing care in several studies. Grillo-Peck and Risner (1995) found no significant difference in medication error rates after restructuring; however, Lengacher et al. (1997) reported a significant increase with the new care delivery model, and Seago (1999) found a decrease. Blegen et al. (1998) and Blegen and Vaughn (1998) found that when the staff mix was higher (up to 85% to 87%), the medication administration error rates were lower. Medication error rates are most usefully calculated at the patient care unit level; however, the accuracy of these rates are quite suspect given the small proportion of administration errors that are reported by the staff. Patient discharge data typically include only those errors that directly caused patient injury.

There are several nationwide efforts to collect data about medication safety. Reporting to national repositories of errors made or near errors caught and the circumstances surrounding each provides a rich source of information. The U.S. Pharmacopeia collects medication error data through a national database called MEDMARX®. These data provide the basis for reports about medication safety and analysis to identify areas for which interventions could be developed (MEDMARX, 2005). The Institute for Safe Medication Practices (ISMP) (2005) operates the Medication Errors Reporting Program, a project that collects national voluntarily submitted data. Using these data, the ISMP creates reports about incidence and related factors for medication errors and near misses.

It is difficult to link these data back to the actual nurse staffing levels; but submitters often comment about staffing levels in the factors related to the error.

Patient Falls and Injuries

Prevention of patient falls is a frequently used indicator of the quality of nursing care. The rate of patient falls at the patient care unit level is usually measured using voluntary reports from staff. Kustaborder and Rigner (1983), Morse, Tylko, and Dixon (1987), and Tutuarini, de Hann, and Limburg (1993) found no relationship between patient fall rates and the number of nurses or the patient to nurse ratios. Fall rates declined with restructuring that reduced staff mix RNs (from 80%–60%) (Grillo-Peck & Risner, 1995) and with the introduction of differentiated practice (Malloch, Milton, & Jobes, 1990). However, Lengacher and colleagues (1997) reported an increase in the rate of falls with the Partners in Patient Care model; and Seago (1999) reported no significant change after the introduction of patient-focused care.

Relatively consistent results have been produced in more recent research, with higher nurse staffing levels on patient care units associated with lower fall rates (Blegen & Vaughn, 1998; Dunton, Gajewski, Taunton, & Moore, 2004; Potter et al., 2003; Sovie & Jawad, 2001). Patient injuries from falls have also been measured using patient discharge data. One recent study (Unruh, 2003) found that the hospital rates of injuries from falls were lower when the nursing hours per day were higher.

Skin Breakdown

One of the primary goals of nursing care for hospital patients with reduced mobility is the prevention of skin breakdown. More intervention studies are reported in nursing in regard to preventing pressure ulcers than preventing the other adverse outcomes. Most report success in reducing the incidence of pressure ulcers (Arikian, Kingery, Beall, & Abbott, 1990; Frye, 1986; Hunter et al., 1995; Kartes, 1996; Moody et al., 1988).

Data for skin breakdown have also been derived from several sources in studies of the effect of nurse staffing and restructuring. Studies that used occurrence reporting or quality management data derived directly from the hospitals reported that higher levels of nurse staffing were associated with lower rates of skin breakdown (Blegen, Goode, & Reed, 1998; Sovie & Jawad, 2001). Studies using skin breakdown data from patient discharge summaries produced inconsistent results, with two reporting that higher nurse staffing reduced skin breakdown (ANA, 1997; Unruh, 2003) and two showing no effect of nurse staffing on skin breakdown (Cho et al., 2003; Needleman et al., 2002).

Hospital Acquired Infections

Patient characteristics explain much of the infection incidence (Larson, Oram, & Henrick, 1988), but several studies have shown that environment and staffing factors also play an important role in the incidence of infection. Although the staffing variable has been measured many different ways in these studies, there is more standardization of outcome variables for measuring infection than other outcomes measured in hospitals. A great deal of the work linking nurse staffing levels to decreased nosocomial infections has been carried out on ICUs, with hospital data collection efforts providing the specific infection rates. These include studies of specific organisms, such as methicillin-resistant staphylococcus aureas (Farrington, Trundle, Redpath, & Anderson, 2000; Grundmann, Hori, Winter, Tami, & Austin, 2002; Haley & Bergman, 1982; Vicca, 1999), enterobacter cloacae (Harbarth Sudre, Sharan, Cadenas, & Pittet, 1999), and gram negative organisms (Isaacs, Catterson, Hope, Moxon, &Wilkinson, 1988). This work has also addressed the beneficial effects from nurse staffing on specific routes such as blood stream infections (Fridkin Pear, Williamson, Galgianai & Jarvis, 1996; Robert et al., 2000).

There are also a significant number of studies that relate nurse staffing to less-specific hospital infection rates from patient discharge data or hospital quality data. These include respiratory infections and UTIs (Amaravadi et al., 2000; Cho, 2003; Kovner & Gergen, 1998; Kovner et al., 2001; Needleman et al., 2002; Sovie & Jawad, 2001; Unruh, 2003). Overall infection rates were shown to be higher when units were short-staffed (Behner et al., 1990; Flood & Diers, 1988), and when skill mix was lower (ANA, 1997; Blegen et al., 1998). In contrast, Grillo-Peck and Risner (1995) reported lower rates of infections when nursing staff were restructured and the staff mix changed from 80% to 60% RNs.

Mortality Rates/Failure to Rescue

Mortality rates at the hospital level, adjusted for expected mortality given patient characteristics, have been used in multiple outcomes studies during the past two decades. Nurse staffing levels have been linked to lower mortality rates in numerous studies (Aiken, Clark, et al., 2003; Aiken, Smith, et al., 1994; Estabrook et al., 2005; Person et al., 2004; Pronovost et al., 1999; Tourangeau et al., 2002); while others have not found the linkage to be statistically significant (Needleman et al., 2002). While recognizing the importance of nursing care to patient outcomes, living or dying may not be the most sensitive outcome from nursing care. More recently, failure to rescue (mortality rates following the development of complications) has been used along with the overall mortality rate. One of the main roles played by nurses in hospitals is to monitor patients for their responses to treatments and to detect complications early. Therefore, death following a complication may be a more sensitive indicator of nursing care. Studies have included this variable and found that higher nurse staffing levels were associated with a lower failure to rescue rate (Aiken et al., 2003; Needleman et al., 2002).

Several patient outcome indicators have been linked to nurse staffing levels. As indicated in Tables 5.1 and 5.2 and in the reviews by Lang et al. (2004) and Blegen (2004), however, there are many studies that have found nonsignificant results for this same set of indicators. The crucial question is whether these inconsistencies are due only to problems with data and level of measurement or whether there are true differences in the influence of nurse staffing on patient safety.

FUTURE RESEARCH NEEDED

The research reported since 1996, when the IOM concluded that we knew little about the relationship between nurse staffing and the quality of care, has contributed greatly to our knowledge in this area. Unfortunately, researchers have continued to find inconsistent results. A rigorous review of this literature (Lang et al., 2004) concluded that "the literature offers no support for specific nurse-patient ratios" (p. 9). Further, these investigators suggest that there is limited support for the relationship between nurse staffing and mortality rates, failure to rescue rates, and shorter hospital stays. And there is little to no support for relationships between nurse staffing and pneumonia, UTIs, pressure ulcers, falls, and nosocomial infections. Blegen's review (2004) suggested stronger, though still inconsistent, support for the effect of nurse staffing on pneumonia, failure to rescue, UTIs, pressure ulcers, and falls.

Overall, knowledge has grown. There remain some areas about which we know little. Hospital studies have examined all units together and therefore tell us little about the staffing levels on different kinds of units (e.g., medical, surgical, intensive care). Most of the unit-level studies have looked only at medical and surgical units, or only ICUs and often studied only a limited number of units, making it difficult to produce recommendations to guide nursing administrators.

In 2003, the IOM published another set of recommendations regarding patient safety in relation to nursing care. In this they acknowledge the strides that have been made and noted in particular the need for more accurate and reliable staffing data and the need for more research on specific types of patient care units (p. 9). Not mentioned in the IOM report, but equally important, is the need for a standardized way to adjust for the acuity of the patients being cared for on the specific types of units. At this point, there is no accepted way to account for patient risk related to nursing-sensitive outcomes.

There is reasonable agreement regarding the best measure of nurse staffing (hppd). Unfortunately, these data are only available at the patient care unit level, requiring time-consuming primary data collection. The time RNs spend caring for patients should be separated from the time used for education, administration, or other support functions. In order to capture a complete picture of patient care, the hours of patient care from LPNs and NAs must also be captured at the patient care unit level and included in data sets. Finally, there is little agreement about reliably measuring nurse competency. Competency may be partially accessed using education, experience, and certification; however, these data are also not reliably measured or readily available.

CONCLUSION

Research linking nurse staffing to the quality of patient care has increased markedly since the 1996 IOM report on nursing staff (Wunderlich et al., 1996). However, the results of these recent research projects do not yet provide a thorough and consistent foundation for producing solutions to the crisis (Blegen, 2004; Heinz, 2004; Lang et al., 2004; Seago, 2001). These inconsistencies are largely due to differing units of analysis (hospital, patient, care unit), the variability in measures of nurse staffing, the variety of quality indicators chosen, the difficulty in finding accurate measures of these indicators, and the difficulty in creating risk-adjustment strategies for the indicators most sensitive to nursing care.

Conducting the research needed to bring clarity to the state of the science regarding nurse staffing and patient safety requires a national effort to produce standardized data sets of patient outcomes and nurse staffing information at the patient care unit level. The data on nurse staffing must include all providers of nursing care (RN, LPN, CNA) and must separate direct caregiver hours from support hours. The data on patient safety must include indicators sensitive to nursing care and adjusted for patient risk.

REFERENCES

Abdellah, F. G. & Levine, E. (1958). Effect of nursing staffing on satisfaction with nursing care. *Hospital Monograph Series*, No. 4.

Agency for Healthcare Research and Quality. (2002). *Measures of patient safety based on hospital administrative data—the patient Safety indicators*. Technical Review 5, Agency for Healthcare Research and Quality Publication No. 02-0038.

Aiken, L. H. (2005). The unfinished patient safety agenda. Agency for Healthcare Research and Quality WebM&M. Retrieved August 2005 from http://webmm.ahrq.gov/perspective.aspx

Aiken, L. H., Clarke, S. P., Sloane, D. M., Sochalski, J., & Silber, J. (2002). Hospital nurse staffing and patient mortality, nurse burnout and job dissatisfaction. *Journal of the American Medical Association*, 288(16), 1987–1993.

Aiken, L. H., Clarke, S. P., Cheung, R., Sloane, D., & Silber, J. (2003). Educational levels of hospital nurses and surgical patient mortality. *Journal of the American Medical Association, 290*(12), 1617–1623.

Aiken, L., Smith, H., & Lake, E. T. (1994). Lower medicare mortality among a set of hospital known for good nursing care. *Medical Care, 32*(8), 771–787.

Amaravadi, R. K., Dimick, J. B., Pronovost. P. J., & Lipsett, P. A. (2000). ICU nurse-to-patient ratio is associated with complications and resource use after esophagectomy. *Intensive Care Medicine, 26*, 1857–1862.

American Nurses Association. (1997). *Implementing Nursings' Report Card: A study of RN staffing, length of stay and patient outcomes.* Washington, DC: American Nurses Publishing.

Arikian, V., Kingery, C., Beall, K., & Abbott, R. (1990). Education and QA: A model for continuous improvement in skin integrity. *Journal of Nursing Quality Assurance, 5*(1), 1–7.

Aydelotte, M. K. & Tener, M. E. (1960). *An investigation of the relation between nursing activity and patient welfare.* Ames, IA: The State University of Iowa.

Behner, K. G., Fogg, L., Frankenbach, J. & Robertson, S. (1990). Nursing resource management: Analyzing the relationship between costs and quality in staffing decisions. *Health Care Management Review, 15*(4), 63–71.

Bernreuter, M. E. & Cardona, S. (1997). Survey and critique of studies related to unlicensed assistive personnel from 1975 to 1998, Part II. *Journal of Nursing Administration, 27*(7/8), 49–55.

Blegen, M. A. (2004, October). Nurse staffing relationships with patient care quality and safety. Paper presented at the National Congress on the State of the Science in Nursing Research, Washington, DC.

Blegen, M. A., Goode, C. J., & Reed, L. (1998). Nurse staffing and patient outcomes. *Nursing Research, 47*(1), 43–50.

Blegen, M. A., & Vaughn, T. (1998). A multisite study of nurse staffing and patient outcomes. *Nursing Economics, 16*(4), 196–203.

Blegen, M. A., Vaughn, T. E., & Goode C. J. (2001). Nurse experience and education: Effect on quality of care. *Journal of Nursing Administration, 31*(1), 33–39.

Bostrom, J. & Zimmerman, J. (1993). Restructuring nursing for a competitive health care environment. *Nursing Economics, 11*(1), 35–41, 54.

Bostrom, J., Tisnado, J., Zimmerman, J., & Lazar, N. (1994). The impact of continuity of nursing care personnel on patient satisfaction. *Journal of Nursing Administration, 24*(10), 64–68.

Budreau, G., Balakrishnan, R., Titler, M., & Hafner, M. (1999). Caregiver-patient ratio: Capturing census and staffing variability. *Nursing Economics, 17*(6), 317–324.

Cho, S. H., Ketefian, S., Barkauskas, V., & Smith, D. (2003). The effects of nurse staffing on adverse events, morbidity, mortality, and medical costs. *Nursing Research, 52*(2), 71–79.

Dang, D., Johantgen, M., Pronovost, P., Jenckes, M., & Bass, E. (2002). Postoperative complications: Does intensive care unit staff nursing make a difference? *Heart and Lung, 31*(3), 219–228.

DesHarnais, S., McMahon, L. F., Wroblewski, R. T., & Hogan, A. J. (1990). Measuring hospital performance. *Medical Care, 28*(12), 1127–1141.

Dimick, J. B., Swoboda, S. M., Pronovost. P. J., & Lipsett, P. A. (2001). Effect of nurse-to-patient ratio in the intensive care unit on pulmonary complications and resource use after hepatectomy. *American Journal of Critical Care*, 40(6), 376–382.

Dunton, N., Gajewski, B., Taunton, R., & Moore, J. (2004). Nurse staffing and patient falls on acute care hospital units. *Nursing Outlook*, 52(1), 53–59.

Estabrooks, C. A., Midodzi, W. K., Cummings, G., Ricker, K. L., & Giovannetti, P. (2005). The impact of hospital nursing characteristics on 30-day mortality. *Nursing Research*, 54(2), 74–84.

Farrington, M., Trundle, C., Redpath, C., & Anderson, L. (2000). Effects on nursing workload of different methicillin-resistant Staphylococcus aureus (MRSA) control strategies. *Journal of Hospital Infection*, 46, 118–123.

Flood, S. D., & Diers, D. (1988). Nurse staffing, patient outcome and cost. *Nursing Management*, 19(5), 34–43.

Fridkin S. K., Pear, S. M., Williamson, T. H., Galgianai, J. N., & Jarvis, W. R. (1996). The role of understaffing in central venous catheter-associated bloodstream infections. *Infection Control and Hospital Epidemiology*, 17, 150–158.

Frye, B. (1986). A cost of many colors: A program to reduce the incidence of hospital-originated pressure sores. *Rehabilitation Nursing*, 11(1), 24–25.

Gardner, K. (1991). A summary of findings of a five-year comparison study of primary and team nursing. *Nursing Research*, 40(2), 113–117.

Goode, C. J., Pinkerton, S. E., McCausland, M., Southard, P., Graham, R., & Krsek, C. (2001). Documenting chief nursing officers' preference for BSN-prepared nurses. *Journal of Nursing Administration*, 31, 55–59.

Grillo-Peck, A. M. & Risner, P. B. (1995). The effect of a partnership model on quality and length of stay. *Nursing Economics*, 13(6), 367–374.

Grundmann, J., Hori, S., Winter, B., Tami, A., & Austin, D. (2002). Risk factors for the transmission of methicillin-resistant staphylococcus aureus in an adult intensive care unit: Fitting a model to the data. *The Journal of Infectious Diseases*, 185, 481–488.

Haley, R. & Bergman, D. (1982). The role of understaffing and overcrowding in recurrent outbreaks of staphylococcal infection in a neonatal special-care unit. *The Journal of Infectious Diseases*, 145, 875–885.

Hall, L. M., Doran, D., Baker, G. R., Pink, G, Sidani S., O'Brien-Pallas, L., et al. (2003). Nurse staffing models as predictors of patient outcomes. *Medical Care*, 41(9), 1096–1109.

Hall, L. M. (1997). Staff mix models: Complementary or substitution roles for nurses. *Nursing Administration Quarterly*, 21(2), 31–39.

Harbarth, S., Sudre, P., Sharan, S., Cadenas, M., & Pittet, D. (1999). Outbreak of enterobacter cloacae related to understaffing, overcrowding, and poor hygiene practices. *Infection Control and Hospital Epidemiology*, 20, 598–603.

Hegyvary, S. T. (1991). Issues in outcomes research. *Journal of Nursing Quality Assurance*, 5(2), 1–6.

Heinz, D. (2004). Hospital nurse staffing and patient outcomes. *Dimensions of Critical Care Nursing*, 23(1), 44–50.

Hinshaw, A. S., Scofield, R., & Atwood, J. R. (1981, November/December). Staff, patient, and cost outcomes of all-registered nurse staffing. *Journal of Nursing Administration*, 11, 30–36.

Hunter, S., Langemo, D., Olson, B., Hanson, D., Cathcart-Silververg. T., Burd, C., et al. (1995). The effectiveness of skin care protocols for pressure ulcers. *Rehabilitation Nursing, 20,* 250–255.

Huston, C. L. (1996). Unlicensed assistive personnel: A solution to dwindling health care resources or the precursor to the apocalypse of Registered Nursing. *Nursing Outlook, 44,* 67–73.

Institute of Medicine. (2003). *Keeping patients safe: Transforming the work environment of nurses.* Washington, DC: National Academy Press.

Institute for Safe Medication Practices. (2005). U.S. Pharmacopeia Institute for Safe Medication Practices Medication Errors Reporting Program . Retrieved October, 2005, from www.ismp.org

Isaacs, D., Catterson, J., Hope, P. L., Moxon, E. R., & Wilkinson, A. R. (1988). Factors influencing colonisation with gentamicin resistant gram negative organisms in the neonatal unit. *Archives of Disease in Childhood, 63,* 533–535.

Jones, K. R. (1993). Outcomes analysis: Methods and issues. *Nursing Economics, 11*(3), 145–152.

Kartes, S. K. (1996). A team approach for risk assessment, prevention, and treatment of pressure ulcers in nursing home patients. *Journal of Nursing Care Quality, 10*(3), 34–45.

Kovner, C. & Gergen, P. J. (1998). Nurse staffing levels and adverse events following surgery in U.S. hospitals. *Image: Journal of Nursing Scholarship, 30*(4), 315–321.

Kovner, C., Jones, C., Zhan, C., Gergen, P., & Basu, J. (2002). Nurse staffing and postsurgical adverse events: An analysis of administrative data from a sample of U.S. hospitals, 1990–1996. *Health Services Research, 37,* 611–629.

Krapohl, G. L., & Larson, E. (1996). The impact of unlicensed assistive personnel on nursing care delivery. *Nursing Economics, 14*(2), 99–110.

Kustaborder, M., & Rigner, M. (1983). Interventions for safety. *Journal of Gerontological Nursing, 9*(3), 159–162, 173, 182.

Lang, T., Hodge, M., Olson, V., Romano, P., & Kravitz, R. (2004). Nurse-patient ratios: A systematic review of the effects of nurse staffing on patients, nurse employee, and hospital outcomes. *Journal of Nursing Administration, 34,* 326–337.

Larson, E., Oram, L. F., & Hedrick, E. (1988). Nosocomial infection rates as an indicator of quality. *Medical Care, 26*(7), 676–684.

Lengacher, D. A., Mabe, P. R., Heinemann, D., VanCott, M. L., Swymer, S., & Kent, K. (1996). Effects of the PIPC model on outcome measures of productivity and costs. *Nursing Economics, 14*(4), 205–213.

Lengacher, D. A., Mabe, P. R., Heinemann, D., VanCott, M. L., Kent, K., & Swymer, S. (1997). Collaboration in research: Testing the PIPC model on clinical and nonclinical outcomes. *Nursing Connections, 10*(1), 17–30.

Lichtig, L. K., Knauf, R. A., & Milholland, D. K. (1999). Some impacts of nursing on acute care hospital outcomes. *Journal of Nursing Administration, 29,* 25–33.

Maas, M., Johnson, M., & Moorhead, S. (1996) Classifying nursing-sensitive patient outcomes. *IMAGE: Journal of Nursing Scholarship, 28*(4), 295–301.

Malloch, K. M., Milton, D. A., & Jobes, M. O. (1990). A model for differentiated nursing practice. *Journal of Nursing Administration, 20*(2), 20.

Mark B. A., Salyer, J., & Wan, T. (2003). Professional nursing practice: Impact on organizational and patient outcomes. *Journal of Nursing Administration, 33*(4), 224–234.

MEDMARX®. (2005). U.S. Pharmacopeia. Retrieved October 2005 from www.usp.org

Moody, B., Fanale, J., Thompson, M., Vaillancourt, D., Symonds, G., & Bonasoro, C. (1988). Impact of staff education on pressure sore development in elderly hospitalized patients. *Archives of Internal Medicine, 148*, 2241–2243.

Morse, J., Tylko, S., & Dixon, H. (1987). Characteristics of the fall-prone patient. *The Gerontologist, 27*(4), 516–522.

National Quality forum. (2004). *National voluntary consensus standards for nursing-sensitive performance measures: An initial performance measure set.* National Quality Forum, Washington, DC.

Needleman, J., Buerhaus, P., Mattke, S., Stewart, M., & Zelevinsky, K. (2002). Nurse-staffing levels and the quality of care in hospitals. *New England Journal of Medicine, 346*(22), 1715–1722.

Neidlinger, S., Bostrom, J., Stricker, A., Hild, J., & Zhang, J. (1993). Incorporating nursing assistive personnel into a nursing professional practice model. *Journal of Nursing Administration, 23*(3), 29–37.

Person, S. D., Allison, J. J., Kiefe, C. I., Weaver, M. T., Williams, O. D., Centor, R. M., et al. (2004). Nurse staffing and mortality for medicare patients with acute myocardial infarction. *Medical Care, 42*, 4–12.

Pierce, S. (1997). Nurse sensitive healthcare outcomes in acute care settings: An integrative analysis of the literature. *Journal of Nursing Care Quality, 11*(4), 60–72.

Potter, P., Barr, N., McSweeney, M., & Sledge, J. (2003). Identifying nurse staffing and patient outcomes relationships: A guide for change in care delivery. *Nursing Economics, 21*(4), 158–166.

Prescott, P. (1993). Nursing: An important component of hospital survival under a reformed health care system. *Nursing Economics, 11*(4), 192–198.

Pronovost, P. J., Dimick, J. B., Swoboda, S. M., & Lipsett, P. A. (2001). Effect of nurse-to-patient ratio in the intensive care unit on pulmonary complications and resource use after hepatectomy. *American Journal of Critical Care, 40*(6), 376–382.

Pronovost, P. J., Jenckes, M., Dorman, T., Garrett, E., Breslow, M., Rosenfeld, B., et al. (1999). Organizational characteristics of intensive care units related to outcomes of abdominal aortic surgery. *Journal of the American Medical Association, 281*(14), 1310–1317.

Robert, J., Fridkin, S. K., Blumberg, H. M., Anderson, B., White, N., Ray, S. M., et al. (2000). The influence of the composition of the nursing staff on primary blood stream infections rates in a surgical intensive care unit. *Infection control and Hospital Epidemiology, 21*, 12–17.

Rogers, A. E., Hwang, W. T., Scott, L. D., Aiken, L. H., & Dinges, D. F. (2004). The working hours of hospital staff nurses and patient safety. *Health Affairs, 23*, 202–212.

Safford, B. J. & Schlotfeldt, R. M. (1960). Nursing service staffing and quality of nursing care. *Nursing Research, 9*(3), 149–154.

Seago, J. A. (1999). Evaluation of a hospital work redesign. *Journal of Nursing Administration, 29*(11), 31–38.

Seago, J. A. (2001). Nurse staffing, models of care delivery, and interventions. Chapter 39 in Shojania et al. (Eds.), *Making health care safer: A critical analysis of patient safety practices* (pp. 427–450). Rockville, MD: Agency for Healthcare Research and Quality.

Sovie, M. D. & Jawad, A. F. (2001). Hospital restructuring and its impact on outcomes. *Journal of Nursing Administration, 31*(12), 588–600.

Tourangeau, A. E., Giovannetti, P., Tu, J. V., & Wood, M. (2002). Nursing-related determinants of 30 day mortality for hospitalized patients. *Canadian Journal of Nursing Research, 33*(4), 71–88.

Tutuarini, J., de Haan, R., & Limburg, M. (1993). Number of nursing staff and falls: A case-control study on falls by stroke patients in acute-care settings. *Journal of Advanced Nursing, 18,* 1101–1105.

Unruh, L. (2003). Licensed nurse staffing and adverse events in hospitals. *Medical Care, 41,* 142–152.

Verran, J. A. (1996) Quality of care, organizational variables, and nursing staffing. In Wunderlich, G., Sloan, F., & Davis, C. (Eds.), *Nursing Staff in Hospitals and Nursing Homes* (pp. 308–332). Washington, DC: National Academy Press.

Vicca, A. F. (1999). Nursing staff workload as a determinant of methicillin-resistant Staphylococcus aureus spread in an adult intensive therapy unit. *Journal of Hospital Infection, 43,* 109–113.

Wachter, R. (2005). In conversation with Barbara A. Blakeney, MS,RN. AHRQ WebM&M. http://webmm.ahrq.gov/perspective.aspx accessed August, 2005.

Wunderlich, G. S., Sloan, F. A., & Davis, C. K. (Eds.). (1996). *Nursing staff in hospitals and nursing homes*. Washington, DC: Institute of Medicine National Academy Press.

Chapter 6

Medication Safety Within the Perioperative Environment

Linda J. Wanzer* and Rodney W. Hicks

ABSTRACT

With the widespread patient safety movement comes an increased public awareness of the risks inherent within the health care setting. More specifically, the highly publicized medication error cases that hit the media demonstrate the effect mediation errors have on patient safety within the perioperative environment. This awareness, however, has triggered limited research across the continuum of care within this complex environment. A current review of the state of the science related to medication safety within this setting reveals research primarily focused on the anesthesia domain of practice. Although application to the perioperative environment can be extrapolated from this research, there is a notable lack of nursing-initiated research that focuses on improved systems or processes related to medication safety within the perioperative continuum of care. This knowledge gap in the literature presents an excellent opportunity for

---

* The views expressed are those of the author and do not reflect the official policy or position of the Uniformed Services University of the Health Sciences, the Department of Defense, or the United States government.

nursing to grow a research program to improve medication safety within the perioperative environment in support of evidence-based practice.

Keywords: patient safety, nursing, medication, perioperative

The United States has the world's most technologically advanced health care delivery system, and it includes a highly dedicated and skilled work force, a wide range of pharmacological agents, and state-of-the-art facilities that provide perioperative services (Gabel & Fitzner, 2003). These desirable attributes have helped transform care of the surgical patient over the past several decades. The United States also has the world's most expensive health care delivery system (Anderson, Hussey, Frogner, & Waters, 2005). And although it has the capacity to produce the finest health care services in the world, failures in the delivery system have been widely reported and the failures occur with some regularity (Becher & Chassin, 2001). Medical errors, including medication errors, represent one such failure that injures patients, erodes public confidence, and increases health care costs (Bates et al., 1997; Kohn, Corrigan, & Donaldson, 2000). Medication errors have also been associated with increases in morbidity and mortality (Fortescue et al., 2003; Kaushal, Jaggi, Walsh, Fortescue, & Bates, 2004; Kohn et al., 2000). Simply put, medication errors strike at the heart of the health care system—the responsibility to do good and avoid harm (Mayo & Duncan, 2004).

BACKGROUND

In 1859, Florence Nightingale emphasized the importance of the medical tenet in *Notes on Nursing* when she wrote, "It may seem a strange principle to enunciate as the first requirement in a hospital that it should do the sick no harm" (Nightingale, 1859/1970). This tenet is a part of our medical culture, for we are the patient's advocate. It is now clear that an institution that professes as its primary creed to "first and foremost, do no harm," actually becomes an instrument of death.

In 1999, the Institute of Medicine's (IOM) report *To Err Is Human: Building a Safer Health System* catapulted patient safety to national attention. The IOM asserted that the U.S. health care system could annually expect as many as 98,000 individuals to become the victims of fatal medical errors, a number that exceeds the combined annual deaths from motor vehicle accidents, HIV/AIDS, and breast cancer (Kohn et al., 2000). Iatrogenic injuries became the eighth leading cause of death in America, and it is estimated that as many as 7,000 of these deaths were from medication errors (Kohn et al.). This IOM report emphasized that "People working in health care are among the most educated and dedicated work force in any industry. The problem is not bad people; the problem is that the system needs to be safer" (Kohn et al., p. 49). The report further explored the human element of mistakes, identifying that mistakes will continue to happen unintentionally until road blocks to prevent their occurrence are erected (Kohn et al.). Because of the report, health care providers, payers, and policymakers are now more aware of the effect that human error and process weaknesses have within the world's most complex health care system.

In July 2004, Health Grades, Inc., released a study that suggested the IOM report may have underestimated the number of deaths by half, and a truer number of medical error deaths is closer to 198,000 deaths each year (Health Grades, Inc., 2004). These errors know no boundaries, for they occur at epidemic rates across the health care system and within all clinical areas (Health Grades, Inc., 2004, 2005; Zhan & Miller, 2003), including the perioperative continuum.

The IOM challenged professional organizations to set performance standards and expectations for patient safety (Kohn et al., 2000). Health care organizations received notice to "incorporate well-understood safety principles" and implement patient safety programs that were "strong, clear, and visible" (Kohn et al., p. 14). The report also advanced the previously underdeveloped discipline of patient safety by challenging existing practices, contributing to the development of new theories, spurring additional scientific inquiries, increasing significant funding opportunities, and identifying national targets for error reduction. The IOM also called for participation in voluntary event-reporting programs.

The United States Pharmacopeia (USP) has more than three decades of experience in event-reporting programs. USP is a nongovernmental, nonprofit standards-setting organization that has advanced public health since it's founding in 1820. USP, through expert committee consensus, develops legally enforceable standards that address the strength, purity, and quality of pharmaceutical products (Santell, 2005). It operates two national medication error databases: the Medication Errors Reporting (MER) Programs and MEDMARX®. MER is a voluntary program open to all clinicians in all settings. This database, which is operated in cooperation with the Institute for Safe Medication Practices, collects information and provides data to regulatory agencies, professional organizations, and the pharmaceutical industry in an effort to educate others about adverse drug events and their prevention (Santell).

MEDMARX, launched in 1998, is an Internet-accessible, anonymous, subscription-based, medication error database used by hospitals and health systems as part of their ongoing quality improvements efforts and is aimed at safe medication use. MEDMARX offers participants an opportunity to review errors reported by other facilities and to learn from their mistakes, in hopes of preventing future similar occurrences (Santell, 2005). Although slightly more than 5% of U.S. facilities (approximately 850) participate in MEDMARX, the program has amassed the largest repository of medication error data currently available in the

TABLE 6.1   MEDMARX Reports by Calendar Year, 1999–2004

Year	Number of reports	Number of facilities
1999	6,224	56
2000	41,296	164
2001	105,603	368
2002	192,477	482
2003	235,159	570
2004	248,733	616

Source: Hicks, R. W., Santell, J. P., Cousins, D. D., and Williams, R. L. (2004); Santell, J. P., Hicks, R. W., & Cousins, D. D. (2005)

world and now has more than 800,000 case reports (Table 6.1). The MEDMARX program only consists of reported errors; the actual number of medication errors is an unknown figure, and there is general believe that such events are vastly under-reported.

Researchers have studied the relationship of actual errors versus reported errors. In a landmark study, researchers extrapolated a ratio of slightly more than 1,400 actual errors for every reported event (Flynn, n.d.). In a more recent study, the errors detected to errors reported ratio was 300 to 1 (Flynn, Barker, Pepper, Bates, & Mikeal, 2002), indicating that the majority of errors go undetected. Estimates suggest that medication errors occur at an astounding rate.

Purpose

The purpose of this paper is to review selected studies related to medication errors originating in the perioperative environment, which was defined as same day surgery, pre-operative holding area, operating room (including anesthesia), and postanesthesia care unit (PACU).

Methods

A literature review was conducted using the Cumulative Index to Nursing and Allied Health Literature and PubMED databases. Key search words/medical subject headings were *medication errors, perioperative care, perioperative nursing, anesthesia, surgery, ambulatory surgery, outpatient surgery, same day surgery, postanesthesia care unit, medication systems, drug administration, and operating rooms.* Initially, there were 257 citations, abstracts, and articles identified related to medication errors from the perioperative setting for further review with no date limitations. The final review excluded newsletters, articles describing case studies, editorials, and

TABLE 6.2   NCC MERP Taxonomy of Medication Errors

Taxonomy elements
Patient information
Setting
Event
Patient outcome
Product information
Personnel involved
Types
Causes
Contributing factors

Source: National Coordinating Council for Medication Error Reporting and Prevention, 1988–2001 (www.nccmerp.org)

medication errors occurring outside the perioperative environment. The eligible articles were further examined using the National Coordinating Council for Medication Error Reporting and Prevention's (NCC MERP's) Taxonomy for Medication Errors (National Coordinating Council for Medication Error Reporting and Prevention [NCC MERP], 1998–2001). The NCC MERP taxonomy spans 10 major elements that are useful for recording and tracking medication errors (Table 6.2). The taxonomy also provides standard language and structure useful in analyzing medication error summaries (NCC MERP). For purposes of this review, the analysis was organized into major themes utilizing the NCC MERP taxonomy elements: patient outcome, products, types of errors, causes of errors, contributing factors, and personnel involved. To complete the review process, three other variables (themes) were examined that were not present in the NCC MERP taxonomy: the medication use process (MUP), error reduction strategies, and level of care rendered as a result of the error.

Findings

Table 6.3 identifies the articles that were audited. As an emerging program of research, medication safety within the perioperative environment is in the early stages of development. Current research within this environment suggests a national focus is coalescing; however, even in the early phases, the nursing profession has conducted only limited research. The early stages of this new science are taking the form of systematic reviews of the literature, descriptive/prospective studies, secondary data analysis, and randomized clinical evaluations to enhance patient safety within the perioperative environment.

TABLE 6.3   Studies Reporting Perioperative Errors

Author (year)	Setting	Design	Sample
Abeysekera et al. (2005)	Anesthesia	Descriptive	$n = 896$
Beyea et al. (2003a)	Same day surgery	Descriptive	$n = 610$
Beyea et al. (2003b)	Operating room	Descriptive	$n = 731$
Currie et al. (1993)	Anesthesia	Descriptive	$n = 144$
Fasting et al. (2000)	Anesthesia	Prospective design with intervention	$n = 55,426$
Hicks et al. (2004)	Postanesthesia care unit	Descriptive	$n = 645$
Jenson et al. (2004)	Anesthesia	Review article	$n = 98$
Khan et al. (2005)	Anesthesia	Descriptive	$n = 768$
Liu et al. (2003)	Anesthesia	Survey	$n = 116$
Orser et al. (2004)	Anesthesia	Secondary analysis	$n = 232$
Webster et al. (2004)	Anesthesia	Randomized clinical evaluation	$n = 15$
Wheeler et al. (2005)	Anesthesia	Review article	$n = 221$

The literature revealed inconsistencies regarding the definition of a medication error. An early definition stated that a medication error is an act of variance from the physician's original order (Flynn, n.d.). Another definition is an error in the prescription, dispensing, or administration of a medication with the result that the patient fails to receive the correct drug or the indicated proper drug dosage (Wheeler & Wheeler, 2005). One of the most widely recognized definitions of a medication error was developed by the NCC MERP. NCC MERP is an independent group composed of 22 national organizations, including the American Hospital Association, American Medical Association, American Society of Health-System Pharmacists (ASHP), American Nurses Association, the Food and Drug Administration, the Joint Commission on Accreditation of Healthcare Organizations (JCAHO), the National Patient Safety Foundation, the Veterans Administration, the Department of Defense, and the USP. NCC MERP's definition of a medication error is

> . . . *any preventable event that may cause or lead to inappropriate medication use or patient harm while the medication is in the control of the health care professional, patient, or consumer. Such events may be related to professional practice, health care products, procedures, and systems, including prescribing; order communication; product labeling, packaging, nomenclature; compounding; dispensing; distribution; administration; education; monitoring; and use* (NCC MERP 1998–2001).

Patient Outcome

Measures for patient outcome varied between the studies. A common measure of patient outcome, established by the NCC MERP's *Index of Categorizing Medication Errors* (Table 6.4), was present in three of the studies. Two studies used descriptive terminology to indicate patient outcome, while the remaining seven studies did not sufficiently address patient outcomes as a result of the medication error (Table 6.5).

For medication errors originating on the day surgery setting, a descriptive study conducted by researchers reviewed 610 medication error records from 166 facilities and concluded that 3.9% were harmful errors, based on the NCC MERP *Index of Categorizing Medication Errors* (Beyea, Hicks, & Becker, 2003a). In a secondary analysis of medication errors in the operating room, researchers examined 731 reported medication errors from 189 facilities and concluded that 10% were harmful (Beyea, Hicks, & Becker, 2003b). For medication errors originating in the PACU, researchers reviewed 645 error reports from 189 facilities and found 6.9% were harmful (Hicks, Becker, Krenzischeck, & Beyea, 2004).

One Australian study included a review of 896 anaesthesia reports (Abeysekera, Bergman, Kluger, & Short, 2005). The researchers reported 73.5% of the errors as not having any untoward outcome, and 0.3% were unspecified. The remaining outcomes consisted of anaesthesia awareness (4.4%), death (0.3%), minor morbidity (11.7%), major morbidity (4.7%), and prolonged hospitalization (5%).

Researchers in Norway conducted a prospective, direct observational study over a period of 36 months and documented 55,426 anesthetic procedures from which drug errors were assessed. The results of the study revealed 63 drug errors, ranging from moderately severe to serious, of which 30 (0.05%) resulted in some form of harm (Fasting & Gisvold, 2000).

Products

Eight of the 12 medication error studies included discussions about the products involved in the error (Table 6.6). Some studies provided detailed information pertaining to the number of unique products involved (Beyea et al., 2003a, 2003b; Fasting & Gisvold, 2000; Hicks, Becker et al., 2004), while others recorded therapeutic classification (Abeysekera et al., 2005; Currie et al., 1993; Fasting & Gisvold, 2000; Khan & Hoda, 2005; Wheeler & Wheeler, 2005).

The anesthesia articles identified neuromuscular blocking agents, vasopressors, inhalational agents, and reversal agents as being involved in the errors. Common to all perioperative areas were antimicrobial agents, intravenous solutions, opioid analgesia and other analgesia agents. Anti-coagulant errors occurred both in the operating room and in the PACU. Ophthalmic preparations were limited to same day surgery.

TABLE 6.4 NCC MERP Index of Categorizing Medication Errors

Category B: An error occurred but the error did not reach the patient	**Category A:** Circumstances or events that have the capacity to cause error	
	Category C: An error occurred that reached the patient but did not cause patient harm	**Category D:** An error occurred that reached the patient and required monitoring to confirm that it resulted in no harm to the patient and/or required intervention to preclude harm
Category E: An error occurred that may have contributed to or resulted in temporary harm to the patient and required intervention	**Category F:** An error occurred that may have contributed to or resulted in temporary harm to the patient and required initial or prolonged hospitalization	**Category G:** An error occurred that may have contributed to or resulted in permanent patient harm
	Category I: An error occurred that may have contributed to or resulted in the patient's death	**Category H:** An error occurred that required intervention necessary to sustain life

Category A: No error (e.g., two patients with the same last name)
Category B–D: Error, no harm (e.g., giving a medication late or medication omitted)
Category E–H: Error, harm (e.g., resuscitation or defibrillation to sustain life)
Category I: Error, death

Source: National Coordinating Council for Medication Error Reporting and Prevention, 1998–2001 (www.nccmerp.org)

TABLE 6.5   Studies Reporting Patient Outcome

Author (year)	Setting	Major findings
Beyea et al. (2003a)	Same day surgery	3.9% harmful[1]
Beyea et al. (2003b)	Operating room	10% harmful[1]
Hicks et al. (2004)	Postanesthesia care unit	6.9% harmful[1]
Abeysekera et al. (2005)	Anesthesia	26.1% harmful[2]
Fasting et al. (2000)	Anesthesia	0.05% harmful[3]

[1] Based on National Coordinating Council for Medication Error Reporting and Prevention
[2] Based on Australian Incident Monitoring Study and included minor morbidity, majority morbidity, death, unplanned high dependency care, prolonged stay, awareness
[3] Used classifications as serious and moderate severity

Types of Error

The type of medication error is a textual expression of the event—that is to say, how does the error manifest itself regardless of cause. Using the NCC MERP taxonomy element, *Type*, 8 of the 12 articles provided sufficient information to describe the error's effect. Omission errors (not the giving the medication) were common in each of the clinical areas (Table 6.7), as was improper dose/quantity (i.e., wrong amount) and wrong drug errors. Wrong drug errors, especially those involving anesthesia, were the result of syringe swaps or labeling errors (Abeysekera et al., 2005; Fasting & Gisvold, 2000; Khan & Hoda, 2005). Other types of errors consistent with NCC MERP taxonomy include wrong time, wrong patient, extra dose, wrong route, wrong dosage form, prescribing errors, and wrong administration technique. Errors reported, but not covered by the NCC MERP taxonomy, include drug not effective, miscellaneous, and drug in inappropriate location (Khan & Hoda).

Causes of Error

The why and how behind a medication error's occurrence is the cause of the event and represents proximal risk conditions that precipitate the error. Multiple frameworks exist for evaluating causes of errors. One of the prevailing approaches, the human factors model, is an applied science that acknowledges the universal nature of human fallibility by evaluating strengths and weakness and then compensating for the limitations (Schneider, 2002). This approach identifies and separates active human error from latent or systems-related error and, thus, becomes an effective means to design tools, systems, or tasks to reduce risk or minimize the occurrence of error.

TABLE 6.6   Studies Reporting Product Information

Author (year)	Setting	Major findings
Abeysekera et al. (2005)	Anesthesia	*Product Classification* -benzodiazepines -local anesthetics -neuromuscular blocking agents -opioids -reversal agents -vasopressors
Beyea et al. (2003a)	Same day surgery	*Product Classification*[1] -antimicrobials -ophthalmic preparations -analgesics and sedatives -intravenous solutions
Beyea et al. (2003b)	Operating room	*Product Classification*[2] -antimicrobials -intravenous solution -analgesics and sedatives -local anesthetics -anticoagulants
Currie et al. (1993)	Anesthesia	*Product Classification* -neuromuscular blockers
Fasting et al. (2002)	Anesthesia	*Product Classification* -neuromuscular blockers -opioids -neostigmine -local anesthesia -antimicrobials
Hicks et al. (2004)	Postanesthesia care unit	*Product Classification*[3] -antimicrobials -intravenous solution -analgesics and sedatives -anticoagulants
Khan et al. (2005)	Anesthesia	*Product Classification* -neuromuscular blockers -miscellaneous -induction agents -inhalation agents -local anesthetics -narcotics -intravenous fluids -sedatives
Wheeler et al. (2005)	Anesthesia	*Product Classification* -inhalation agents

[1] Spans 143 unique products
[2] Spans 147 unique products
[3] Spans 131 unique products

TABLE 6.7   Studies Reporting Types of Errors

Author (year)	Setting (n)	Major findings
Abeysekera et al. (2005)	Anesthesia (n = 452)	Ampoule labeling (41%) Syringe swap (37%) Omission (14%) Incorrect dose (11%) Wrong route of administration
Beyea et al. (2003a)	Same day surgery (n = 610)	Omission error (24.9%) Improper dose/quantity (23.8%) Unauthorized medication (15%) Prescribing error (10.5%) Wrong time (5.6%) Wrong administration technique (5.2%) Wrong medication (4.3%) Wrong patient (3.6%) Extra dose (3.2%) Wrong route (2.7%) Wrong dosage form (1.1%)
Beyea et al. (2003b)	Operating room (n = 731)	Omission error (26.5%) Unauthorized medication (16%) Prescribing error (14.4%) Improper dose/quantity (12.9%) Wrong medication (9.4%) Wrong time (6.6%) Wrong administration technique (4%) Extra dose (3.9%) Wrong route (3.3%) Wrong patient (1.9%) Wrong dosage form (0.9%)
Currie et al. (1993)	Anesthesia (n = 144)	Wrong drug (7.2%)
Fasting et al. (2000)	Anesthesia (n = 63)	Syringe swaps (44%) Ampoule swaps (14%) Wrong drug (13%) Wrong dose (29%)
Hicks et al. (2004)	Postanesthesia care unit (n = 645)	Improper dose/quantity (24%) Omission error (20%) Prescribing error (15%) Unauthorized drug (14%) Extra dose (6%) Wrong drug preparation (5%)

(continued)

TABLE 6.7 (*continued*)

Author (year)	Setting (*n*)	Major findings
		Wrong administration technique (5%)
		Wrong time (3%)
		Wrong patient (2%)
		Wrong route (1%)
		Wrong dosage form (1%)
Jenson et al. (2004)	Anesthesia	Omission
		Wrong drug
Khan et al. (2005)	Anesthesia (*n* = 165)	Underdosage of drug (*n* = 35)
		Known drug side effects/reaction (*n* = 29)
		Syringe swap (*n* = 26)
		Overdosage of drug (*n* = 23)
		Wrong drug given/timing (*n* = 15)
		Drug not effective (*n* = 12)
		Problems with labeling (*n* = 10)
		Miscellaneous (*n* = 10)
		Drug in inappropriate location (*n* = 5)
Liu et al. (2003)	Anesthesia (*n* = 116)	Wrong drug/dose (28.4%)

The identification of active errors, such as performance deficit, errors in calculations, inattention, not following established policies and procedures, erroneous transcription, failure to verify correct medication or inadequate monitoring, was present in 10 of the articles reviewed (Table 6.8) and were evident in each of the clinical areas. Systems-related errors (e.g., similar packaging, erroneous use of pre-printed order forms, equipment design, lack of standardization, and manufacturer's label) were also present in the studies.

Errors involving infusion devices and vaporizers were recorded in the operating room, anesthesia unit, and PACU (Abeysekera et al., 2005; Beyea et al., 2003a and b; Hicks, Becker, et al., 2004). Errors that occurred during the setup of the pump were active errors, and equipment failure were system errors. Nine of the 10 articles identified communication as a cause of error, a finding that may have applicability to active failure, latent failure, or both.

Contributing Factors

Nine articles reported contributing factors (Table 6.9), those events that influence the error's occurrence and, thus, are one-step (or more) removed from the direct cause of error. Contributing factors can be situational, organizational,

TABLE 6.8   Studies Reporting Causes of Errors

Author (year)	Setting	Major findings
Abeysekera et al. (2005)	Anesthesia	Infusion pumps and vaporizers (misuse, malfunction, lack of standardization) Communication Misuse of intravenous access Failure to check equipment Performance deficit
Beyea et al. (2003a)	Same day surgery (n = 574)	Performance deficit (39.9%) Procedure/protocol not followed (22.1%) Communication (18.1%) Equipment design (11%) Knowledge deficit (10.5%) Documentation (7.5%) Contraindicated, allergy (7%) Written order (3.7%) Monitoring inadequate/lacking (3.1%) Transcription inaccurate/missing (3.1%) Medication distribution system (3%) Preprinted medication order form (3%) Verbal order (3%) Similar packaging/labeling (2.4%) Dispensing device involved (2.1%) Calculation error (1.9%) Handwriting illegible/unclear (1.9%) Dosage form confusion (1.6%) Label (manufacturer's) design (1.6%) System safeguards (1.6%)
Beyea et al. (2003b)	Operating room (n = 731)	Performance deficit (42.5%) Procedure/protocol not followed (23.7%) Communication (21.8%) Documentation (9.9%) Contraindicated medication allergy (9.1%) Knowledge deficit (9%) Package/container design (4.9%) Similar packaging/labeling (4.8%) System safeguard(s) (3.9%) Dispensing device involved (3.3%) Medication distribution system (3.3%) Facility labeling (3.1%) Oral order (3%) Monitoring inadequate/lacking (2.8%) Transcription inaccurate/omitted (2.7%)

(continued)

TABLE 6.8   (*continued*)

Author (year)	Setting	Major findings
		Written order (2.2%)
		Calculation order (2.1%)
		Preprinted medication order form (1.8%)
		Pump, improper use (1.6%)
		Dose form confusion (1.5%)
Currie et al. (1993)	Anesthesia	Package (similar in appearance)
		Failure to communicate
		Haste
		Inattention
Hicks et al. (2004)	Postanesthesia care unit ($n = 645$)	Performance deficit (45.6%)
		Procedure/protocol not followed (23.8%)
		Communication (17.2%)
		Documentation (13.1%)
		Knowledge deficit (11.3%)
		Contraindicated medication allergy (6.6%)
		Dispensing device involved (6.6%)
		Written order (6.2%)
		Pump, improper use (5.2%)
		Transcription inaccurate/omitted (5.2%)
		Monitoring inadequate/lacking (5.1%)
		Calculation order (3.9%)
		System safeguard(s) (3.6%)
		Preprinted medication order form (3.1%)
		Verbal order (3.1%)
		Dose form confusion (3%)
		Drug distribution system (3%)
		Computer entry (2.1%)
		Equipment design (2%)
		Package/container design (2%)
Jenson et al. (2004)	Anesthesia	Failure in communication
		Contraindicated medication allergy
		Performance deficit
Khan et al. (2005)	Anesthesia	Human error/Performance deficit (56%)
		Known drug side effect/complication (21%)
		System error (19%)
		Equipment failure (4%)
		Latent errors:
		-communication
		-labeling of medications
		-inadequately labeled syringe
		-medication not in standardized location

TABLE 6.8   (*continued*)

Author (year)	Setting	Major findings
Liu et al. (2003)	Anesthesia	Performance deficit (failure to check equipment)
Orser et al. (2004)	Anesthesia	Performance Communication Delay/misdiagnosis of problem/complication Administration (transcription issues/policies- procedures) Conduct
Wheeler et al. (2005)	Anesthesia	Misuse of intravenous access Performance deficit Equipment failure Equipment design Knowledge deficit Failure to check drugs before administration Lack of communication Inadequate monitoring Lack of standardization of labels/protocols

environmental, or personal in nature; and it is recognized that there can be overlap (Hicks, Santell, Cousins, & Williams, 2004).

Situational factors, such as distractions or haste were those most commonly reported and present in multiple articles (Abeysekera et al., 2005; Beyea et al., 2003a, 2003b; Currie et al., 1993; Hicks, Becker et al., 2004; Orser & Byrick, 2004; Webster, Merry, Gander, & Mann, 2004). Other situational events include emergency situations, fatigue, communication breakdown, workload increase, not having access to patient information at the time it was needed, and inattention to detail.

Organizational factors ranged from issues involving staffing (staffing insufficient, agency or temporary staff, shift change, cross-coverage, and off-hour assignment) to not having sufficient workspace, the lack of 24-hour pharmacy support, and scheduling. Environmental factors included poor lighting. Personal factors included fatigue, as well as the mention of age-induced changes in the provider's eyesight (Webster et al., 2004).

Staff

The scope of medication errors leads to the conclusion that multiple disciplines can be involved in an error. Identifying the discipline involved in the error, rather

TABLE 6.9 Studies Reporting Contributing Factors

Author (year)	Setting	Major findings

Abeysekera et al. (2005)	Anesthesia	*Syringe or drug preparation errors (n = 452)*
		  -haste (34%)
		  -inattention to detail (47%)
		  -drug labeling (32%)
		  -distraction (24%)
		  -communication (10%)
		  -fatigue (11%)
		  -failure to check equipment (10%)
		Equipment errors (n = 234)
		  -failure to check equipment (37%)
		  -inattention (31%)
		  -haste (14%)
		  -unfamiliar environment or equipment (10%)
		Communication errors (n = 35)
		  -inattention (28%)
		  -staff inexperience (20%)
		Route of administration error (n = 126)
		  -fault of technique (19%)
		  -error in judgment (14%)

Beyea et al. (2003a)	Same day surgery (n = 179)	Distractions (56.4%) Staff, inexperienced (14.5%) Workload increase (11.2%) Staffing, insufficient (8.4%) Cross coverage (7.3%) No access to patient information (6.1%) Staff, float (5%) Emergency situation (3.9%) Shift change (1.7%) No 24-hour pharmacy (1.1%) Poor lighting (1.1%) Emergency situation (0.6%) Staff, agency/temporary (0.6%)
Beyea et al. (2003b)	Operating room (n = 731)	Distractions (48.5%) Staff, inexperienced (17%) Workload increase (11.5%) Emergency situation (7.3%) No access to patient information (6.1%) Staffing, insufficient (4.8%) Poor lighting (3%)

TABLE 6.9 (*continued*)

Author (year)	Setting	Major findings
		Shift change (3%)
		Staff, floating (2.4%)
		Code situation (1.8%)
		No 24-hour pharmacy (1.8%)
		Staff, agency/temporary (1.8%)
		Staffing, alternative hours (0.6%)
Currie et al. (1993)	Anesthesia	Haste Inattention
Hicks et al. (2004)	Postanesthesia care unit (n = 645)	Distractions (47.2%) Workload increase (15.5%) Staff, inexperienced (14.9%) No access to patient information (8.7%) Shift change (8.7%) Cross coverage (8.1%) Emergency situation (4.3%) Staffing, insufficient (4.3%) Staff, floating (3.1%) No 24-hour pharmacy (2.5%) Staff, agency/temporary (1.9%) Poor lighting (0.6%)
Jenson et al. (2004)	Anesthesia	Failure in communication Inattention Haste Distractions Fatigue
Liu et al. (2003)	Anesthesia	*Human factors*: -inattention -haste -failure to check equipment
Orser et al. (2004)	Anesthesia	Fatigue Staff aging Disabilities of care providers (e.g., eyesight with age)
Webster et al. (2004)	Anesthesia	Overcrowding of anaesthetic workspace Case scheduling problems Communication breakdown Equipment malfunction

than the name of the staff member, supports the nonpunitive nature of learning from mistakes in hopes of preventing future errors. Of the 12 studies, 9 focused on anesthesia errors, which would implicate anesthesia providers as having been involved in the error. The other three studies (Table 6.10) more broadly identified other disciplines involved in errors, a finding consistent with the broad reporting of medication errors from multiple facilities. From these studies, most of the errors were associated with registered nurses (RNs). The articles also identify other staff as having made the initial error, including physicians, anesthesia providers, pharmacy staff, and support staff.

Medication Use Process

The MUP depicts the five-steps from medication orders to administration of a product and subsequent monitoring. Table 6.11 outlines the steps: prescribing, documenting/transcribing, dispensing, administering, and monitoring. Each step involves various discipline-specific activities, inclusive of generally accepted standards of practice. For example, nurses are most familiar with the five rights of administering a medication (right drug, right patient, right time, right route, and right dose). The five rights serve as a legal standard for safe practice and offer protection and guidance against medication errors; however, they narrowly focus on the single task of administering a medication rather than the entire medication use process (Hicks, Becker et al., 2004).

Six of the articles designated the administration point, the fourth step in the five-step medication use process, as the origin of the error. It is during this phase that the patient/product interface occurs. The studies reviewed (Table 6.12) lend credence to the idea that the five rights, once thought of as a mantra for medication administration, are no longer the fail-safe system to eliminate or control medication errors within organizations (Hicks Becker et al., 2004; Stetina, Groves & Pafford, 2005). However, strict adherence to the medication use process provides a broad, multidisciplinary systems approach to safe medication delivery as an effective strategy to improve patient safety (Stetina et al.).

Level of Care

Two studies reviewed describe the level of care rendered to the patient following the error. This is noteworthy for two reasons. First, the level of care should be internally consistent with the error category or severity. As the severity increases, so should the level of care rendered. Second, the level of care is one means of documenting the resources expended as a direct result of an error. Such documentation supports the accepted principle that medication errors cost the health care system valuable resources.

TABLE 6.10   Studies Reporting Staff Involved in the Initial Error

Author (year)	Setting	Major findings
Beyea et al. (2003a)	Same day surgery ($n = 588$)	*Providers involved:* -nurse, registered (76.2%) -physician (11.7%) -nurse, licensed vocational/practical (3.4%) -unit secretary/clerk (2.2%) -pharmacist (1.9%) -anesthesiologist (1.5%) -nurse anesthetist (1.5%) -pharmacy technician (0.5%) -patient/caregiver (0.3%) -dentist (0.2%) -radiology technician (0.2%) -respiratory therapist (0.2%) -student (0.2%)
Beyea et al. (2003b)	Operating room ($n = 731$)	*Providers involved:* -nurse, registered (64.1%) -physician (20.9%) -nurse anesthetist (9.2%) -anesthesiologist (7.3%) -pharmacist (3.2%)
Hicks et al. (2004)	Postanesthesia care unit ($n = 645$)	*Providers involved:* -nurse, registered (68%) -physician (19.4%) -anesthesiologist (2.7%) -pharmacist (2.5%) -nurse anesthetist (2.1%) -unit clerk (2.1%) -pharmacy technician (1.4%) -respiratory therapist (0.6%) -nurse, licensed practical/vocational (0.5%) -physician assistant (0.3%) -student (0.2%) -nursing assistant/aide (0.2%)

TABLE 6.11   Phases in the Medication Use Process

Phase	Definition
Prescribing	The phase in the medication use process that involves an action of legitimate prescriber to issue a medication order.
Documenting/ Transcribing	The phase in the medication use process that involves anything related to the act of transcribing an order (by someone other than the prescriber) for order processing either electronically or manually in the patient's record.
Dispensing	The phase in the medication use process that begins with a pharmacist's assessment of a medication order and continues to the point of releasing the product for use by another health care professional. In the perioperative environment, dispensing processes can vary, as items may be obtained from open stock or automated dispensing–type systems with little or no pharmacy interaction.
Administering	The phase in the medication use process where the drug product and patient interface. If follows the documenting/transcribing and/or dispensing phase and precedes the monitoring phase and includes the five rights and informing the patient about the medication.
Monitoring	The phase in the medication use process that involved evaluating the patient's physical, emotional, and/or psychological response to the medication and then recording such findings.

Source: Hicks, R. W., Santell, J. P., Cousins, D. D., and Williams, R. L. (2004)

In an operating room study, Beyea et al. (2003b) reported the level of care following an error (Table 6.13). Of the 11 selections, the most common (57%) documented that the patient had an increase in observation. In 48% of the reports, there was evidence that an initial or change of medication treatment plan occurred. Prolonged hospitalization was present in 5% of the reports. In a PACU study, Hicks, Becker et al. (2004) reported similar results.

Error Reduction Strategies

Reducing medication errors is an international goal, and many authors propose recommendations that could lead to the development of better practices based on the evidence from their respective study (Table 6.14). The recommendations and conclusions drawn from these articles ranged from general discussions to specific interventions. Practice changes were suggested, including double checks,

TABLE 6.12   Studies Reporting the Medication Use Process

Author (year)	Setting	Major findings
Beyea et al. (2003a)	Same day surgery (n = 610)	Administering (68.4%) Prescribing (13.6%) Documenting (10.8%) Dispensing (6.1%) Monitoring (1.1%)
Beyea et al. (2003b)	Operating room (n = 731)	Administering (62%) Prescribing (18.1%) Dispensing (9.4%) Documenting (8.8%) Monitoring (1.5%)
Hicks et al. (2004)	Postanesthesia care unit (n = 645)	Administering (59.5%) Prescribing (22.5%) Documenting (10.7%) Dispensing (5.9%) Monitoring (1.2%)
Jenson et al. (2004)	Anesthesia	Administering
Webster et al. (2004)	Anesthesia	Administering
Wheeler et al. (2005)	Anesthesia	Administering Prescribing Transcribing

applying medication labels, discarding unlabeled products, and color-coding syringes (Beyea et al., 2003b; Currie et al., 1993; Jenson, Merry, Webster, Weller, & Larsson, 2004). Systems-level changes recommended by several authors (Beyea et al., 2003a, 2003b; Currie et al., 1993; Hicks, Becker et al., 2004; Jenson et al.; Orser & Byrick, 2004; Webster et al., 2004) spanned forcing functions, redundancy safeguards, standardization of strengths and dosages, standardizing drug storage and inventory, and implementing point of care pharmacists in the perioperative setting. Other system-level changes include reporting and reviewing all medication error events and barcoding. Many of these system-level changes reported are consistent with the human factors approach to designing safer systems.

CONCLUSION

The health care industry currently faces multiple challenges, ranging from increased pressure to control costs, an aging work force, recurring periodic

TABLE 6.13   Studies Reporting Level of Care

Author (year)	Setting	Major findings
Beyea et al. (2003b)	Operating room	*Level of care:* -observation initiated/increased (57%) -medication therapy initiated/changed (48%) -vital sign monitoring initiated/increased (30%) -laboratory tests performed (16%) -antidote administered (15%) -oxygen administered (9%) -airway established/patient ventilated (6%) -hospitalization prolonged: 1–5 days (5%) -transferred to a higher level of care (3%) -surgery performed (2%) -CPR performed (2%)
Hicks et al. (2004)	Postanesthesia Care Unit	*Level of care:* -drug therapy initiated/changed (64%) -observation initiated/increased (61%) -vital sign monitoring initiated/increased (33%) -laboratory tests performed (13%) -antidote administered (5%) -transferred to a higher level of care (5%) -airway established/patient ventilated (2%) -narcotic antagonist administered (2%) -CPR administered (1%) -oxygen administered (1%) -hospitalization prolonged: 1–5 days (1%)

shortages of qualified health care workers, and compliance with expanding regulatory requirements to exponential growth and utilization of technology. It is estimated that 1 out of every 5 doses given, or 2 out of every 100 admissions, experience a preventable medication error or adverse drug event (ADE) (Alaris Medical Systems, n.d.; Morgan, 2005). In 1995, researchers estimated that each adverse ADE cost the institution approximately $4,700 (Bates et al., 1997). A 700-bed teaching hospital could conceivably incur costs of $2.8 million dollars annually, directly attributed to ADEs. Estimates for the national cost of medication errors could easily exceed $2 billion annually. With double-digit health care inflation since 1995, the cost for ADEs in today's dollars would be more than double the 1995 values. Cost containment, coupled with ever-changing patterns

TABLE 6.14   Studies Reporting Error Reduction Strategies

Author (year)	Setting	Major findings
Beyea et al. (2003a)	Same day surgery	*Discussion of strategies/interventions:* -forcing function -system redundancy -centralizing error prone processes -screening new products for risk
Beyea et al. (2003b)	Operating room	*Discussion of strategies/interventions:* -dose and strength standardization -labeling protocol—on and off the sterile field -double checks of medications/labels during hand-offs -unlabeled medications to be discarded -define system for allergy alerts -system solution to timely administration of preop antibiotics -medication administration competency -periodic systems analysis for process changes
Currie et al. (1993)	Anesthesia	*Strategies/intervention for improvement:* -rechecking syringe or ampoule before giving the drug -staff education -color-coding selected drug class of medications (syringes/ampoules) -standardize drug storage -standardize process for labeling -establish checking protocols
Hicks et al. (2004)	Postanesthesia care unit	*Discussion of strategies/interventions:* -point of care pharmacists -address high-alert products concerns -system redundancies -centralizing error-prone processes -review medication storage procedures -standardize dosing -review pre-printed order forms
Jenson et al. (2004)	Anesthesia	*12 strategies for minimizing drug administration errors:* -reading and checking the label on ampoule or syringe -labels to be legible -label all syringes -standardize drug drawers and workspace

(continued)

TABLE 6.14   (*continued*)

Author (year)	Setting	Major findings
		-labels should be checked by a second person or device prior to drug being drawn up or administered -review near misses and errors reported -inventory management -alert to drugs that sound-alike/look-alike -use prefilled syringes when possible -provider who will administer the drug is to draw up and label the medication -color-code labels by classification -coding of syringe
Orser et al. (2004)	Anesthesia	*Strategies/intervention for improvement:* -development of unambiguous drug labels -infusion pump safety -voluntary medication error-reporting program -bilingual drug labels
Webster et al. (2004)	Anesthesia	*Strategies/intervention for improvement:* -administration system for injectable drugs

Note: visual (color-coding/labeling) and auditory (bar-coding and computer verification) processes for prefilled syringes containing common anesthesia agents.

of reimbursement, remains at the forefront of many hospital administrators concerns (American College of Healthcare Executives, 2005). Today's climate provides institutions with an opportunity to explore the effect medication errors have on patient safety in an effort to understand the depth, breadth, and scope of the problem while containing health care costs. Nursing research is one vehicle that contributes solutions to these perplexing problems.

Research that documents the effects of needed ergonomic changes (e.g., larger print for medication labels, sufficient printing on pre-filled syringes, allowing more time to perform activities, adopting visual and auditory cues related to medication delivery) in the perioperative environment and their effect on patient safety, as well as staff safety, are now becoming essential as the nursing population ages. Nurse researchers must consider human factors when designing studies, planning for interventions, or evaluating outcomes.

Periodic health care worker shortage is not a new phenomenon to nursing, but current worker shortages are more profound and have deeper implications for education and practice. As institutions recruit talented workers educated out-side the United States, new threats to patient safety may result from language barriers, cultural barriers, or deficits in knowledge about products. A professional nurse shortage opens the possibility of replacing the perioperative specialist with a different type of health care worker, one with less formal education and possessing only technical skills. Through nursing research, the value of fur-ther role delineation of the professional perioperative nurse will become more evident.

Compliance with ever-expanding regulatory and/or accreditation standards is a professional expectation. Regulations can arise from licensure requirements that are legally mandated. Hospitals and other health care entities (such as nurs-ing homes or outpatient centers) are among the most heavily regulated insti-tutions in the United States (Miller & Hutton, 2000). Licensed health care providers, such as physicians, nurses, or pharmacists, also face a burdensome num-ber of regulations. Statutory, administrative, and public laws are commonplace in the health care system. Administrative agencies are the outcome of legisla-tive enactments and these agencies have the ability to legislate and adjudicate (Pozgar, 2004). Legally mandated regulations draw on the authority of a govern-ment's (either federal or state) administrative agency to compel compliance with adopted standards, provided the standards are within the scope of authority of the agency. Accreditation, on the other hand, invokes voluntary standards put forth by an accrediting body (Miller & Hutton, 2000). Accrediting bodies for health care professionals may be professional associations or similar entities. JCAHO, an independent, not-for-profit organization, is the largest accrediting body for hospitals, long-term care facilities, and many other health-related organizations (Chen, Rathore, Radford, & Krumholz, 2003; Joint Commission on Accredi-tation of Healthcare Organizations, 2005). JCAHO's accreditation process has been prominent in the United States since the landmark legislation of 1965 that decreed hospitals had to satisfy federal guidelines as a condition of partic-ipation in the Medicare system. JCAHO's philosophy is that compliance with more than 50 quality and patient safety standards would likely achieve favor-able outcomes. JCAHO is the quasi-regulatory organization found to be the primary driver of hospitals' patient safety initiatives (Devers, Pham, & Liu, 2004).

The IOM called on hospitals and health system to participate in voluntary event-reporting programs to reduce morbidity and mortality (Kohn et al., 2000). Such programs collect information about adverse events, errors, or both for the primary purpose of learning from experience (Leape, 2002). A successful report-ing program would be nonpunitive in nature, confidential, independent, able to deliver expert analysis of the reports in a timely fashion, and able to provide systems-oriented recommendations (Leape). Reporting is achieved by means of an interface, either through questionnaires (which is the most common), interviews, or automation (Nyssen, Aunac, Faymonville, & Lutte, 2004).

Quantitative and qualitative research should guide the creation of a critical incident self-reporting process specifically focused on perioperative continuum variables related to the medication delivery process. Integrating this information into existing documents would eliminate the need for additional forms and reduce extra workload. The development of a simple method of recording data could provide the evidence needed to quantify the frequency and cause of medication errors and ADEs within the medication use process, thereby changing practices and institutional policies for safe medication delivery.

There is extensive research published about medication safety within other specialty environments (e.g., intensive care units, emergency departments, or pharmacies); however, there is a dearth of studies within the perioperative continuum of care. As the science of medication safety emerges within this specialty area, the nursing profession should take the lead in defining practice to eliminate or reduce the severity of medication errors. Although medication errors within the perioperative environment threaten patient safety and are associated with high rates of harm, nursing research could set the stage for providing evidenced-based processes that drive practice and result in advancing patient safety within this specialty area. Nursing research also recognizes the need to explore the linkages between the multiple areas of perioperative care as a whole continuum rather than in isolation.

Wheeler and Wheeler's (2005) general review of the literature examined medication errors in anaesthesia and critical care and identified a need to develop studies to highlight the improvement needed in education related to medication errors and the medication delivery process. Supporting this need, research focused on interventional studies should examine how drug education will effect both practitioners and medication delivery. Current technology (patient simulators) could be used to assist in the process of evaluating educational interventions for use in clinical settings.

Because "safety does not reside in a person, device, or department, but emerges from interactions of components of a system" (Kohn et al., 2000, p. 57), exploring a process that focuses on educational competencies for the entire team (e.g., administrative clerk, nurse assistant, surgical technologist, respiratory therapist, pharmacy technician, pharmacist, physician/surgeon, and RN) could be the key to optimizing medication safety within this complex environment. A multidisciplinary team approach to determine and maintain medication administration competencies to improve patient safety is a unique approach to staff education that warrants further study.

Safe medication use in the perioperative environment is a reasonable expectation from patients and providers alike. Understanding the unique characteristics of the medication use process within this environment and the conditions from the complex health care system that contribute to medication errors will direct the necessary science to achieve this goal.

REFERENCES

Abeysekera, A., Bergman, I. J., Kluger, M. T., & Short, T. G. (2005). Drug error in anaesthetic practice: A review of 896 reports from the Australian Incident Monitoring Study database. *Anaesthesia, 60*(3), 220–227.

Alaris Medical Systems. (n.d.). Medication error statistics. Retrieved October 8, 2005, from www.alarismed.com/alariscenter/stats.html

American College of Healthcare Executives. (2005). Top issues confronting hospitals: 2004. Retrieved January 8, 2005, from www.ache.org/pugs/research/ceoissues.cfm

Anderson, G. F., Hussey, P. S., Frogner, B. K., & Waters, H. R. (2005). Health spending in the United States and the rest of the industrialized world. *Health Affairs, 24*(4), 903–914.

Bates, D. W., Spell, N., Cullen, D. J., Burdick, E., Laird, N., Petersen, L. A., et al. (1997). The costs of adverse drug events in hospitalized patients. Adverse Drug Events Prevention Study Group. *Journal of the American Medical Association, 277*(4), 307–311.

Becher, E. C., & Chassin, M. R. (2001). Improving quality, minimizing error: Making it happen. *Health Affairs, 20*(3), 68–81.

Beyea, S. C., Hicks, R. W., & Becker, S. C. (2003a). Medication errors in the day surgery setting. *Surgical Services Management, 9*(1), 65–70, 73–76.

Beyea, S. C., Hicks, R. W., & Becker, S. C. (2003b). Medication errors in the OR—a secondary analysis of MEDMARX. *AORN Journal, 77*(1), 122, 125–129, 132–124.

Chen, J., Rathore, S. S., Radford, M. J., & Krumholz, H. M. (2003). JCAHO accreditation and quality of care for acute myocardial infarction. *Health Affairs, 22*(2), 243–254.

Currie, M., Mackay, P., Morgan, C., Runciman, W. B., Russell, W. J., Sellen, A., et al. (1993). The Australian Incident Monitoring Study. The "wrong drug" problem in anaesthesia: An analysis of 2000 incident reports. *Anaesthesia Intensive Care, 21*(5), 596–601.

Devers, K. J., Pham, H. H., & Liu, G. (2004). What is driving hospitals' patient-safety efforts? *Health Affairs (Millwood), 23*(2), 103–115.

Fasting, S., & Gisvold, S. E. (2000). Adverse drug errors in anesthesia, and the impact of coloured syringe labels. *Canadian Journal of Anaesthesia, 47*(11), 1060–1067.

Flynn, E. A. (n.d.). A brief history of medication errors. Retrieved November 17, 2005, from www.nmshp.org/med%20errors%20and%20questions.pdf

Flynn, E. A., Barker, K. N., Pepper, G. A., Bates, D. W., & Mikeal, R. L. (2002). Comparison of methods for detecting medication errors in 36 hospitals and skilled-nursing facilities. *American Journal for Health-System Pharmacists, 59*(5), 436–446.

Fortescue, E. B., Kaushal, R., Landrigan, C. P., McKenna, K. J., Clapp, M. D., Federico, F., et al. (2003). Prioritizing strategies for preventing medication errors and adverse drug events in pediatric inpatients. *Pediatrics, 111*(4), 722–729.

Gabel, J., & Fitzner, K. (2003). New evidence to explain rising healthcare costs. *The American Journal of Managed Care, 9*(Special Issue 1), SP1–SP2.

Health Grades, Inc. (2004). *Patient safety in American hospitals.* Lakewood, CO.

Health Grades, Inc. (2005). *Patient safety in American hospitals. Second annual report.* Lakewood, CO.

Hicks, R. W., Becker, S. C., Krenzischeck, D., & Beyea, S. C. (2004). Medication errors in the PACU: A secondary analysis of MEDMARX findings. *Journal Perianesthesia Nursing*, 19(1), 18–28.

Hicks, R. W., Santell, J. P., Cousins, D. D., & Williams, R. L. (2004). *MEDMARX 5th anniversary data report. A chartbook of 2003 findings and trends 1999–2003*. Rockville, MD: The United States Pharmacopeia Center for the Advancement of Patient Safety.

Jenson, L., Merry, A., Webster, C., Weller, J., & Larsson, L. (2004). Evidence-based strategies for preventing drug administration errors during anaesthesia. *Anaesthesia*, 59, 493–504.

Joint Commission on Accreditation of Healthcare Organizations. (2005). A journey through the history of the Joint Commission. Retrieved January 13, 2005, from www.jcaho.org/about+us/history/index.htm

Kaushal, R., Jaggi, T., Walsh, K., Fortescue, E. B., & Bates, D. W. (2004). Pediatric medication errors: What do we know? What gaps remain? *Ambulatory Pediatrics*, 4(1), 73–81.

Khan, F. A., & Hoda, M. Q. (2005). Drug related critical incidents. *Anaesthesia*, 60, 48–52.

Kohn, L. T., Corrigan, J. M., & Donaldson, M. S. (2000). *To err is human: Building a safer health system*. Washington, DC: National Academy Press.

Leape, L. L. (2002). Reporting of adverse events. *New England Journal of Medicine*, 347(20), 1633–1638.

Liu, E. H. & Koh, K. F. (2003). A prospective audit of critical incidents in anaesthesia in a university teaching hospital. *ANNALS Academy of Medicine Singapore*, 32(6), 814–820.

Mayo, A. M., & Duncan, D. (2004). Nurse perceptions of medication errors: What we need to know for patient safety. *Journal of Nursing Care and Quality*, 19(3), 209–217.

Miller, R. D., & Hutton, R. C. (2000). *Problems in health care law* (8th ed.). Rockville, MD: Aspen Publishers, Inc.

Morgan, S. (2005). Medication error statistics. *The Prescription*, 1(1), 1.

National Coordinating Council for Medication Error Reporting and Prevention. (1998–2001). What is a medication error? Retrieved February 25, 2005, from www.nccmerp. org/

Nightingale, F. (1970). *Notes on nursing*. Princeton, NJ: Brandon/System Press. (Original work published 1859).

Nyssen, A. S., Aunac, S., Faymonville, M. E., & Lutte, I. (2004). Reporting systems in healthcare from a case-by-case experience to a general framework: An example in anaesthesia. *European Journal of Anaesthesiology*, 21(10), 757–765.

Orser, B. A., & Byrick, R. (2004). Anesthesia-related medication error: Time to take action. *Canadian Journal of Anaesthesia*, 51(8), 756–760.

Pozgar, G. D. (2004). *Legal aspects of health care administration* (9th ed.). Sudbury, MA: Jones and Bartlett Publishers, Inc.

Santell, J. P. (2005). Medication errors: Experience of the United States Pharmacopeia (USP). *Joint Commission Journal on Quality and Patient Safety*, 31(2), 114–119.

Santell, J. P., Hicks, R. W., & Cousins, D. D. (2005). *MEDMARX data report: A chartbook of 2000–2004 findings from intensive care units and radiological services*. Rockville, MD: The United States Pharmacopeia Center for the Advancement of Patient Safety.

Schneider, P. J. (2002). Applying human factors in improving medication-use safety. *American Journal of Health-System Pharmacists*, 59, 1155–1159.

Stetina, P., Groves, M., & Pafford, L. (2005). Managing medication errors—a qualitative study. *Medsurg Nursing, 14*(3), 174–178.

Webster, C., Merry, A., Gander, P., & Mann, N. (2004). A prospective, randomised clinical evaluation of a new safety-oriented injectable drug administration system in comparison with conventional methods. *Anaesthesia, 59*, 80–87.

Wheeler, S. J., & Wheeler, D. W. (2005). Medication errors in anaesthesia and critical care. *Anaesthesia, 60*, 257–273.

Zhan, C., & Miller, M. R. (2003). Excess length of stay, charges, and mortality attributable to medical injuries during hospitalization. *Journal of the American Medical Association, 290*(14), 1868–1874.

Chapter 7

Nurse Home Visit Programs for the Elderly

Karen Dorman Marek and Carol Dean Baker

ABSTRACT

Nurses are the largest professional provider of health care services in the home setting. However, nurse home visit programs are diverse. The purpose of this review was to examine the many factors that influence the effectiveness of nurse home visit programs for older adults. Donebedian's Quality Assessment Model was used to organize the review using the components of structure, process, and outcome. A total of 60 home visit studies were identified that met the following criteria: (1) nurses were a major or only provider of the intervention, (2) the intervention was delivered by home visits, and (3) the study included a comparison group. This review demonstrates the complexity of variables that determine the effectiveness of home visit interventions. Many studies demonstrated lower overall health care costs for the intervention group with either improved or at least no change in clinical outcomes.

Keywords: patient safety, nursing, home health

Nurses have a long history of providing care in the patient's home. As the largest professional provider of home care services, nurses have a significant influence in the development of home-based health care programs, and the programs vary in purpose and type of interventions provided. Within the context of patient safety, which includes errors of omission and commission, the purpose of this review is to examine the many factors that influence the effectiveness of nurse home visit programs for older adults.

Preventive home visits are an important component in the care of the frail elderly. There is a growing interest in coordination across sites of care delivered to older adults. In addition, care that once only was provided in the acute setting is now becoming more commonplace in the home setting. To create programs that support the frail elderly, attention must be paid not only to preventive care, but to care that integrates preventive care with interventions tailored to treat specific diseases and/or chronic conditions.

Several recent systematic reviews were conducted on home visit programs designed to care for the elderly. However, the conclusions from the reviews were mixed related to the effectiveness of these programs. A review conducted by van Haastregt, Diederiks, van Rossum, de Witte, and Crebolder (2000) examined 15 studies that consisted of home visits to person's 65 and older living in the community. The authors concluded there was no clear evidence to support preventive home visits for the elderly. However, a more rigorous review using meta-analysis of 15 studies examining home visit programs was conducted (Elkan et al., 2001), and the authors concluded that home visit programs to older people can reduce mortality and admissions to long-term institutional care. In addition, another group of researchers conducted a meta-analysis of 18 randomized controlled trials to evaluate the effect of preventive home visits on functional status, nursing home admission, and mortality (Stuck, Egger, Hammer, Minder, & Beck, 2002). These studies demonstrated that preventive home visitation programs were effective if a multidimensional geriatric assessment and multiple follow-up visits were conducted. In addition, young-old populations had higher survival than old-old populations. Nurses were the predominant provider in the studies reviewed. Finally, Hallberg and Kristersson (2004) reviewed preventive home care of frail older people that used case management. The authors concluded that the most successful programs targeted frail older people using a comprehensive geriatric assessment as a base and nurses trained in gerontological practice.

To conduct this review, a search of PubMed, the Cumulative Index to Nursing & Allied Health Literature, Cochrane Database of Systematic Reviews, HealthStar, ISI Web of Science, Social Service Abstracts, Database of Abstracts of Reviews of Effectiveness, and Internet searches for citations occurring from January 1990 to August 2005, the time when the search was conducted. Key search terms used alone and in combination included home nursing, professional; community health nursing; nursing process; nursing interventions; home care services; frail elderly; aged; outcomes; cost benefit analysis; cost effectiveness; polypharmacy; medication management; chronic illness; and chronic disease as well as individual types of chronic illness. All searches were limited to patients aged 65 and older and Web sites conducted in the English language. The ISI Web of Science was used to track citations to major works and article references were reviewed for inclusion.

Criteria for inclusion in the review included the following: (1) nurses were a major or only provider of the intervention, (2) the intervention was delivered by visits to the subject's home, and (3) the study design included a comparison group. A total of 165 possible articles were identified from the literature, with 60 meeting the study criteria. To provide a framework for the examination of the different variables influencing nurse home visit programs, Donabedian's Quality Assessment Evaluation model was used. This model is based on the three major components: structure, process, and outcome (Donabedian, 1980). It has long served as unifying framework for examining health services. From the standpoint of patient safety, the model permits an examination of how risk and hazards embedded within the structure of care and the resulting processes have the potential to negatively or positively affect patient outcomes. The major question to be addressed is, what are the major structure, process, and outcome characteristics that contribute to successful nurse home visit programs?

STRUCTURE OF CARE

Structural items are the variables that provide inputs to the system. The structural items influencing home visit program are characteristics of clients and providers, as well as attributes of the setting of care (Donabedian, 1980). The following discussion will present the structural characteristics of the studies reviewed.

Client Characteristics

Home visit programs were based on a variety of client characteristics. Several programs were designed for the general care of frail older adults, with age as the major criteria to receive the home visit intervention (McEwan, Davison, Forster, Pearson, & Stirling, 1990; Pathy, Bayer, Harding, & Dibble, 1992; Stuck et al., 2000; van Rossum et al., 1993). General measures of frailty, such as multiple chronic conditions (Bernabei et al., 1998; Hebert, Robichaud, Roy, Bravo, & Voyer, 2001; Leveille et al., 1998; Nicolaides-Bouman, van Rossum, Kempen, & Knipschild, 2004; Siu et al., 1996; Stessman et al., 1996; Tibaldi et al., 2004) and/or limitations in activities of daily living (ADL), also were used as to determine participants (Bula et al., 1999; Cummings et al., 1990; Dalby et al., 2000; Gagnon, Schein, McVey, & Bergman, 1999; Landi et al., 1999; Miller, Hornbrook, Archbold, & Stewart, 1996; Robertson, Devlin, Gardner, & Campbell, 2001). In addition, several studies focused on subjects who were nursing home–eligible based on preexisting criteria set by governmental programs (Fabacher et al., 1994; Marek et al., 2005; Oktay & Volland, 1990).

Clinical condition is often the focus of nurse home visit programs. Several intervention programs using home visits were focused on specific medical diagnoses. The largest number of programs (11) were organized around the medical diagnosis of chronic obstructive pulmonary disease (COPD)(Cotton et al., 2000; Davies, Wilkinson, Bonner, Calverley, & Angus, 2000; Hermiz et al., 2002; Hernandez et al., 2003; Kwok et al., 2004; Neff, Madigan, & Narsavage, 2003; Nicholson et al., 2001; Oh, 2003; Skwarska et al., 2000; Smith et al., 1999; Strijbos, Postma, van Altena, Gimeno, & Koeter, 1996a), followed closely by heart failure (HF), with 10 studies reported (Benatar, Bondmass, Ghitelman, & Avitall, 2003; Feldman, Murtaugh, Pezzin, McDonald, & Peng, 2005; Johnston, Wheeler, Deuser, & Sousa, 2000; Naylor et al., 2004; Padula & Yeaw, 2001; Rich et al., 1995; Scott, Setter-Kline, & Britton, 2004; Stewart & Horowitz, 2002; Stewart, Marley, & Horowitz, 1999; Thompson, Roebuck, & Stewart, 2005). Other cardiac-related diagnoses included a program based on care of older adults with atrial fibrillation (Inglis et al., 2004), myocardial infarction (Frasure-Smith et al., 1997), hypertension (Garcia-Pena, Thorogood, Wonderling, & Reyes-Frausto, 2002), and cardiac surgery (Penque, Petersen, Arom, Ratner, & Halm, 1999). Other conditions used to define home visit programs were depression (Banerjee, Shamash, Macdonald, & Mann, 1996), stroke (Boter, 2004; Fjaertoft, Indredavik, Johnsen, & Lydersen, 2004), cancer surgery (de Wit & van Dam, 2001; McCorkle et al., 2000), diabetes (Huang, Wu, Jeng, & Lin, 2004), Parkinson disease (Hurwitz, 1989), and dementia (Tibaldi et al., 2004). Finally, three nurse home visit evaluations were found based on the nursing diagnoses of pain (de Wit & van Dam, 2001), fall risk (Huang, Wu et al.,) and medication management (Meredith et al., 2002).

Provider Characteristics

In more than half of the studies evaluated (37 of 60) nurses were the sole provider of the home visit intervention. Nurse-led teams were identified in five studies (Inglis et al., 2004;. Leveille et al., 1998; Neff et al., 2003; Rich et al., 1995; Thompson, Roebuck, & Stewart, 2005). Advanced practice nurses (APNs) were the major intervention provider in 10 studies (Bula et al., 1999; Leveille et al., 1998; McCorkle et al., 2000; Naylor et al., 2004; Naylor et al., 1994; Naylor et al., 1999; Neff et al., 2003; Nicholson et al., 2001; Siu et al., 1996; Stuck et al., 1995), and advanced training related to the condition treated was provided to nurse providers in four studies (Boter, 2004; de Wit & van Dam, 2001; Kwok et al., 2004; Thompson et al., 2005).

Another interesting finding in the review was the different combination of providers used in the home visit intervention. There were the traditional teams found in home care, consisting of nurses, physicians, physical therapists, occupational therapists, and social workers. However, provider pairs including pairings between nurses and pharmacists (Meredith et al., 2002; Stewart, Pearson, & Horowitz, 1998; Stone, Curran, & Bakken, 2002), occupational therapists (Penque et al., 1999), or physiotherapists (Strijbos et al., 1996a) were also tested in the home visit interventions. Home visit programs that used a team of disciplines were more successful in achieving significant improvement in clinical and cost outcomes.

Setting of Care

Multiple characteristics of the setting of care influence the process and outcome of health care interventions. Health care systems vary widely by country, and often it is the national health care policy that determines the type, amount, and site of care delivered. Studies included in this review originated from more than 15 countries, with 51 of 60 studies from western industrialized countries. A literature review of nursing care of the chronically ill in six western industrialized countries identified that integrated care innovations such as hospital-at-home and advanced nursing practice are implemented predominantly in primary care–oriented countries (Temmink, Francke, Hutten, Van Der Zee, & Abu-Saad, 2000). In the United States, several of the nurse home visit programs were designed around a specific payer source such as Medicaid (Marek et al., 2005) and the Veterans Administration (Cummings et al., 1990; Fabacher et al., 1994). Investigators in several other countries addressed high-cost problems within national health system with universal health coverage (Farrero, Escarrabill, Prats, Maderal, & Manresa, 2001; Nicholson et al., 2001).

PROCESS

Process items represent the content or configuration of care (Donabedian, 1980). Structural variables influence the process of care or the type and amount of intervention delivered. Home visit programs varied in specificity of protocols and integration with other health care delivery sites. In reviewing the nurse home visit studies, the following process categories of hospital-to-home, early hospital discharge, transitional care, and disease-specific protocols will be discussed.

Hospital-to-Home

These programs are referred to as the "substitution of care" phenomenon, where care is provided by the most appropriate professional at the lowest cost level (Temmink et al., 2000). For purposes of this review, the programs presented are home visit programs that replace hospitalization. In these programs the providers are generally interdisciplinary teams. Although nurses deliver the majority of home visits, physician home visits are common. (Cummings et al., 1990; Farrero et al., 2001; Fjaertoft et al., 2004; Leff et al., 1999; Stessman et al., 1996; Tibaldi et al., 2004).

Emergency department (ED) diversion programs also were used to identify patients for whom intense home care services could be substituted for acute care hospitalization. Several programs provided clients the option of intense home-based services instead of admission to the hospital. For example, in one study subjects with dementia requiring hospitalization were provided similar services in their home. The study results found less agitation and better clinical outcomes in the group receiving home-based services when compared to subjects who were hospitalized (Tibaldi et al., 2004).

Early Hospital Discharge

Instead of diverting hospital admissions, several research teams instituted an early hospital discharge program, substituting nurse home visits in substitution for hospital care (Cotton et al., 2000; Hernandez et al., 2003; Penque et al., 1999). Common to these programs was a visit to the acute care setting by a nurse to begin discharge planning and follow up by the same nurse once the client was discharged from the hospital.

Transitional Care

The transition from hospital to home is a focus of care delivered in several of the studies. Transitional care includes a combination of services and environments designed to promote the safe and timely transfer of patients from one level of care to another or one setting to another (Brooten & Naylor, 1999). Similar to early discharge programs, in transitional care programs, care is begun in the hospital by the same nurse provider who coordinates and visits the subjects in their home. Naylor (2002) has conducted seminal work in this area using APNs to conduct discharge planning in the acute care setting and follow up home care visits. This model was expanded by Neff et al. (2003), who used APNs to direct the program and home health care registered nurses and licensed practical nurses to provide the nursing services. Transitional care programs are time limited, ending usually about 3 months after hospital discharge.

Disease-Specific Protocols

As discussed earlier, several programs were based on specific clinical conditions, with COPD and HF as the most common focuses for home visit studies. The disease-specific protocols addressed areas such as medication management, counseling, telehealth, rehabilitation, exercise, diet, self care, and preventive monitoring.

Medication management. Several programs included interventions focused on the management of medication. Meredith et al. (2002) implemented a pharmacy review program conducted by a nurse and pharmacist of newly admitted home health care patients. No differences in clinical outcomes were achieved; however, the intervention group experienced a significant decrease in therapeutic duplication of medications, which could have a longer-term effect in both cost and clinical outcomes of older adults. Another group of investigators examined the effectiveness of a nurse and pharmacist visit to focus on pharmacotherapy of congestive heart failure (CHF) patients compared to standard care (Stewart et al., 1998). The researchers found significantly ($p = 0.03$) fewer rehospitalizations in the intervention group. Monitoring of medication compliance was identified in 17 other studies as a component of the study protocol (Benatar et al., 2003; Cotton et al., 2000; Davies et al., 2000; Feldman et al., 2004; Flaherty et al., 1998; Hernandez et al., 2003; Huang, Wu et al., 2004;. Huang & Acton, 2004; Inglis et al., 2004; Kwok et al., 2004; Naylor et al., 2004; Oktay & Volland, 1990; Rich et al., 1995; Skwarska et al., 2000; Smith et al., 1999; Stessman et al., 1996; Stewart et al., 1999).

Counseling. Mental health counseling was a major focus of several home visit programs specifically designed to address specific clinical conditions such as depression (Banerjee et al., 1996; Flaherty et al., 1998), myocardial infarction (Frasure-Smith et al., 1997), HF (Scott et al., 2004) and post–breast cancer surgery (Wyatt, Donze, & Beckrow, 2004). In these programs nurses were specially trained in counseling interventions specific to a clinical condition.

Telehealth. Use of technology to substitute for nurse visits is a growing area of home care. Two studies were identified that compared nurse home visit programs with programs that used telehealth technology such as blood pressure, weights, and stethoscopes (Benatar et al., 2003; Johnston et al., 2000). Both research teams demonstrated lower cost and no significant difference in clinical outcomes when the group with the telehealth intervention was compared to the group with only traditional nurse home visits.

Rehabilitation. Two studies were identified that focused on pulmonary rehabilitation for persons with chronic lung disease. These programs consisted of education, inspiratory muscle training, exercise training, and relaxation exercises (Oh, 2003; Strijbos, Postma, van Altena, Gimeno, & Koeter, 1996b). Both programs demonstrated significantly better clinical outcomes in the intervention group; however, both studies had small sample sizes.

Exercise. Similar to the exercises identified in the rehabilitation programs, several researchers included interventions designed to improve exercise tolerance beyond basic ADLs (Hermiz et al., 2002; Huang, Wu et al., 2004; Naylor et al., 2004; Penque et al., 1999; Robertson et al., 2001; Smith et al., 1999; Stewart et al., 1999). There was limited information related to the specific exercises included in the exercise intervention, or the frequency and duration of the exercise activity.

Diet. Interventions focused on teaching and monitoring diet were included in several disease-specific protocols for CHF (Feldman et al., 2004; Rich et al., 1995), hypertension (Garcia-Pena et al., 2002), diabetes (Huang, Wu et al., 2004), and COPD (Hernandez et al., 2003). Although diet interventions were included in the discussion of the protocol, more descriptive information related to the diet interventions would be useful. Inclusion of information such as subject adherence or number of times diet was addressed in home visits would enhance our understanding of this type of intervention.

Self care. For purposes of this review, self care will include interventions related to supporting ADLs. Interventions focused on promoting the client's ability to perform ADLs were present in several disease-specific protocols. (Feldman et al., 2004; Garcia-Pena et al., 2002; Hermiz et al., 2002; Tinetti et al., 2002). Using a restorative home care model highly focused on self care, Tinnetti et al. demonstrated a reduction in ED visits and increase in mobility in the intervention group when compared to the control group.

Preventive monitoring. Several researchers followed older adults for time periods of 1 to 3 years, with the goal of early identification of problems and referral or provision of the appropriate care as soon as a problem was identified. Programs that included comprehensive geriatric assessment and at least four nurse visits per year were more successful in demonstrating a positive effect on the intervention group's clinical and utilization outcomes (Bernabei et al., 1998; Fabacher et al., 1994; Landi et al., 1999; Marek et al., 2005; McEwan et al., 1990; Stuck et al., 1995; Stuck et al., 2000; van Rossum et al., 1993).

However, several programs with similar characteristics did not produce significant differences in clinical outcomes. Two Canadian older adult visit programs were unsuccessful in identifying differences in outcomes. Authors of both studies identified insufficient statistical power as a limitation (Dalby et al., 2000; Gagnon et al., 1999). Also, the lack of power or authority to control use of other services was identified. Low intervention dose is another possible reason for insignificant findings; for example, in one study the intervention consisted of one nurse visit with follow-up phone calls (Hebert et al., 2001).

OUTCOME

The final component of the quality assessment model is the outcome—the procedural end point or effect of the process component. Both process items and structural items can influence outcomes, which are categorized into four areas: (1) clinical health outcomes, or measures of the client's health status at a designated point in time; (2) utilization outcomes, or measures of clients' use of health care services; (3) cost outcomes, or measures of expenditures on health care services; and (4) client satisfaction or perceptions of the quality of the care delivered (Marek, 1997).

Clinical Outcomes

Quality of life (QOL). The QOL was the most common clinical outcome measured in the studies reviewed. Of the 20 studies that measured QOL, 8 identified a significant ($p < 0.05$) difference between the intervention and control groups in at least one component if not all components of the QOL instrument (Boter, 2004; Fjaertoft et al., 2004; Hernandez et al., 2003; Naylor et al., 2004; Oh, 2003; Rich et al., 1995; Scott et al., 2004; Stewart et al., 1998) and 11 had no significant differences in any component of QOL between groups (Benatar et al., 2003; Farrero et al., 2001; Feldman et al., 2004; Gagnon et al., 1999; Hermiz et al., 2002; Huang, Wu et al., 2004; Meredith et al., 2002; Penque et al., 1999; Siu et al., 1996; Thompson et al., 2005; Wyatt et al., 2004). A total of nine instruments were used to measure QOL: Some were disease specific, and others were more general measures.

Two instruments, St. George's Respiratory Questionnaire and the Chronic Respiratory Disease Questionnaire (CRQ), were developed to measure QOL of persons with chronic lung disease (Guyatt, Berman, Townsend, Pugsley, & Chambers, 1987; Jones, 1992). Hernandez et al. (2003) tested a home hospitalization program for COPD patients and found a significant ($p = 0.05$) difference in QOL between the intervention and control groups using St. George's instrument. However, no significance difference was found in QOL in the same study when the more general SF-12 QOL measure was used. Hermiz et al. (2002) found no difference between intervention and control groups' QOL in COPD patients posthospitalization using the St. George's measure. However, the intervention Hermiz et al. tested was less intense (two nurse home visits) than that examined by Hernandez et al. In the latter study, the intervention was a hospitalization diversion program that included more intensive home services and more acutely ill subjects. Oh (2003), using the CRQ, found significant ($p = 0.03$) differences in the QOL between the intervention group that received home-based pulmonary rehabilitation services and the control group. However, a home care program for COPD patients who used oxygen did not find group differences in QOL using the CRQ.

A QOL tool designed specifically for HF patients called the Minnesota Living with Heart Failure (MLHF) was used in four studies (Rector & Cohn, 1992). Using this instrument, Naylor et al. (2004) tested the effectiveness of an APN transitional care program and found a significant ($p < 0.05$) difference between the intervention and control groups at 12 weeks, with the intervention group presenting a higher level of QOL. However, no significant group differences were identified at 26 and 52 weeks. A study by Stewart et al. (1999) using the same instrument, demonstrated significant ($p < 0.05$) differences between groups at 3 months, but not at 6 months. Interestingly, the SF-36 also was used in this study, and the physical health score was significantly different at 3 but not 6 months, similar to the results of the MLHF instrument. However, a home health care program that used a standardized approach for HF patients found no significant group differences in QOL (Feldman et al., 2004). In contrast, one study's finding of no group differences was not viewed as an undesired outcome, because the intervention tested was a less costly telehealth visit that substituted some home nursing visits. The result of no difference in QOL between groups can be viewed as supportive of the tested intervention (Benatar et al., 2003).

In addition, one other QOL instrument specific to HF was identified (Guyatt et al., 1989). The Chronic Heart Failure Questionnaire was used in a study by Rich et al. (1995). In this study, a significant ($p = 0.001$) difference between groups was identified, with the intervention group who received the nurse-directed multidisciplinary intervention having a higher level of QOL when compared to the control group.

Four general QOL instruments were found in the studies reviewed. The SF-36 (Ware & Sherbourne, 1992) was the most prevalent general QOL instrument, present in a total of eight studies (Boter, 2004; Gagnon et al., 1999; Meredith et al., 2001; Scott et al., 2004; Siu et al., 1996; Stewart et al., 1999; Thompson et al., 2005; Wyatt et al., 2004). None of the reviewed studies had significant differences between groups in all eight subscales of the instrument. However, one investigator (Stewart et al., 1999), identified differences in the physical component of the SF-36 at 3 months ($p < 0.05$), and Boter (2004) found group differences in the role emotional subscale ($p < 0.05$), but no group differences were found in the remaining subscales. The SF-12 (a shorter version of the SF-36) was used in one study with no group differences identified (Penque et al., 1999). The lack of significant results using the SF-36 merits further examination of its sensitivity as a clinical outcome measure in nurse intervention studies.

Two other QOL instruments also were identified in this review. The Nottingham Health Profile was used in a study of stroke patients in an early supported discharge intervention (Hunt, McKenna, McEwen, Williams, & Papp, 1981). The group receiving the intervention demonstrated a higher level of QOL ($p = 0.048$) at 52 weeks when compared to the control group. The cardiac version of the Quality of Life Index (QLI) identified significant ($p = 0.01$) group differences using a mutual group goal-setting intervention for HF individuals (Ferrans & Powers, 1992; Scott et al., 2004). A Chinese version of the QLI was used as one measure of clinical outcome in a study of home visits to persons with diabetes; however, no significant group differences were identified (Huang, Wu et al., 2004; Liu, 1993).

Functional status. Functional status is often defined as a rating of independence in ADLs and in some cases instrumental ADLs. In seven studies, the intervention group had significantly ($p < 0.05$) better ADL status when compared to the control group (Bernabei et al., 1998; Bula et al., 1999; Fabacher et al., 1994; Marek et al., 2005; Neff et al., 2003; Strijbos et al., 1996a; Stuck et al., 1995; Tinetti et al., 2002). All of these programs included a comprehensive assessment and at least quarterly home visits for monitoring of potential problems in need of intervention.

Exercise tolerance. In two studies, patient tolerance of vigorous activity was measured by timed stair climbing (Oh, 2003) or treadmill tolerance (Penque et al., 1999). In the study conducted by Oh, individuals who received the pulmonary rehabilitation intervention had significantly ($p = 0.05$) better exercise tolerance at 8 weeks when compared to the control group. There was no significant difference in groups in the study conducted by Penque et al.; however, this study tested an early discharge program for persons after cardiac bypass surgery, so the lack of group difference in exercise tolerance could be considered a good outcome.

Measures of emotions. Concepts such as depression, morale, and anxiety are considered in measures of emotions. These types of clinical phenomena were common clinical outcome measures of nurse visit programs. Significant ($p < 0.05$) group differences in depression, with the intervention group testing as less depressed, were identified in seven studies (Banerjee et al., 1996; Benatar et al., 2003; Bernabei et al., 1998; Cummings et al., 1990; Marek et al., 2005; McEwan et al., 1990; Neff et al., 2003), and no difference was found in four (Fjaertoft et al., 2004; Frasure-Smith et al., 1997;. Huang, Wu et al., 2004; Naylor et al., 2004). McEwan et al. (1990) tested a preventive screening program for older adults and found a significant ($p = 0.05$) difference in morale in the group receiving nurse visits. A significant ($p < 0.05$) group difference in anxiety was identified in two studies (Benatar et al., 2003; Boter, 2004).

Cognition. Measures of cognition focused on short-term memory. Significant ($p < 0.05$) group differences, with the intervention group less cognitively impaired, were identified in two studies (Bernabei et al., 1998; Marek et al., 2005). However, no significant difference was discovered in three studies (Cummings et al., 1990; Fjaertoft et al., 2004; Meredith et al., 2002).

Physiologic outcomes. The disease-specific symptom of dyspnea was measured in two studies of older adults with COPD. In both studies, the group receiving the nurse home visit intervention has significantly ($p < 0.05$) less dyspnea than the control group (Oh, 2003; Strijbos et al., 1996b). Two studies demonstrated significant ($p < 0.05$) group differences in the physiological measures of blood pressure (Garcia-Pena et al., 2002) and hemoglobin A1c (Huang, Wu et al., 2004). In both studies, the intervention group had more favorable physiologic results when compared to the control group.

Utilization Outcomes

Utilization outcomes were the most popular measures identified in this review. These measures address the use of health care services with the number of hospitalizations, hospital days, ED visits, and nursing home admissions being the most frequently occurring items.

Hospitalizations. Admissions and readmissions to the hospital were measured in 29 of the studies reviewed. Eleven of the studies identified significantly ($p < 0.05$) lower hospitalizations during a specific time period following the study intervention (Benatar et al., 2003; Bernabei et al., 1998; Farrero et al., 2001; Flaherty et al., 1998; Landi et al., 1999; Naylor et al., 2004; Naylor et al., 1994; Naylor et al., 1999; Neff et al., 2003; Rich et al., 1995; Stewart & Horowitz, 2002; Thompson et al., 2005). Four studies that identified no difference between the intervention and control groups were actually positive outcomes because the intervention tested was an early discharge to home hospitalization program with lower cost (Cotton et al., 2000; Davies et al., 2000; Hernandez et al., 2003; Skwarska et al., 2000). The number of days spent in the hospital was significantly lower in seven studies that also had significantly lower hospitalizations (Benatar et al., 2003; Farrero et al., 2001; Landi et al., 1999; Naylor et al., 1999; Rich et al., 1995; Stewart & Horowitz, 2002; Thompson et al.). One study that tested early hospital discharge of COPD patients did not find a difference between the intervention and control group in hospitalizations. However, the intervention group did have significantly fewer days in the hospital (Hernandez et al., 2003).

Emergency department visits. A total of five studies identified a significant reduction in ED visits: Two were hospital-based home care of COPD patients (Farrero et al., 2001; Hernandez et al., 2003), one was a transitional care program for COPD patients (Neff et al., 2003), one study tested an integrated case management program for older adults (Bernabei et al., 1998), and the final study tested a rehabilitation model for home care (Tinetti et al., 2002). All five studies were multidisciplinary in approach. In contrast, there was one study that found significantly ($p < 0.05$) more visits to the ED, the opposite of the desired outcome of the home visit intervention (Gagnon et al., 1999).

Nursing home admissions. Seven studies examined nursing home admission as a utilization outcome measure. Only one of the seven found the intervention group to have significantly lower nursing home admissions. One possible reason for this outcome was that the intervention followed the subjects for 3 years. But another study, conducted by van Haastregt et al. (2000), that also was 3 years in duration did not identify a significant difference in nursing home admission between groups. The intervention for this study had a similar number of nurse visits, but the nurses in the van Hasstregt et al. study did not perform physical examinations and did not work in collaboration with a geriatrician. In the Stuck et al. (2002) study, the providers were geriatric nurse practitioners while the van Hasstregt et al. study providers were not APNs.

Other utilization outcomes include physician visits; however in the three studies that measured this outcome no significant differences were identified (Hermiz et al., 2002; Naylor et al., 1999; Smith et al., 1999). One study that used specially trained nurses to provide a home visit posthospitalization for stroke found the intervention group used significantly less rehabilitation services when compared to the control group (Boter, 2004).

Cost of Care

The overriding concern of most nurse home visit programs is the cost effectiveness of the intervention. When examining cost effectiveness, researchers are interested in the investment it takes to provide the intervention and the intervention's ability to improve clinical outcomes at a dollar amount the payer is willing to spend. Alternatively, the impetus to examine the cost effectiveness of an intervention may be to determine whether a lower-cost intervention causes a deterioration in clinical outcomes. In cost-effectiveness analyses, the perspective (e.g., societal, health provider, payer or individual) is an important issue. Of the studies included in this review, 22 included some type of cost examination. Cost perspective appeared to be from the payer in five studies (Benatar et al., 2003; Leff et al., 1999; Naylor et al., 2004;. Naylor et al., 1994; Naylor et al., 1999) and the provider in the remaining 17 (Bernabei et al., 1998; Cummings et al., 1990; Farrero et al., 2001; Garcia-Pena et al., 2002; Hernandez et al., 2003; Johnston et al., 2000; Landi et al., 1999; Miller et al., 1996; Nicholson et al., 2001; Oktay & Volland, 1990; Penque et al., 1999; Rich et al., 1995; Robertson et al., 2001; Skwarska et al., 2000; Stewart et al., 1999; van Rossum et al., 1993). Nine of the studies had statistically significantly lower costs in the intervention group when compared to the control (Benatar et al., 2003; Cummings et al., 1990; Hernandez et al., 2003; Landi et al., 1999; Leff et al., 1999; Naylor et al., 2004; Naylor et al.,

1999; Nicholson et al., 2001; Rich et al., 1995; Stewart et al., 1998). However, an additional seven studies identified lower total cost for the intervention group but did not include and statistical testing. And one study determined costs were higher for the intervention group, but the result was not statistically significant (van Rossum et al., 1993).

Two studies included incremental cost-effectiveness ratios. For example, in a study of a nurse visit intervention for older adults with hypertension it was determined that it cost $1.10 per mm Hg reduction in systolic blood pressure, and $1.00 for every mm Hg reduction in diastolic blood pressure (Garcia-Pena, Thorogood, Wonderling, & Reyes-Frausto, 2002). Another study that tested a fall prevention intervention determined that it cost $NZ155 per fall prevented when hospital costs averted were considered (Robertson et al., 2001).

Patient Satisfaction

The final area of outcome measurement identified in the studies reviewed is the area of patient satisfaction. Eight studies examined the domain of patient satisfaction, with four research teams identifying significantly greater satisfaction in the intervention group (Cummings et al., 1990; Hermiz et al., 2002; Neff et al., 2003) and four detecting no difference (Feldman et al., 2004; Naylor et al., 1999; Penque et al., 1999; Skwarska et al., 2000).

DISCUSSION

The examination of the structure, process, and outcome components of nurse home visit studies provides a picture of the multiple variables that can influence the success of a program. As health care resources become more scarce, attention to factors in each of these components becomes more critical.

There are many structural variables that influence the effectiveness of home visit programs. Programs structured to be condition specific appear to be more effective than those designed to treat more general older populations. Several programs demonstrated that targeting frail patients, age 80 and older, demonstrated a greater influence on subject outcomes. Nurses with advanced preparation or specialized training had a positive affect on outcomes. Studies that were multidisciplinary were the most effective. This is especially true related to utilization and cost outcomes. If the nurses providing the intervention did not have close communication with the patient's primary physician, ED visits and hospitalizations tended to be higher. Also, the organization of the countries' health system influenced the effectiveness of the system. It may be theoretically impossible for home visit programs to decrease ED visits and hospitalizations if the program is not involved in managing acute care, such as gate keeping with respect to access to the ED and discharge from institutional care (Kane, 1988). Gagnon et al. (1999) postulated that one reason for the nonsignificant results in their study of nurse case management of frail older adults was that the nurses lacked authority in the system and often had difficulty reaching the client's primary care physician, therefore requiring an ED visit. Also, the nurses in the study were from the acute care setting and the options for care provision in the community or home may not have been as familiar to them as they would be for nurses who work in the community (Gagnon et al., 1999).

Core to any nurse home visit study is the interventions performed. Programs that had disease-specific protocols for care were more successful in influencing outcomes. In conducting the review, we found it especially difficult to identify the nursing interventions performed in studies that reported on preventive care home visits to the elderly. Although study reports provided descriptions of the interventions, there was no reporting of the actual type and number of interventions delivered. The absence of such data enforces the perception that all nurse visits are the same. Interestingly, one study reported that patients treated by one specific intervention nurse had significantly worse outcomes when compared to the patients treated by the two other intervention nurses. There are no data on the actual interventions performed; however, if there were, it would be useful to determine whether the interventions performed by the nurses were different (Stuck et al., 2000). One study in the review identified the planned and actual interventions delivered, but there was no examination of the relationship of specific interventions performed and the patient outcomes (Banerjee et al., 1996). Examples of follow-up research to identify specific nurse intervention was conducted by Naylor, Bowles, and Brooten (2000), where the Omaha System was used to code APN transitional care interventions. Examination of the relationships between the type and number of interventions performed with the outcomes of care is the next important step in analysis of home visit interventions.

Duration and intensity of the interventions delivered during a home visit is another area that influences the outcomes of care. Programs that are preventive in nature, targeting a less frail population, require more time to determine the effect of the intervention on the outcomes of care. In addition, care for the chronically ill is not time limited. Transitional care appears to lose its effect at about 6 months. Perhaps less-intense provision of care occurring after the transitional period would prolong the effect of the nurse intervention with patient outcomes that would justify the extension of the duration of care. Continuous care management of the chronically ill, with varying intensities and combining elements of transitional care with more traditional nurse case management, may be an effective method to manage the chronically ill.

Most of the home visit programs reviewed provided care at a lower cost. The programs that substituted home care for hospital care were the most effective. Clinical outcomes do not necessarily need to be better in the intervention group to signal success of a home visit program. In substitution programs, where care is provided by less expensive providers in a less expensive environment, the goal is for the clinical outcomes to be as good or better than the group receiving care in the acute care setting, or wherever care would be delivered if the substitution model was not in place.

Many nurse home visit studies identified improvement in clinical outcomes or a reduction in the cost of care, but the results were not statistically significant. A major reason identified was the small sample size causing a loss of power. To adequately measure effectiveness of nurse home visit interventions, studies with larger sample sizes over longer periods of time are needed. Larger studies are expensive to conduct, but the potential improvement in older adults' QOL in conjunction with cost savings may well justify funding such studies.

Nurses are the major professional provider of health care services in the home setting. This review has identified many areas in which nurse home visit programs to older adults have demonstrated lower costs of care while improving clinical outcomes. In addition, there is a large amount of variation in the way programs are structured and the interventions performed by the provider in the home. Within the patient safety framework, this means not offering effective programs could be considered an error of omission.

Given a choice, most older adults choose to live in their own home. The population of older adults in 2030 is expected to be twice as large as it was in the year 2000 (Federal Interagency Forum on Aging and Related Statistics, 2005). Because of this rapid growth, nurses must continue to create safe health care options for older adults that include cost-effective care in the home setting.

REFERENCES

Banerjee, S., Shamash, K., Macdonald, A. J., & Mann, A. H. (1996). Randomised controlled trial of effect of intervention by psychogeriatric team on depression in frail elderly people at home. *British Medical Journal, 313*(7064), 1058–1061.

Benatar, D., Bondmass, M., Ghitelman, J., & Avitall, B. (2003). Outcomes of chronic heart failure. *Archives of Internal Medicine, 163*(3), 347–352.

Bernabei, R., Landi, F., Gambassi, G., Sgadari, A., Zuccala, G., Mor, V., et al. (1998). Randomised trial of impact of model of integrated care and case management for older people living in the community. *British Medical Journal, 316*(7141), 1348–1351.

Boter, H. (2004). Multicenter randomized controlled trial of an outreach nursing support program for recently discharged stroke patients. *Stroke, 35*(12), 2867–2872.

Brooten, D., & Naylor, M. D. (1999). Transitional environments. In A. Hindshaw & S. Feethan (Eds.), *Handbook of clinical nursing research* (pp. 641–653). Thousand Oaks, CA: Sage.

Bula, C. J., Berod, A. Ç., Stuck, A. E., Alessi, C. A., Aronow, H. U., Santos-Eggimann, B., et al. (1999). Effectiveness of preventive in-home geriatric assessment in well functioning, community-dwelling older people: Secondary analysis of a randomized trial. *Journal of the American Geriatrics Society, 47*(4), 389–395.

Cotton, M. M., Bucknall, C. E., Dagg, K. D., Johnson, M. K., MacGregor, G., Stewart, C., et al. (2000). Early discharge for patients with exacerbations of chronic obstructive pulmonary disease: A randomized controlled trial. *Thorax, 55*(11), 902–906.

Cummings, J. E., Hughes, S. L., Weaver, F. M., Manheim, L. M., Conrad, K. J., Nash, K., et al. (1990). Cost-effectiveness of Veterans Administration hospital-based home care. A randomized clinical trial. *Archives of Internal Medicine, 150*(6), 1274–1280.

Dalby, D. M., Sellors, J. W., Fraser, F. D., Fraser, C., van Ineveld, C., & Howard, M. (2000). Effect of preventive home visits by a nurse on the outcomes of frail elderly people in the community: A randomized controlled trial. *Canadian Medical Association Journal, 162*(4), 497–500.

Davies, L., Wilkinson, M., Bonner, S., Calverley, P. M. A., & Angus, R. M. (2000). "Hospital at home" versus hospital care in patients with exacerbations of chronic obstructive pulmonary disease: Prospective randomised controlled trial. *British Medical Journal, 321*(7271), 1265–1268.

de Wit, R., & van Dam, F. (2001). From hospital to home care: A randomized controlled trial of a Pain Education Programme for cancer patients with chronic pain. *Journal of Advanced Nursing, 36*(6), 742–754.

Donabedian, A. (1980). *Exploration in quality assessment and monitoring* (Vol. 1). Ann Arbor Michigan: Health Administration Press.

Elkan, R., Kendrick, D., Dewey, M., Hewitt, M., Robinson, J., Blair, M., et al. (2001). Effectiveness of home based support for older people: Systematic review and meta-analysis. *British Medical Journal, 323*(7315), 719–725.

Fabacher, D., Josephson, K., Pietruszka, F., Linderborn, K., Morley, J. E., & Rubenstein, L. Z. (1994). An in-home preventive assessment program for independent older adults: A randomized controlled trial. *Journal of the American Geriatrics Society, 42*(6), 630–638.

Farrero, E., Escarrabill, J., Prats, E., Maderal, M., & Manresa, F. (2001). Impact of a hospital-based home-care program on the management of COPD patients receiving long-term oxygen therapy. *Chest, 119*(2), 364–369.

Federal Interagency Forum on Aging Related Statistics. (2005). Number of Older Americans. Retrieved December 7, 2005, from www.agingstats.gov/chartbook2004/population.html

Feldman, P. H., Murtaugh, C. M., Pezzin, L. E., McDonald, M. V., & Peng, T. R. (2005). Just-in-time evidence-based e-mail "reminders" in home health care: Impact on patient outcomes. *Health Services Research, 40*(3), 865–885.

Feldman, P. H., Peng, T. R., Murtaugh, C. M., Kelleher, C., Donelson, S. M., McCann, M. E., et al. (2004). A randomized intervention to improve heart failure outcomes in community-based home health care. *Home Health Care Services Quarterly, 23*(1), 1–23.

Ferrans, C. E., & Powers, M. J. (1992). Psychometric assessment of the Quality of Life Index. *Research in Nursing and Health, 15*(1), 29–38.

Fjaertoft, H., Indredavik, B., Johnsen, R., & Lydersen, S. (2004). Acute stroke unit care combined with early supported discharge. Long-term effects on quality of life. A randomized controlled trial. *Clinical Rehabilitation, 18*(5), 580–586.

Flaherty, J. H., McBride, M., Marzouk, S., Miller, D. K., Chien, N., Hanchett, M., et al. (1998). Decreasing hospitalization rates for older home care patients with symptoms of depression. *Journal of the American Geriatrics Society, 46*(1), 31–38.

Frasure-Smith, N., Lesperance, F., Prince, R. H., Verrier, P., Garber, R. A., Juneau, M., et al. (1997). Randomised trial of home-based psychosocial nursing intervention for patients recovering from myocardial infarction. *The Lancet, 350*(9076), 473–479.

Gagnon, A. J., Schein, C., McVey, L., & Bergman, H. (1999). Randomized controlled trial of nurse case management of frail older people. *Journal of the American Geriatrics Society, 47*(9), 1118–1124.

Garcia-Pena, C., Thorogood, M., Wonderling, D., & Reyes-Frausto, S. (2002). Economic analysis of a pragmatic randomised trial of home visits by a nurse to elderly people with hypertension in Mexico. *Salud Pública de México, 44*(1), 14–20.

Guyatt, G. H., Berman, L. B., Townsend, M., Pugsley, S. O., & Chambers, L. W. (1987). A measure of quality of life for clinical trials in chronic lung disease. *Thorax, 42*(10), 773–778.

Guyatt, G. H., Nogradi, S., Halcrow, S., Singer, J., Sullivan, M. J., & Fallen, E. L. (1989). Development and testing of a new measure of health status for clinical trials in heart failure. *Journal of General Internal Medicine, 4*(2), 101–107.

Hallberg, I. R., & Kristerisson, J. (2004). Preventive home care of frail older people: A review of recent case management studies. *Journal of Clinical Nursing, 13*(6B), 112–120.

Hebert, R., Robichaud, L., Roy, P. M., Bravo, G., & Voyer, L. (2001). Efficacy of a nurse-led multidimensional preventive programme for older people at risk of functional decline. A randomized controlled trial. *Age and Ageing, 30*(2), 147–153.

Hermiz, O., Comino, E., Marks, G., Daffurn, K., Wilson, S., & Harris, M. (2002). Randomised controlled trial of home based care of patients with chronic obstructive pulmonary disease. *British Medical Journal, 325*(7370), 938–940.

Hernandez, C., Casas, A., Escarrabill, J., Alonso, J., Puig-Junoy, J., Farrero, E., et al. (2003). Home hospitalisation of exacerbated chronic obstructive pulmonary disease patients. *European Respiratory Journal, 21*(1), 58–67.

Huang, C., Wu, S., Jeng, C., & Lin, L. (2004). The efficacy of a home-based nursing program in diabetic control of elderly people with diabetes mellitus living alone. *Public Health Nursing, 21*(1), 49–56.

Huang, T., Acton, G. J. (2004). Effectiveness of home visit falls prevention strategy for Taiwanese community-dwelling elders: Randomized trail. *Public Health Nursing, 21*(3), 247–256.

Hunt, S. M., McKenna, S. P., McEwen, J., Williams, J., & Papp, E. (1981). The Nottingham Health Profile: subjective health status and medical consultations. *Social Science & Medicine [A] , 15*(3 Pt 1), 221–229.

Hurwitz, A. (1989). The benefit of a home exercise regimen for ambulatory Parkinson's disease patients. *Journal of Neuroscience Nursing, 21*(3), 180–184.

Inglis, S., McLennan, S., Dawson, A., Birchmore, L., Horowitz, J. D., Wilkinson, D., et al. (2004). A new solution for an old problem? Effects of a nurse-led, multidisciplinary, home-based intervention on readmission and mortality in patients with chronic atrial fibrillation. *Journal of Cardiovascular Nursing, 19*(2), 118–127.

Johnston, B., Wheeler, L., Deuser, J., & Sousa, K. H. (2000). Outcomes of the Kaiser Permanente Tele-Home Health Research Project. *Archives of Family Medicine, 9*(1), 40–45.

Jones, P. (1992). *The St. George's Respiratory Questionnaire*. London: St. George's Medical School.

Kane, R. (1988). The noblest experiment of them all: Learning from the national channeling evaluation. *Health Services Research, 23*, 189–198.

Kwok, T., Lum, C. M., Chan, H. S., Ma, H. M., Lee, D., & Woo, J. (2004). A randomized, controlled trial of an intensive community nurse-supported discharge program in preventing hospital readmissions of older patients with chronic lung disease. *Journal of the American Geriatrics Society, 52*(8), 1240–1246.

Landi, F., Gambassi, G., Pola, R., Tabaccanti, S., Cavinato, T., Carbonin, P. U., et al. (1999). Impact of integrated home care services on hospital use. *Journal of the American Geriatrics Society, 47*(12), 1430–1434.

Leff, B., Burton, L., Guido, S., Greenough, W. B., Steinwachs, D., & Burton, J. R. (1999). Home hospital program: A pilot study. *Journal of the American Geriatrics Society, 47*(6), 697–702.

Leveille, S. G., Wagner, E. H., Davis, C., Grothaus, L., Wallace, J., LoGerfo, M., et al. (1998). Preventing disability and managing chronic illness in frail older adults: A randomized trial of a community-based partnership with primary care. *Journal of the American Geriatrics Society, 46*(10), 1191–1198.

Liu, H. (1993). An exploration of the psychometrics of the quality of life index of Chinese family [Chinese]. *Nursing Research (China), 1*(2), 127–136.

Marek, K. D. (1997). Measuring the effectiveness of nursing care. *Outcomes Management for Nursing Practice, 1*(1), 8–12; quiz 13.

Marek, K. D., Popejoy, L., Petroski, G., Mehr, D., Rantz, M., & Lin, W. C. (2005). Clinical outcomes of aging in place. *Nursing Research, 54*(3), 202–211.

McCorkle, R., Strumpf, N. E., Nuamah, I. F., Adler, D. C., Cooley, M. E., Jepson, C., et al. (2000). A specialized home care intervention improves survival among older post-surgical cancer patients. *Journal of the American Geriatric Society, 48*(12), 1707–1713.

McEwan, R. T., Davison, N., Forster, D. P., Pearson, P., & Stirling, E. (1990). Screening elderly people in primary care: A randomized controlled trial. *The British Journal of General Practice, 40*(332), 94–97.

Meredith, S., Feldman, P., Frey, D., Giammarco, L., Hall, K., Arnold, K., et al. (2002). Improving medication use in newly admitted home healthcare patients: A randomized controlled trial. *Journal of the American Geriatrics Society, 50*(9), 1484–1491.

Meredith, S., Feldman, P. H., Frey, D., Hall, K., Arnold, K., Brown, N. J., et al. (2001). Possible medication errors in home healthcare patients. *Journal of the American Geriatrics Society, 49*(6), 719–724.

Miller, L. L., Hornbrook, M. C., Archbold, P. G., & Stewart, B. J. (1996). Development of use and cost measures in a nursing intervention for family caregivers and frail elderly patients. *Research in Nursing & Health, 19*(4), 273–285.

Naylor, M., Brooten, D., Campbell, R., Maislin, G., McCauley, K., & Schwartz, J. (2004). Transitional care of older adults hospitalized with heart failure: A randomized controlled trial. *Journal of the American Geriatrics Society, 52*, 675–684.

Naylor, M., Brooten, D., Jones, R., Lavizzo-Mourey, R., Mezey, M., & Pauly, M. (1994). Comprehensive discharge planning for the hospitalized elderly. A randomized clinical trial. *Annals of Internal Medicine, 120*(12), 999–1006.

Naylor, M. D. (2002). Transitional care of older adults. *Annual Review of Nursing Research, 20*, 127–147.

Naylor, M. D., Bowles, K. H., & Brooten, D. (2000). Patient problems and advanced practice nurse interventions during transitional care. *Public Health Nursing, 17*(2), 94–102.

Naylor, M. D., Brooten, D., Campbell, R., Jacobsen, B. S., Mezey, M. D., Pauly, M. V., et al. (1999). Comprehensive discharge planning and home follow-up of hospitalized elders: A randomized clinical trial. *Journal of the American Medical Association, 281*(7), 613–620.

Neff, D. F., Madigan, E., & Narsavage, G. (2003). APN-Directed Transitional Home Care Model: achieving positive outcomes for patients with COPD. *Home Healthcare Nurse, 21*(8), 543–550.

Nicholson, C., Bowler, S., Jackson, C., Schollay, D., Tweeddale, M., & O'Rourke, P. (2001). Cost comparison of hospital- and home-based treatment models for acute chronic obstructive pulmonary disease. *Australian Health Review, 24*(4), 181–187.

Nicolaides-Bouman, A., van Rossum, E., Kempen, G., & Knipschild, P. (2004). Effects of home visits by home nurses to elderly people with health problems: Design of a randomised clinical trial in the Netherlands. *BMC Health Services Research, 4*, 1–10.

Oh, E. G. (2003). The effects of home-based pulmonary rehabilitation in patients with chronic lung disease. *International Journal of Nursing Studies, 40*(8), 873–879.

Oktay, J. S., & Volland, P. J. (1990). Post-hospital support program for the frail elderly and their caregivers: A quasi-experimental evaluation. *American Journal of Public Health, 80*(1), 39–46.

Padula, C. A., & Yeaw, E. (2001). Inspiratory muscle training: An exploration of a home-based intervention. *Journal of Applied Research, 1*(2), 85–94.

Pathy, M. S., Bayer, A., Harding, K., & Dibble, A. (1992). Randomised trial of case finding and surveillance of elderly people at home. *The Lancet, 340*(8824), 890–893.

Penque, S., Petersen, B., Arom, K., Ratner, E., & Halm, M. (1999). Early discharge with home health care in the coronary artery bypass patient. *Dimensions in Critical Care Nursing, 18*(6), 40–48.

Rector, T. S., & Cohn, J. N. (1992). Assessment of patient outcome with the Minnesota Living with Heart Failure questionnaire: Reliability and validity during a randomized, double-blind, placebo-controlled trial of pimobendan. Pimobendan Multicenter Research Group. *American Heart Journal, 124*(4), 1017–1025.

Rich, M. W., Beckham, V., Wittenberg, C., Leven, C. L., Freedland, K. E., & Carney, R. M. (1995). A multidisciplinary intervention to prevent the readmission of elderly patients with congestive heart failure. *New England Journal of Medicine, 333*(18), 1190–1195.

Robertson, M. C., Devlin, N., Gardner, M. M., & Campbell, A. J. (2001). Effectiveness and economic evaluation of a nurse delivered home exercise programme to prevent falls. 1: Randomised controlled trial. *British Medical Journal, 322*(7288), 697–701.

Scott, L. D., Setter-Kline, K., & Britton, A. S. (2004). The effects of nursing interventions to enhance mental health and quality of life among individuals with heart failure. *Applied Nursing Research, 17*(4), 248–256.

Siu, A. L., Kravitz, R. L., Keeler, E., Hemmerling, K., Kington, R., Davis, J. W., et al. (1996). Postdischarge geriatric assessment of hospitalized frail elderly patients. *Archives of Internal Medicine, 156*(1), 76–81.

Skwarska, E., Cohen, G., Skwarski, K. M., Lamb, C., Bushell, D., Parker, S., et al. (2000). Randomized controlled trial of supported discharge in patients with exacerbations of chronic obstructive pulmonary disease. *Thorax, 55*(11), 907–912.

Smith, B. J., Adams, R., Appleton, S. L., Trott, C. M., Bennett, P. W., Allan, D. P., et al. (1999). The effect of a respiratory home nurse intervention in patients with chronic obstructive pulmonary disease (COPD). *Australian And New Zealand Journal of Medicine, 29*(5), 718–725.

Stessman, J., Ginsberg, G., Hammerman-Rozenberg, R., Friedman, R., Ronen, D., Israeli, A., et al. (1996). Decreased hospital utilization by older adults attributable to a home hospitalization program. *Journal of the American Geriatric Society, 44*(5), 591–598.

Stewart, S., & Horowitz, J. D. (2002). Home-based intervention in congestive heart failure: Long-term implications on readmission and survival. *Circulation, 105*(24), 2861–2866.

Stewart, S., Marley, J. E., & Horowitz, J. D. (1999). Effects of a multidisciplinary, home-based intervention on unplanned readmissions and survival among patients with chronic congestive heart failure: A randomised controlled study. *The Lancet, 354*(9184), 1077–1083.

Stewart, S., Pearson, S., & Horowitz, J. D. (1998). Effects of a home-based intervention among patients with congestive heart failure discharged from acute hospital care. *Archives of Internal Medicine, 158*(10), 1067–1072.

Stone, P. W., Curran, C. R., & Bakken, S. (2002). Economic evidence for evidence-based practice. *Journal of Nursing Scholarship, 34*(3), 277–282.

Strijbos, J. H., Postma, D. S., van Altena, R., Gimeno, F., & Koeter, G. H. (1996a). A comparison between an outpatient hospital-based pulmonary rehabilitation program and a home-care pulmonary rehabilitation program in patients with COPD: A follow-up of 18 months. *Chest, 109*(2), 366–372.

Strijbos, J. H., Postma, D. S., van Altena, R., Gimeno, F., & Koeter, G. H. (1996b). Feasibility and effects of a home-care rehabilitation program in patients with chronic obstructive pulmonary disease. *Journal of Cardiopulmonary Rehabilitation, 16*(6), 386–393.

Stuck, A. E., Aronow, H. U., Steiner, A., Alessi, C. A., Bula, C. J., Gold, M. N., et al. (1995). A trial of annual in-home comprehensive geriatric assessments for elderly people living in the community. *New England Journal of Medicine, 333*(18), 1184–1189.

Stuck, A. E., Egger, M., Hammer, A., Minder, C. E., & Beck, J. C. (2002). Home visits to prevent nursing home admission and functional decline in elderly people: Systematic review and meta-regression analysis. *Journal of the American Medical Association, 287*(8), 1022–1028.

Stuck, A. E., Minder, C. E., Peter-Wuest, I., Gillmann, G., Egli, C., Kesselring, A., et al. (2000). A randomized trial of in-home visits for disability prevention in community-dwelling older people at low and high risk for nursing home admission. *Archives of Internal Medicine, 160*(7), 977–986.

Temmink, D., Francke, A. L., Hutten, J. B., Van Der Zee, J., & Abu-Saad, H. H. (2000). Innovations in the nursing care of the chronically ill: A literature review from an international perspective. *Journal of Advanced Nursing, 31*(6), 1449–1458.

Thompson, D. R., Roebuck, A., & Stewart, S. (2005). Effects of a nurse-led, clinic and home-based intervention on recurrent hospital use in chronic heart failure. *European Journal of Heart Failure, 7*(3), 377–384.

Tibaldi, V., Aimonino, N., Ponzetto, M., Stasi, M. F., Amati, D., Raspo, S., et al. (2004). A randomized controlled trial of a home hospital intervention for frail elderly demented patients: Behavioral disturbances and caregiver's stress. *Archives of Gerontology and Geriatrics. Suppl.* (9), 431–436.

Tinetti, M. E., Baker, D., Gallo, W. T., Nanda, A., Charpentier, P., & O'Leary, J. (2002). Evaluation of restorative care vs usual care for older adults receiving an acute episode of home care. *Journal of the American Medical Association, 287*(16), 2098–2105.

van Haastregt, J. C., Diederiks, J. P., van Rossum, E., de Witte, L. P., & Crebolder, H. F. (2000). Effects of preventive home visits to elderly people living in the community: Systematic review. *British Medical Journal, 320*(7237), 754–758.

van Haastregt, J. C., Diederiks, J. P., van Rossum, E., de Witte, L. P., Voorhoeve, P. M., & Crebolder, H. F. (2000). Effects of a programme of multifactorial home visits on falls and mobility impairments in elderly people at risk: Randomised controlled trial. *British Medical Journal, 321*(7267), 994–998.

van Rossum, E., Frederiks, C. M., Philipsen, H., Portengen, K., Wiskerke, J., & Knipschild, P. (1993). Effects of preventive home visits to elderly people. *British Medical Journal, 307*(6895), 27–32.

Ware, J. E., Jr., & Sherbourne, C. D. (1992). The MOS 36-item short-form health survey (SF-36). I. Conceptual framework and item selection. *Medical Care, 30*(6), 473–483.

Wyatt, G. K., Donze, L. F., & Beckrow, K. C. (2004). Efficacy of an in-home nursing intervention following short-stay breast cancer surgery. *Research in Nursing and Health, 27*(5), 322–331.

Chapter 8

Nursing Home Safety: A Review of the Literature

Jill Scott-Cawiezell and Amy Vogelsmeier

ABSTRACT

The number of older persons in the United States is rapidly growing and, based on this growth projection, the number of consumers needing nursing home (NH) care will likely triple in the next 10 years. Although NHs have been bombarded and scrutinized about the care that they provide, the concept of safety (specifically, error prevention) remains at the margin of most quality improvement efforts. The purpose of this review is to explore what has recently been written (2000–2005) about the evolution of the NH as an organization focused on safety and the most critical clinical processes that must be closely monitored for a safe NH environment to occur. After a thorough review of both organizational and clinical NH literature, 30 organizational studies and 39 clinically based studies were reviewed. The review revealed that, organizationally, teamwork, communication, and leadership all were critical in resident and staff outcomes and clinically, assessment was an important missing process at critical points in the residents' care for prevention and timely treatment of potentially dangerous conditions. The value of the registered nurse (RN) in this setting was clear in the many assessment issues noted and the lack of RN guidance for adherence to recognized practice guidelines. To explicate the role of the RN, first, better outcome measures must be developed that are nurse sensitive. A second clear agenda for NH research is the explication of the role of leadership, particularly nursing leadership, to create an environment where open and accurate communication can be accomplished among all of the diverse NH roles. This will help all members of the team to identify care improvement opportunities. Finally, a new frontier for the NH setting is the use of technology and the need to harness the information that has set in the NH system for years. Information mastery for staff and leadership is a necessary aspect of the organization that must be developed to provide sound information for strategic and focused change to occur.

Keywords: patient safety, nursing, long-term care

The number of older persons in the United States is rapidly growing. This pattern is expected to continue for the next 20 to 30 years and, based on this growth projection, the number of consumers who will need nursing home (NH) care will likely triple in the next 10 years. The increasing demand for NH services comes in the face of continued concern related to NH performance, particularly as it relates to safety or error prevention. NHs provide care to some of our nation's most frail and vulnerable citizens, with whom even relatively minor discrepancies can have negative outcomes (Bates et al., 1995). Many NH practices are considered basic and routine. But in reality, these clinical practices reflect complex interactions of a large number of specific decisions and actions (Kaushal et al., 2001), often performed under less than ideal conditions by staff members representing diverse roles.

Six years after the Institute of Medicine report (1999) galvanized a dramatically expanded level of conversation and concern about patient safety, conversations in many NHs remain focused on meeting regulations and do not stretch to consider the concept of safety or error prevention in a sustained and systemized way. Although NHs have been bombarded and scrutinized about the care that they provide, the concept of safety (specifically, error prevention) remains at the margin of most quality improvement efforts. This marginalization may be the result of the ambiguity that exists between safety as a desired characteristic and the broader issues of quality (Leape & Berwick, 2005). As thinking evolves, the organizational issues have become most evident. For purposes of this discussion, safety was considered broadly and included consideration of both related organizational issues and specific clinical processes related to both the quality and safety NH literature.

AIMS

The review of NH research literature intended to provide an overview and synthesis of the most recent empirical evidence addressing clinical safety and related organizational issues. The primary goal of this review was to determine where evidence existed to guide both organizational and practice changes to improve the safety orientation of the NH environment. A secondary goal of this review was to provide direction as to where research needs to continue to explore and develop evidence in this setting.

METHOD

The evidence reviewed for this chapter was found using a combination of search terms, including nursing homes and long-term care. Beyond that, there were organizational keywords (e.g., work force, leadership, staffing, quality improvement, organizational culture, patient safety) and clinical keywords (e.g., pressure ulcers, falls, restraints [chemical, physical], infections, medication errors, adverse drug events [ADEs], medication safety). The search was restricted to peer review publications between 2000 and 2005 that represented research studies conducted in the United States. The computerized databases searched were Cumulative Index to Nursing and Allied Health Literature, Medline, and Healthstar. In addition, the Agency for Healthcare Research and Quality (AHRQ) website and a recent compendium of patient safety and selected federal reports from the Centers for Medicare & Medicaid Services (CMS) were also explored. Finally, a manual search of selected journals was completed to ensure that our search strategy had been effective. The selected journals included the *Journal of Gerontological Nursing, The Gerontologist, Journal of the American Geriatric Society,* and *Geriatric Nursing.*

Initially, the search focused on studies authored or coauthored by nurses. The search was then expanded to include studies from other health disciplines that affected nursing practice. So, although much of the patient safety research is interdisciplinary and relevant to the discipline of nursing, there are studies that focused specifically on the interventions of other disciplines (such as physicians) that were not included in the review. The search was also limited to evidence that was developed specifically in the NH setting and did not include studies conducted in assisted living or residential settings.

In an attempt to narrow the search to the most recent literature, some of the classic studies from the NH setting are not presented. However, it is assumed that the recent literature built on earlier findings and provided the foundation for the review of these more recent studies (2000–2005).

ORGANIZATIONAL ISSUES IN NURSING HOME SAFETY

CMS's Quality Indicators (QIs) and Quality Measures have monitored NH quality and safety for more than two decades. Despite ongoing monitoring focused on falls, restraints, pressure ulcers, and infections through the QIs and QMs, safety remains a critical concern. However, until recently, most NHs did not see the results of their quality reports nor were these reports integrated into quality improvement efforts or safety discussions. But after 20 years of counting error prevalence and incidence to no avail, NH researchers and policy makers have increased their efforts to explicate what organizational issues may be influencing minimal improvement results. And this research provides the foundation from which to link NHs' organizational elements to future safety practices and error prevention.

Current Nursing Home Capacity to Embrace Safety

Unlike the acute care setting, there has been little specifically written about NH safety or error prevention. The NH setting may be a decade behind in moving toward a culture of safety and an orientation toward error prevention. Acknowledging that the NH industry lags behind in safety discussions, the review had to consider the evolutionary organizational process required to get to a culture of safety. Therefore, the review began with the development of quality improvement efforts (CQI). Because many NHs have not yet embraced basic CQI in their routine operations, Lucas and colleagues (2005) considered how those who adopted CQI were different. Both environmental and organizational predictors discriminated between NHs that adopted CQI principles and those that did not. With minimal CQI activity in the NH setting, few NH studies have associated CQI efforts to improved clinical outcomes (Castle, 2003; Rantz, Hicks, Grando, Petroski, Madsen, Mehr, et al., 2004; Rantz, Popejoy, Petroski, Madsen, Mehr, Zwygart-Stauffacher, et al., 2001). The three studies that did found that performance feedback could significantly improve selected clinical processes. With clinical feedback, Castle (2003) found that physical restraint use was lowered. Rantz and colleagues (2001) found that advanced practice nurses' (APNs') consultation influenced falls and pressure ulcers, and in a related study, Rantz and colleagues (2004) found that team process, active quality improvement programs and tenure of key leadership also influenced the basics of care.

In addition to linking CQI efforts to improved NH performance, three other studies linked various organizational aspects to resident outcomes. Castle (2001) found that administrative turnover was associated with higher than average pressure ulcer rates and restraint use. Anderson, Issel, and McDaniel (2003) found a relationship between the tenure of the director of nursing (DON) and selected management practices that facilitated openness of communication, participation in decision-making, and relationship-based leadership to improved restraint use and decreased complications of immobility and fractures. Scott-Cawiezell, Main, Vojir, Jones, Moore, Nutting, et al. (in press) considered a broader set of working conditions measures and organizational performance and found that high-performing NHs emphasized staff, good communication, teamwork, and .clear standards and expectations.

The studies presented thus far suggest that organizational elements affect CQI efforts and clinical performance. Therefore, understanding the status of such organizational elements is also important as the NH industry attempts to build the necessary organizational capacity to sustain improvement and look toward a more mindful environment focused on error prevention. Additional studies described key elements of the NH organization such as empowerment (Campbell, 2003), shared values, and the role of leaders (Swagerty, Lee, Smith, & Taunton, 2005).

Two studies specifically explored the nursing assistants' (NAs) perceptions of the NH and how this influenced their ability to provide high-quality care. Pennington, Scott, and Magilvy (2003) found that leadership, teamwork, a clean environment, and a need for respect were related to productivity and meaningful work. Curry, Porter, Michalski, and Gruman (2000) had similar findings when NAs were asked about their ability to provide individualized care. In addition, their study found that work environment flexibility and supervisor assistance with challenging residents facilitated NA work, and inadequate staffing, poor staff attitude, and lack of knowledge and training were perceived barriers.

Summary of Findings Related to the Current Capacity of the Nursing Home to Embrace Safety

Current organizational literature linking the organizational elements of the NH to CQI efforts and performance suggests four key elements to be addressed for sustained organizational improvement: teamwork, communication, leadership, and information mastery. Evidence shows that teams that included frontline staff members with an active voice were important to the performance of the NH and directly influenced resident outcomes (Anderson et al., 2003; Campbell, 2003; Curry et al., 2000; Lucas, Avi-Itzhak, Robinson, Morris, Koren, & Reinhard, 2005; Pennington et al., 2003; Rantz et al., 2004; Scott-Cawiezell et al., in press). The importance of good communication structures and strategies and their influence on performance was noted across many studies (Anderson et al., 2003; Curry et al., 2000; Lucas et al., 2005; Scott-Cawiezell et al., in press). Proper communication was essential in sharing information about errors, near misses, and system issues that are setting staff members up to make mistakes. In an ongoing study, leadership has been found to have great influence in staff members' desire to take the risk to share procedural concerns, errors, and near misses (Scott-Cawiezell, unpublished raw data).

The influence of leadership, through stability and style, was also frequently noted to be associated with resident outcomes (Anderson, et al., 2003;

Castle, 2001; Curry et al., 2000; Pennington et al., 2003; Rantz et al., 2004; Scott-Cawiezell et al., in press; Swagerty et al., 2005). A final theme was the importance of information mastery (using data to drive decision-making) and its influence on improvement efforts (Castle, 2003; Rantz et al., 2001).

Nursing Home Work Force

Teamwork, communication, and leadership not only influence the care of residents, but these organizational elements also have an effect on the staff. In addition to providing direct care to residents, staff members provide ongoing surveillance for a safer environment. A critical staff outcome is turnover. Castle and Engberg (2005) reported NA and licensed practical nurse (LPN) annual turnover rate at 85.5% and RN turnover rate at 55.4% in a study of 354 facilities in four states. Brannon, Zinn, Mor, and Davis (2002) specifically explored NA turnover and discovered a wide variation among 360 facilities in eight states, with a mean for the sample of 51% for a 6-month period and a standard deviation of almost 54%.

Although turnover of clinical staff influences the ongoing surveillance of residents, it has been inconsistently linked to a decreased quality of care (Castle & Engberg, 2005). Several studies prior to this review, cite the belief that staff turnover influences resident outcomes; nonetheless, based on current and past empiric studies specific to the NH setting, this appears to be a premature association (Castle & Engberg). Based on these inconsistencies, Brannon and colleagues (2002) proposed an alternative model to turnover in their exploration of NA turnover. The study proposed that both high and low turnover is an issue. The study hypothesized that turnover is not a linear function and was influenced by many factors. Low turnover was associated with supervisors who lacked management training and union activity, RN turnover was associated with both low and high NA turnover, and high turnover was associated with the NH being a training site and investor ownership.

Although there are inconsistencies in the attempt to associate turnover with resident outcomes, Zimmerman, Gruber-Baldini, Hebel, Sloane, and Magaziner (2002) found an association between RN turnover and resident infections and hospitalization. Horn, Bender, Ferguson, Smout, Bergstron, Taler, et al. (2004) found that an LPN turnover rate of less than 25% was associated with a reduction of stage one pressure ulcers. And several other studies found organizational elements to be associated with turnover. Higher levels of open and accurate communication explained lower LPN and NA turnover. Longer tenure of the DON was also predictive of turnover (Anderson, Corazzini, & McDaniel, 2004; Castle, 2005). Castle suggests that leadership turnover begets staff turnover, again emphasizing the importance of leadership in this setting. Harrington and Swan

(2003) found higher total hours of care per resident day were also associated with lower turnover rates.

Turnover was considered specifically as it relates to the NA role. Bowers, Esmond, and Jacobson (2003) found that appreciation and valuing minimizes NA turnover. However, recognition and appreciation were also associated with the most dissatisfying aspects of the NA role in a study by Parsons, Simmons, Penn, and Furlough (2003) when the NAs did not feel that they had been recognized or appreciated for the contribution, suggesting that recognition and appreciation can be both a powerful satisfier and dissatisfier. In addition, supervision and participation in decision-making were also found to be associated with the most dissatisfying aspects of the NA role (Parsons et al., 2003).

Staffing

As evidence develops related to turnover and the association to resident outcomes, evidence related to adequate staffing also continues to evolve. Many studies have explored the effect of staffing using different NH outcome measures. Three studies reviewed suggested that staffing levels do not influence resident outcomes independent of other issues. Zhang and Grabowski (2004) explored the effect of the NH Reform Act (NHRA) and improved staffing levels for more than 5,000 NHs. The study did not find a significant association between increased staffing and resident outcomes, particularly as it related to those that were deficient prior to the NHRA changes. Harrington, Zimmerman, Karon, Robinson, and Buetel (2000) found that facility characteristics and NH location were stronger predictors of deficiencies than staffing hours and resident characteristics. Moseley and Jones (2003) also had mixed findings about the significance of staffing, particularly RN staffing. They suggested that their insignificant findings may be related to minimal variation in staffing across facilities or mediating organizational variables. Further consideration should also be made to the sensitivity of the outcome measures that were considered (Mueller & Karon, 2004).

The American Nurses Association (ANA) has defined nurse-sensitive outcomes in the NH setting, and these include skill mix of RNs, LPNs, and unlicensed staff members, and total hours provided per resident day (Mueller & Karon, 2004). Harrington (2005a) recently reported that almost one-half of all states in the United States had higher licensed nurse requirements (which may or may not include the RN or the DON according to the state) than the federal minimum requirements, and 64.5% of all states had requirements for NAs when the federal government did not. Twenty-five percent of all states had increased staffing standards between 1999 and 2001. Harrington (2005b) also reported that the actual median nurse staffing levels were substantially higher than each state's standard (2.32 hours per resident day is the average state standard, compared to 3.16 hours per resident day of actual staffing).

Despite the inability to find consistent associations between staffing measures and resident outcomes, four studies did produce significant associations using nurse-sensitive outcome measures. Dorr, Horn, and Smout (2005) demonstrated that an annual net societal benefit of $3,191 per resident per year in high-risk NHs that employed sufficient nurses achieved 30 to 40 minutes of RN direct care per resident per day when compared to NHs that provided less than 10 minutes of direct RN time. Bates-Jensen, Schnelle, Alessi, Al-Samarrai, and Levy-Storms (2004) explored the relationship of staffing to the number of residents who remained in bed. Lower-staffed NHs were six times more likely to have 50% of their observations result in residents remaining in bed regardless of their functional status. Bostick (2004) found a significant relationship between RN and NA hours and pressure ulcer rates; however, the study also found contradictory findings about LPN staffing hours.

Although exploration of staffing routinely addressed the proportion of RNs, LPNs, and NAs, Ryden, Snyder, Gross, Savik, Pearson, Krichbaum, et al. (2000) explored adding an APN to work with newly admitted residents to facilitate evidence-based practice protocols. Residents with APN consultation ($n = 86$) experienced greater improvement or less decline. In addition to exploring associations between staffing variables and resident outcomes, McCarty and Drebing (2002) attempted to link staffing variables to staff members' perceptions of the work and the environment. They considered caregiver burden on an Alzheimer Unit and found that a 5% reduction in staffing levels significantly increased perceived burden.

Summary of Nursing Workforce Findings

It is evident from the literature that turnover is a problem. However, there is wide variation in reported turnover statistics (Brannon et al., 2002; Castle & Engberg, 2005). Although there appears to be great variation in turnover, staffing appeared to be more consistent, with almost one-half of the states exceeding federal licensed nurse requirements minimums and 64.5% of states having minimum standards for NA staffing levels (Harrington, 2005a).

The limitations of minimal variation must be addressed statistically; however, what outcomes should be used to determine the effect of nursing must be further explored. Many of the studies used outcomes that were derived from the federal data sets, such as deficiencies. These data are easily accessible, but both the consistency of these measures across states (Winzelberg, 2003) and the sensitivity of these measures to nursing care are areas for concern. The reality is that NH performance is a complex, multidimensional phenomenon that has eluded current performance measures (Mor, Berg, Angelleli, Gifford, Morris, & Moore, 2003). NH outcome measures must be "tightly linked to clinical actions and accountable for a substantial degree of variation in resident outcomes" (Berg, Mor, Morris, Murphy, Moore, & Harris, 2002; Kerr, Smith, Hogan, Hofer, Krein, Bermann, et al., 2003; Mor et al.). To improve the sensitivity of the measures, researchers should look to studies that considered alternative outcome measures that produced significant results and are directly linked to nursing care. Dorr and colleagues (2005) considered societal benefit in terms of additional dollars spent in unnecessary care and complications, and Bates-Jensen, Cadogen, Osterweil, Levy-Storms, Jorge, Al-Samarrai, et al. (2005) observed the number of residents who remained in bed as a proxy measure of many of the basics of care. Both studies focused on outcome measures that were directly linked to nursing.

An important study that must set the stage for future research is the model proposed by Brannon and colleagues (2002). The model suggested that turnover is not a linear function and that low turnover does not equal a good NH. This is a critical conceptual shift in the exploration of turnover and should be further explored. By explicating the job and organizational factors associated with low turnover, much can be learned about the problems in NH staffing that often go unnoticed or misunderstood. When one considers that extreme staff stability may reflect an absence of functional management, the concept of considering turnover at both extremes becomes more meaningful (Brannon et al.).

SUMMARY OF NURSING HOME ORGANIZATIONAL STUDIES

Several studies alluded to the complex relationship between the organization, the resident, and staffing measures (Harrington et al., 2000; Moseley & Jones, 2003; Zhang & Grabowski, 2004). This suggests that these relationships are challenging to study and articulate with many of the current performance measures. Looking across all the organizational studies, teamwork, communication, and leadership, all are critical in resident and staff outcomes (Table 8.1). Teamwork was found in both the organizational and work force studies to be an important ingredient in affecting both resident and staff outcomes (Anderson et al., 2003; Campbell, 2003; Curry et al., 2000; Lucas et al., 2005; Pennington et al., 2003; Rantz et al., 2004; Scott-Cawiezell et al., in press). Of particular note were the discussions related to participation in decision-making (Anderson et al., 2003; Parsons, Simmons, Penn, & Furlough, 2003).

Communication was also noted to be an important organizational element in considering both resident and staff outcomes. Communication encompassed the openness, accuracy, and respectfulness of the message (Anderson et al., 2003; Anderson et al., 2004; Curry et al., 2000; Lucas et al., 2005; Scott-Cawiezell

TABLE 8.1 Organizational Nursing Home Studies 2000–2005

Author(s), date of publication	Methods	Selected findings
Anderson, Issel, & McDaniel (2003)	Design: exploratory, cross-sectional interviews Sample: NH (n = 164) Variables of interest: communication, decision-making, organization formalization Outcome measure(s): secondary data of 1995 Medicaid cost reports and MDS data	Better resident outcomes were associated with DON tenure and management practices that facilitated openness of communication, participation in decision-making, and relationship-based leadership
Campbell (2003)	Design: exploratory interviews Sample: NH (n = 1) Interviews focused on empowerment and disempowering experiences in their lives and work	Empowering included education, communication, relationships with staff and residents
Castle (2003)	Design: intervention study Sample: NHs (n = 120) Intervention: provision of outcome information Outcome measure(s): restraint use, pressure ulcers, quality of care deficiencies	Clinical feedback reduced use of restraints and quality of care deficiencies
Castle (2001)	Design: descriptive, cross-sectional, secondary data analysis Sample: NHs (n = 420) Variables: NHA turnover, NH ownership status Outcome measure(s): catheterization rates, pressure ulcers, quality of care deficiencies	NHA turnover was associated with higher pressure ulcers, quality of care deficiencies and pressure rates

Source	Design and Sample	Variables/Measures	Findings
Curry, Porter, Mickalski, & Gruman (2000)	Design: descriptive, cross-sectional survey Sample: NAs (n = 254)	Variable of interest: current beliefs about individualizing care	Facilitators included scheduling flexibility, supervisor assistance, participation in care planning, and supervisors open to NA suggestion Barriers included staffing, poor communication, and staff attitudes
Lucas, Avi-Itzhak, Robinson, Morris, Koren, & Reinhard (2005)	Design: descriptive, cross-sectional survey Sample: NHAs (n = 159)	Variables of interest: measures of the environment, organization, NH size Outcome measure(s): adoption of CQI	Predictors to adopting CQI processes included regulation, competition, teamwork, communication, priority, and training
Pennington, Scott, & Magilvy (2003)	Design: descriptive, cross-sectional interviews and observations Sample: NHs (n = 6)	Interviews and observation to examine experiences of NAs; engagement in the work force and what keeps them in the workforce	Important issues: job enrichment, personal growth, recognition, responsibility, and sense of achievement
Rantz, Hicks, Grando, Petroski, Madsen, et al. (2004)	Design: three-group randomized exploratory observational study Sample: NHs (n = 92)	Variables of interest: care delivery processes	Facilities strong in providing the basics of care had active teams, CQI, and leaders with longer tenure
Rantz, Popejoy, Petroski, Madsen, Mehr et al. (2001)	Design: randomized controlled trial Sample: NHs (n = 13)	Intervention: expert clinical consultation Outcome measure(s): selected QIs (23)	Falls, pressure ulcers improved with an expert nurses consultant

(continued)

TABLE 8.1 (*continued*)

Author(s), date of publication	Methods	Selected Findings
Scott-Cawiezell, Main, Vojir, Jones, Moore et al. (in press)	Design: descriptive, cross-sectional survey, interviews, observations, and secondary data analyses Sample: NHs (n = 32) Variables of interest: communication, leadership, teamwork, culture, environment Outcome measure(s): QIs, QMs, perceived effectiveness, state survey citations	High performing homes had leaders with positive view of staff, good communication systems, strong sense of team, and focused internally on standards and setting expectations
Swagerty et al. (2005)	Design: qualitative emergent case study Sample: NHs (n = 3) Interviews and observations focused on contextual factors that integrate or fragment nursing care	Integrating factors included shared values, role of leaders, and family influence Fragmenting factors included competing demands, task orientation, and external accountability
Turnover		
Anderson, Corazzini, & McDaniel (2004)	Design: descriptive, cross-sectional survey Sample: NHs (n = 164) Variables of interest: communication, tenure Outcome measure(s): turnover	Higher levels of communication explained lower turnover of LVN and NA Adequate staffing and longer tenure of DON predicted lower staff turnover
Bowers, Esmond, & Jacobson (2003)	Design: grounded dimensional analysis Sample: NAs (n = 41) Interviews focused on exploring reasons why NAs leave their jobs	NAs perceived that they are underappreciated and undervalued

Reference	Design/Sample	Variables and outcome measures	Findings
Brannon, Zinn, Mor, & Davis (2002)	Design: descriptive, cross-sectional survey Sample: NHs (n = 360)	Variables of interest: job, organization and environmental factors through a high/low turnover model Outcome measure(s): NA turnover	Lower turnover was associated with untrained supervisors, lower RN turnover, and the presence of a NA union Higher turnover was associated with higher RN turnover; being a training site, and investor owned
Castle (2005)	Design: descriptive, cross-sectional survey Sample: NHs (n = 470)	Variables of interest: top management turnover Outcome measure(s): staff turnover	10% increase in top management turnover is associated with an increased probability that NAs and licensed nurse turnover will be high
Castle & Engberg (2005)	Design: descriptive, cross-sectional survey Sample: NHs (n = 526)	Variables of interest: staff turnover Outcome measure(s): restraint use, pressure ulcers, deficiency citations	Some improvement in QMs was associated with RN turnover (particularly moving from low to moderate turnover) and NA and LPN turnover (particularly moderate to high turnover)
Harrington & Swan (2003)	Design: descriptive, cross-sectional Sample: NHs (n = 1,155)	Variables of interest: facility characteristics Outcome measure(s): staffing levels, turnover rates, resident case mix	Total nurse and RN staffing hours were negatively associated with turnover and positively associated with resident case mix Higher total hours per resident day were associated with lower rates
Horn, Bender, Ferguson, Smout, Bergstrom, et al. (2004)	Design: retrospective cohort study Sample: NHs (n = 95)	Variables of interest: resident characteristics, treatment characteristics, staffing Outcome measure(s): prevalence of pressure ulcers	RN hours of 0.025 per day, NA hours of 2 per day, and less than 25% LPN turnover were associated with decreased likelihood of developing stage 1 pressure ulcers

(continued)

TABLE 8.1 (*continued*)

Author(s), date of publication	Methods	Selected Findings
Parsons, Simmons, Penn, & Furlough (2003)	Design: descriptive, cross-sectional survey Sample: NA (n = 550) Variables of interest: NA job satisfaction, work characteristics, work issues Outcome measure(s): turnover	Personal opportunity is the most important variable for predicting turnover
Zimmerman, Gruber-Baldini, Hebel, Sloane, & Magaziner (2002)	Design: descriptive Sample: NHs (n = 59) Variables of interest: turnover, organizational characteristics Outcome measure(s): infection, hospitalization	RN turnover is associated with increased risk of infection and hospitalization
Staffing Levels and Staffing Mix		
Bates-Jensen, Schnelle, Alessi, Al-Samarrai, & Levy-Storms (2004)	Design: descriptive, cross-sectional observation Sample: NH (n = 34) Variables of interest: staffing levels, resident characteristics Outcome measure(s): time in bed for the resident	Staffing levels were associated with time observed in bed for residents
Bostick (2004)	Design: descriptive, cross-sectional Sample: NHs (n = 413) Variables of interest: staffing hours Outcome measure(s): physical restraints and pressure ulcers (MDS data and OSCAR)	Mixed results included higher RN and NA hours associated with lower pressure ulcer prevalence and higher LPN hours associated with higher prevalence of pressure ulcers
Dorr, Horn, & Smout (2005)	Design: retrospective cost study Sample: NHs (n = 82) Variables of interest: costs of care, RN time Outcome measure(s): pressure ulcers, urinary tract infections, hospitalizations	Annual net societal benefit of $3,191 per resident per year in a high-risk, long-stay nursing home that can achieve 30 to 40 minutes of RN direct care time per resident per day

	Design/Sample	Variables of interest/Outcome measures	Findings
Harrington, Zimmerman, Karon, Robinson, & Beutel (2000)	Design: descriptive, cross-sectional Sample: NHs (n = 13,770)	Variables of interest: staffing hours Outcome measure(s): pressure ulcers and deficiencies	Total deficiencies and quality of care deficiencies were associated with fewer NA and RN hours
Harrington (2005a)	Design: descriptive, cross-sectional survey and secondary data analyses Sample: NHs (n = 12,209)	Variables of interest: state minimum and actual staffing levels	Compared to the federal licensed nurse staffing minimum, 24 states had higher standards, and 10 states had lower standards Fifteen states had more RN hours required than the federal standard
Harrington (2005b)	Design: descriptive, cross-sectional secondary data analyses Sample: NHs (n = 12,209)	Variables of interest: state minimum staffing and actual staffing levels	Median nurse staffing levels per resident per day was higher than the average state standard
McCarthy & Debring (2002)	Design: exploratory, longitudinal Sample: NH staff (n = 42) and (n = 34)	Variables of interest: staffing Outcome measure(s): caregiver burden	Professional Caregiver Burden scores increased significantly following 5% reductions in staffing levels
Moseley & Jones (2003)	Design: exploratory, cross-sectional Sample: NHs (n = 28)	Variables of interest: RN staffing Outcome measure(s): deficiencies	Higher RN hours were associated with more quality of life deficiencies Facilities with relatively fewer RNs per LPN had more total and resident assessment deficiencies

(continued)

TABLE 8.1 (*continued*)

Author(s), date of publication	Methods	Selected Findings
Mueller & Karon (2004)	Design: expert survey Sample: LTC experts ($n = 106$)	The majority of experts agree that ANA nurse-sensitive indicators were relevant to LTC; however, some modifications were proposed related to RN influence
Ryden, Snyder, Gross, Savik, Pearson, Krichbaum, et al. (2000)	Intervention: APN implementation of evidence-based protocols Outcome measure(s): pressure ulcers	APN treatment group experienced significantly greater improvements (or less decline)
Zhang & Grabowski (2004)	Variables of interest: staffing Outcome measure(s): pressure ulcers and restraint use	Increased staffing did not directly relate to improvement in quality

Variables of interest: ANA nurse-sensitive QIs

Design: quasi-experimental Sample: NHs ($n = 3$)

Design: descriptive, cross-sectional Sample: NHs ($n = 5,092$)

NH = Nursing Home, NHA = Nursing Home Administrator

et al., in press). Finally, leadership also was noted to be a key element across studies. The tenure of leadership was found to be associated with both resident (Anderson et al., 2003; Castle, 2001; Rantz et al., 2004) and staff outcomes (Anderson et al., 2004; Castle, 2005). Although the tenure of leadership was found to be important, leadership was also articulated as emphasized on staff, clear in expectations and setting high standards, trained and skilled as a leader, involved in day-to-day activities, and appreciative of staff efforts (Brannon et al., 2002; Curry et al., 2000; Pennington et al., 2003; Scott-Cawiezell et al.; Swagerty et al., 2005).

CLINICAL CHALLENGES IN NURSING HOME SAFETY

Understanding what needs to be present in the NH for sustained improvement is critical. Yet changing the organization without a clear understanding of the evidence to make the right improvements leaves NHs at continued risk of providing unsafe care. Although the ANA has proposed pressure ulcers and falls as nurse-sensitive measures in this area, NH researchers and policy makers have focused on five clinical conditions and related processes in the provision of safe NH care: pressure ulcers and falls, limited use of physical and chemical restraints, infections, and medication safety practices (Table 8.2).

As with the NH organizational safety literature, few studies focused on specific safety issues. Many are descriptive and have addressed prevalence and associated factors, while other studies have considered adherence to practice guidelines. Guidelines do exist for the prevention and treatment of pressure ulcers (Agency for Health Care Policy and Research, 1992, 1994), the prevention of falls (American Geriatrics Society, 2001), the control of infections (American Medical Directors Association, 2004; Smith & Rusnak, 1997) and the provision of safe medication administration (Association of Health Systems Pharmacists, 2005). These guidelines provide guidance across settings.

Pressure Ulcers

The first step to providing a safer environment is to be mindful of residents who are at risk so that timely and appropriate prevention and treatment can be completed. Several of the articles in the review of pressure ulcer literature addressed the issue of pressure ulcer prevalence and how risk-adjusted models were explicating the characteristics of residents who should be carefully monitored (Berlowitz, Bezzera, Brandies, Kader, & Anderson, 2000; Berlowitz, Brandies, Anderson, Ash, Kader, Morris, et al., 2001; Berlowitz, Brandies, Morris, Ash, Anderson, Kader, et al., 2001; Coleman, Martau, Lin, & Kramer, 2002; Dellefield, 2004; Horn et al.,

TABLE 8.2 Clinical Challenges in Nursing Home Safety 2000–2005

Author(s), date of publication	Methods	Selected Findings
Pressure Ulcers		
Bates-Jensen, Alessi, Al-Samarrai, & Schnelle (2003)	Design: randomized controlled trial Sample: NHs (n = 4) Intervention: received exercise and incontinence care four times a day and five times a week Outcome measure(s): skin health outcomes	Intervention participants improved in four risk factors; however, there were no differences in the rate of pressure ulcers
Bates-Jensen, Cadogan, Osterweil, Levy-Storms, Jorge, et al. (2003)	Design: descriptive cohort observational and survey Sample: NHs (n = 16) Variables of interest: related care processes Outcome measure(s): 16 QIs related to pressure ulcers, continence, nutrition	There was no difference between high- and low-performing NHs for pressure ulcers on most care processes and neither group routinely repositioned residents every 2 hours despite documentation indicating that repositioning was done
Bates-Jensen, Cadogan, Jorge, & Schnelle (2003)	Design: descriptive observation Sample: NHs (n = 8) Intervention: standardized protocol for pressure ulcers (checklist) and thigh monitoring Outcome measure(s): nine QIs related to pressure ulcer assessment, management	More problems were noted related to the completion of the protocol and documentation for those residents before the pressure ulcer was detected than after detection
Baumgarten, Margolis, van Doorn, Gruber-Baldini, Hebel, et al. (2004)	Design: prospective cohort Sample: NHs (n = 59) Variables of interest: race, other resident characteristics Outcome measure(s): first occurrence of a Stage 2, 3, or 4 pressure ulcer	Incidence of pressure ulcer was 0.38 per resident per year, with the rate for black residents significantly higher when controlling for both resident and organizational characteristics

Study	Design/Sample	Variables/Outcome Measures	Findings
Bergstrom & Braden (2002)	Design: descriptive, longitudinal. Sample: NH residents (n = 843)	Variables of interest: race. Outcomes measure(s): prevalence of pressure ulcers	White residents had a significantly higher incidence of pressure ulcer than did black residents. A score of 18 predicted risk for both groups
Berlowitz, Bezzera, Brandies, Kader, & Anderson (2000)	Design: descriptive, longitudinal. Sample: NHs (n = 107)	Variables of interest: Resident characteristics. Outcome Measure(s): Prevalence of pressure ulcer	A decline of 25% in the incidence of pressure ulcer development was noted over five years with the proportion of new ulcers stage 3 or stage 4 declining
Berlowitz, Brandies, Morris, Ash, Anderson, et al. (2001)	Design: perspective observational. Sample: NHs (n = 100)	Variables of interest: resident characteristics. Outcome measure(s): prevalence of pressure ulcers	17 resident characteristics were found to be associated with pressure ulcer development
Berlowitz Brandies, Anderson, Ash, Kader, et al. (2001)	Design: retrospective. Sample: NHs (n = 108)	Variables of interest: resident characteristics. Outcome measure(s): prevalence of pressure ulcers	Risk adjustment model for pressure ulcer development was validated
Clever, Smith, Bowser, & Monroe (2002)	Design: retrospective. Sample: NH (n = 1)	Intervention: skin cleansing/protectant product. Outcome measure(s): prevalence of pressure ulcers	The observed decrease in the prevalence of pressure ulcers suggests a significant association with consistent application of skin protectant
Coleman, Martau, Lin, & Kramer (2002)	Design: cross-sectional comparison. Sample: NHs (n = 92)	Variables of interest: resident characteristics. Outcome measure(s): pressure ulcer prevalence, stage of pressure ulcers	Unadjusted prevalence rates and prevalence rates for stage two or greater did not differ for two time periods, 5 years apart

(continued)

TABLE 8.2 (*continued*)

Author(s), date of publication	Methods	Selected Findings
Dellefield (2004)	Design: descriptive cross-sectional Sample: NHs (n = 883) Variables of interest: risk factors Outcome measure(s): prevalence of pressure ulcers	Pressure ulcer on admission, difficulty eating independently, difficulty walking, independent transfer, and restraints were all associated with an increased prevalence of pressure ulcers
Geyer, Brienza, Karg, Trefler, & Kelsey (2001)	Design: randomized controlled trial Sample: NHs (n = 2) NH residents (n = 32) Intervention: seating evaluation with pressure mapping and seating prescription using either foam or pressure-reducing mattress Outcome measure(s): prevalence of pressure ulcers, days to ulceration, peak interface pressure	There were no differences between the two devices for prevalence, days to ulceration or peak interface pressure. Pressure was more effective in preventing sitting acquired (ischial) pressure ulcers
Graumlich, Blough, McLaughlin, Milbrandt, Calderon, et al. (2003)	Design: randomized controlled trail Sample: NHs (n = 11) Intervention: collagen and hydrocolloid dressings Outcome measure(s): complete healing, time to heal, area healed	There were no differences in the outcomes, and the collagen is a more expensive alternative
Horn, Bender, Ferguson, Smout, Bergstrom, Taler, et al. (2004)	Design: retrospective cohort Sample: NHs (n = 95) Variables of interest: resident and facility characteristics Outcome measure(s): prevalence of pressure ulcers	Resident characteristics associated with pressure ulcer incidence include initial severity of illness, history of recent pressure ulcer, significant weight loss, oral eating problems, use of catheters, and use of positioning devices

Hunter, Anderson, Hanson, Thompson, Langemo, & Klug (2003)	Design: quasi experimental pretest/posttest Sample: NH residents (n = 136)	Intervention: body wash and skin protectant, early intervention Variables of interest: resident characteristics Outcome measure(s): prevalence of pressure ulcers, use of skin protocol	Significant decrease in skin breakdown (31.6% pre-intervention to 21.3% post-intervention) Significant decrease in stage I and II incidence
Ochs, Horn, van Rijswijk, Pietsch, & Smout (2005)	Design: retrospective Sample: NH residents (n = 664)	Variables of interest: support surfaces Outcome measure(s): healing rates, hospitalization, ED visits	Air fluidized support surfaces represent greater healing potential when compared to static overlays or low-air-loss beds
Vap & Dunaye (2000)	Design: descriptive Sample: NHs (n = 8)	Variables of interest: resident characteristics Outcome measure(s): prevalence of pressure ulcers	MDS had greater predictive ability identifying 311 at risk, resulting in an accurate prediction of 62 of the 66 pressure ulcers, while the Braden Scale only found 172 at risk and predicted only 46 of the 66 pressure ulcers
Viamontes, Temple, Wytall, & Walker (2003)	Design: 5-year retrospective descriptive Sample: NHs (n = 30)	Variables of interest: resident characteristics, wound regiments, assessment processes, product used Outcome measure(s): pressure ulcer stage, rate of healing	There were no differences in rate of healing between adhesive hydrocellular form dressings and self-adherent, soft silicone foam dressings
Wipke-Tevis, Williams, Rantz, Popejoy, Madsen, et al. (2004)	Design: retrospective Sample: NHs (n = 362)	Variables of interest: pressure ulcer prevention and treatment practices Outcome measure(s): pressure ulcer QIs	No relationship was found between the number of prevention strategies or the number of treatment strategies and the pressure ulcer QI scores

(continued)

TABLE 8.2 *(continued)*

Author(s), date of publication	Methods	Selected Findings
	Falls & Restraints	
Avidan, Fries, James, Szafara, Wright, & Chervin (2005)	Design: secondary analysis Sample: NH (n = 437) Variables of interest: insomnia, use of hypnotics, other resident characteristics Outcome measure(s): falls, hip fractures	A history of insomnia predicted falls Hypnotic use did not predict falls
Capezuti, Maislin, Strumpf, & Evans (2002)	Design: prospective, clinical trial Sample: NHs (n = 3) Variables of interest: physical restraint usage, side rail usage, cognitive status Outcome measure(s): bed-related falls	Bilateral side rail use increased and did not reduce the likelihood of falls, recurrent falls, or serious injury Education and RN consultation did not affect the rate of side rail use
Castle (2000)	Design: descriptive Sample: NHs (n = 15,455) and (n = 16,533) Variables of interest: organizational characteristics Outcome measure(s): physical restraint use	Staffing levels of rehabilitative services and chain membership were associated with increases in restraint use
Castle (2002)	Design: longitudinal descriptive Sample: national sample of NHs Variables of interest: resident and organizational characteristics Outcome measure(s): restraint related deficiencies	Persistent poor quality in the use of restraints was negatively associated with higher staffing levels and positively associated higher ADL levels

Source	Design and Sample	Variables and Outcome Measures	Findings
Dunn (2001)	Design: ex post facto descriptive Sample: NH residents (n = 97)	Variables of interest: use of restraints Outcome measure(s): falls, injuries	There were no significant changes in falls rates, but falls that occurred after the reduction of restraints resulted in less injury
Harrison, Booth, & Algase (2001)	Design: cross-sectional Sample: NH residents (n = 67)	Variables of interest: risk factors for falls, mental assessments Outcome measure(s): falls, injuries	Number of falls increased as cognitive ability decreased; however, residents without dementia fell more often than those without dementia
Miceli, Strumpf, Reinhard, Zanna, & Fritz (2004)	Design: descriptive, cross-sectional Sample: NHs (n = 149)	Variables of interest: post-assessment fall tools	Approaches to post-fall assessment are inconsistent and do not reflect use of the guidelines
Ooi, Hossain, & Lipsitz (2000)	Design: descriptive, cohort Sample: NHs (n = 40)	Variables of interest: orthostatic blood pressure Outcome measure(s): recurrent falls	A history of falls and orthostatic hypotension suggested an increased risk of recurrent falls
van Doorn, Gruber-Baldini, Zimmerman, Hebel, Port, et al. (2003)	Design: prospective, cohort Sample: NHs (n = 59)	Variables of interest: dementia, Outcome measure(s): falls, injuries	Residents with dementia had a greater number of falls compared to residents without dementia Falls occurring to residents with dementia were no more likely to result in injury than falls to those without dementia
Barry, Brown, Esker, Denning, Kruse, & Binder (2002)	Design: descriptive, cross-sectional Sample: NHs (n = 12)	Variables of interest: facility characteristics Outcome measure(s): prevalence assessment with acute change	Only 52% of residents identified as acutely ill received some type of physical assessment

(continued)

TABLE 8.2 (continued)

Author(s), date of publication	Methods	Selected Findings
Infections		
Bockvar, Gruber-Baldini, Burton, Zimmerman, May, & Magaziner (2005)	Design: descriptive Sample: NHs ($n = 59$) Variables of interest: hospital transfer, infection, resident and nursing home characteristics Outcome measure(s): outcomes of infection that included pressure ulcers and death	Residents with infections who received an early hospital transfer had higher mortality rates
Longo, Young, Mehr, Lindbloom, & Salerno (2004)	Design: qualitative Sample: NHs ($n = 4$) What is the process of illness identification and initiating management in episodes of acute infection?	Four distinct stages to illness recognition: sign and symptom recognition, illness identification, physician notification, and treatment Barriers to timely care: failure of communication, evening or weekend illness and difficulty in contacting the on-call physician, and communication of inappropriate or inaccurate information
Trick, Weinstein, DeMarais, Tomaska, Nathan, et al. (2004)	Design: quasi-experimental Sample: NH residents ($n = 156$) Intervention: glove use, isolation precautions Outcome measure(s): resident acquisition of four resistant organisms	Resident acquisition of antimicrobial-resistant organisms was no different in the glove use and isolation-precautions sections

Barker, Flynn, Pepper, Bates, & Mikeal (2002)	Design: prospective cohort Sample: hospitals (n = 24) NHs (n = 12)	Outcome measure(s): prevalence of medication error	19% of total doses in error of which 43% were wrong time, 30% were omitted, 17% were wrong doses, and 4% were unauthorized 7% were potential ADEs
Boockvar, Fishman, Kyriacou, Monias, Gavi, & Cortes (2004)	Design: descriptive, Sample: NH (n = 4)	Variables of interest: hospital to nursing homes transfers Outcome measure(s): Medication changes, ADEs	ADEs attributable to medication changes occurred during 20% of bi-directional transfers
Briesacher, Limcango, Simoni-Wastila, Doshi, & Gurwitz (2005)	Design: quasi-experimental, longitudinal Sample: national sample of NH residents (n = 2,242)	Variables of interest: drug use review Outcome measure(s): prevalence and incidence of use of 38 potentially inappropriate medications	Multivariate results detected no differences in inappropriate drug usage between NHs mandated to review and assisted living facilities who were not mandated to review
Gurwitz, Field, Avron, McCormick, Jain, Eckler, et al. (2000)	Design: descriptive, cohort Sample: NHs (n = 18)	Variables of interest: categories of medications, drug related incidents, symptoms related to potential ADEs, medication process Outcome measure(s): ADEs	546 ADEs and 188 potential ADEs 51% were judged to be preventable Errors resulting from preventable ADEs occurred most often with prescribing and monitoring

(continued)

TABLE 8.2 (continued)

Author(s), date of publication	Methods	Selected Findings
Gurwitz, Field, Judge, Rochon, Harrold, Cadoret, et al. (2005)	Design: cohort, case control nested within the prospective study Sample: NH residents ($n = 1,247$) Variables of interest: categories of medications, medication process Outcome measure(s): ADEs, severity of events	815 ADEs were found, of which 42% were judged to be preventable Errors associated with ADEs occurred most often at the stage of prescribing and monitoring Residents taking medications in several drug classes were most at risk
Perri, Menon, Deshpande, Shinde, Jiang, et al. (2005)	Design: cohort Sample: NHs ($n = 15$) Variables of interest: prevalence of inappropriate medications by Beers's criteria Outcome measure(s): ADEs, hospitalization, ED visits, death	Total number of medications increases likelihood of receiving an inappropriate medication which, in turn, increased the likelihood of an ADE Diagnosis of dementia decreased the likelihood of receiving an inappropriate medication Propoxyphene (Darvocet) was significantly associated with the occurrence of an ADE
Vogelsmeier, Scott-Cawiezell, & Zellmer (in press)	Design: qualitative focus groups and key informant interviews Sample: NHs ($n = 5$) What are your current concerns related to medication administration processes in the NH?	Common themes included issues related to communication, competing demands, and the challenges of a paper based system Concerns were often associated with the timeliness and accuracy of the current medication administration process

2004). Seventeen resident characteristics were tested and validated in two studies that considered almost 28,000 residents and pressure ulcer development. Key characteristics included dependence in mobility and transferring, diabetes mellitus, peripheral vascular disease, urinary incontinence, lower body mass index, and end-stage disease (Berlowitz, Brandies, Anderson et al.; Berlowitz, Brandies, Morris et al.). Race was explored as another risk factor, and it was noted that black residents have a higher incidence of pressure ulcers than white residents (Baumgarten, Margolis, van Doorn, Gruber-Baldini, Hebel, Zimmerman, et al., 2004). In addition, Horn and colleagues (2004) found higher severity of illness, history of a recent pressure ulcer, weight loss, oral eating problems, and the use of catheters or positioning devices were also associated with an increased prevalence of pressure ulcers. Factors associated with a decreased prevalence of pressure ulcers were nutritional interventions and use of antidepressants and disposable briefs.

Both the Braden Scale (a widely used resident skin risk assessment tool) and the minimum data set (MDS) standardized pressure ulcer assessment were further explored as risk assessment tools. One study compared the Braden Scale's predictive validity to the MDS (Vap & Dunaye, 2000), and another studied the predictive ability of the Braden Scale among both white and black residents (Bergstorm & Braden, 2002). The Braden Scale's predictive ability was brought into question with the MDS, predicting 62 of 66 residents who developed pressure ulcers, while the Braden Scale only predicted 46 of the 66 residents. A later study found no differences in the Braden Scale's predictive abilities between black and white residents and indicated that a score of 18 can be used to identify risk in both races (Bergstorm & Braden). Further exploration of the MDS pressure ulcer assessment found that the standardized assessment (nine related QIs) provided explicit scoring that was useful for both the external survey process and internal quality improvement efforts (Bates-Jensen, Cadogan, Jorge, & Schnelle, 2003).

The pressure ulcer guidelines supported by AHRQ have been available for more than a decade, and they consider assessment a critical component of the pressure ulcer prevention and treatment. Bates-Jensen, Cadogan, Jorge, et al. (2003) found that only after pressure ulcers were detected did adherence to the protocol and documentation improve. Similar findings were noted by Wipke-Tevis, Williams, Rantz, Popejoy, Madsen, Petroski, et al. (2004) who found that pressure ulcer risk assessment tools were under-used and that evidence-based guidelines were rarely implemented.

Several studies tested different aspects of pressure ulcer care. Interventions with no differences between groups included exercise and incontinence care (Bates-Jensen, Alessi, Al-Samarrai, & Schnelle, 2003), alternative sitting devices (Geyer, Brienza, Karg, Trefler, & Kelsey, 2001), and various dressing supplies (Graumlich, Blough, McLaughlin, Milbrandt, Claderon, Agha, et al., 2003; Viamontes, Temple, Wytall, & Walker, 2003). There were decreases in the prevalence of pressure ulcers noted with the use of skin protectant and cleansing

(Clever, Smith, Bowser, & Monroe, 2002; Hunter, Anderson, Hanson, Thompson, Langemom & Klug, 2003) and air fluidized support surfaces (Ochs, Horn, van Rijswijk, Pietsch, & Smout, 2005). In addition to exploring particular interventions, Bates-Jensen, Cadogan, Osterweil, et al. (2003) looked at the differences in practice between high and low performing NHs. There was no difference between high- and low-performing NHs for pressure ulcers on most care processes and neither routinely repositioned residents every two hours despite documentation indicating that repositioning was done.

Falls and Restraints

The fall and restraint literature is limited for the past 5 years. The studies that exist focused on prevalence, associated risk factors, and the interaction of restraint usage and fall prevalence. Capezuti, Maislin, Strumpf, and Evans (2002) found that the use of bilateral side rails had significantly increased over the 1-year study and did not significantly reduce the likelihood of falls, recurrent falls, or serious injury. This affirms that bilateral side rails do not promote a safer environment for the resident. Dunn (2001) found that falls that occurred after the reduction of restraints resulted in less injury.

Assessment of risk factors and identification of associated risk factors were explored in four studies. Miceli, Strumpf, Reinhard, Zanna, and Fritz (2004) found that, despite recommendations in the geriatric literature about post-fall assessment, these assessments were inconsistent. Three other studies explored associated risk factors. Harrison, Booth, and Algase (2001) found a decline in cognition was associated with more falls; yet residents with mild dementia had a lower number of falls than those who did not have dementia, suggesting that the relationship between cognition and falling was not linear. Contrary to this, van Doorn, Gruber-Baldini, Zimmerman, Hebel, Port, Baumgarten, et al. (2003) found that residents with dementia had increased falls. Ooi, Hossain, and Lipsitz (2000) found that orthostatic hypotension was not associated with subsequent falls. However, there was increased risk for recurrent falls among residents with a history of previous falls who had orthostatic hypotension. Avidan, Fries, James, Szafara, Wright, and Chervin (2005) found that insomnia predicted future falls, but the use of hypnotics did not, and that untreated insomnia and those who remained unresponsive to hypnotic-treated insomnia also had more falls.

Two studies exclusively focused on restraints. Castle looked at the difference in restraint usage and organization characteristics (2000) and NHs with persistent deficiencies in restraint usage (2002). Both studies found that, despite policy changes that should be driving the use of restraints to a minimum, usage in some NHs was actually going up.

Infections

The literature for the review on infections was limited, and no articles addressed the prevalence of infections. The four studies considered a broad range of interventions related to residents with acute infections. The interventions ranged from early hospital transfer, which was found to have a higher mortality rate for NH residents (Boockvar, Gruber-Baldini, Burton, Zimmerman, May, & Magaziner, 2005), to glove or contact isolation use, which produced no differences in the acquisition of resistant infections (Trick, Weinstein, DeMarais, Tomaska, Nathan, McAllister, et al., 2004). Barry, Brown, Esker, Denning, Kruse, and Binder (2002) addressed the issue of limited physical assessments related to acute changes in residents with infection, finding only 52% of the residents were assessed. Longo, Young, Mehr, Lindbloom, and Salerno (2004) determined that there were four stages to illness recognition and action for NH staff: sign and symptom recognition, illness identification, physician notification, and treatment. They also found that there were consistent barriers to treatment for residents with acute infection, which included failure of communication with inappropriate and inaccurate information and evening or weekend illness and led to on-call physicians who did not know the resident.

Medication Administration

Medication administration literature was the only body of NH literature to truly address the concept of error and the related adverse drug events (ADEs). Barker, Flynn, Pepper, Bates, and Mikeal (2002) identified the prevalence of medication errors in 36 hospitals and NHs and found no differences in the setting-specific error rates. Across the settings, 19% of the doses were given in error, with 43% of the medication errors being wrong time errors. The study also found that 7% of the errors were judged to be potential ADEs.

Two additional studies explored the prevalence of ADEs in the NH setting. Gurwitz, Field, Judge, Rochon, Harrold, Cadoret, et al. (2005) found an ADE rate of 9.8 per 100 resident months, and 42% of the ADEs were judged as preventable. In an earlier study by Gurwitz, Field, Avorn, McCormick, Jain, Eckler, et al. (2000), the ADE rate was found to be 1.89 per 100 resident months, and 51% of those ADEs were judged as preventable. In both studies, ADEs were associated with ordering and monitoring of medications and the delivery of psychoactive and anticoagulant medications. Boockvar, Fishman, Kyriacou, Monias, Gavi and Cortes (2004) considered the effect of transfer between acute and long-term care facilities and ADEs. Among the 72 bidirectional transfers, ADEs attributable to medication changes occurred during 20% of the transfers.

The standard of care has been established, and a regulation has been created to perform monthly reviews of residents' medications to assess for inappropriate medications for the elderly (Beers, 1997). Briesacher, Limcango, Simoni-Wastila, Doshi, and Gurwitz (2005) detected no differences in inappropriate drugs ordered between NHs mandated to review and assisted living facilities, which were not mandated to review, suggesting that despite policy changes, the use of inappropriate medications in the elderly continues. Perri, Menon, Deshpande, Shinde, Jiang, Cooper, et al. (2005) found that 46.5% of residents reviewed had received at least one inappropriate medication, resulting in 143 ADEs. The total number of medications that residents received increased the likelihood that they would receive an inappropriate medication, while dementia decreased the likelihood that they would receive an inappropriate medication. Only one study considered the nursing staff members' perspective on the provision of safe medication administration. Vogelsmeier, Scott-Cawiezell, and Zellmer (in press) explored the barriers to safe medication administration across the five nodes of the medication process. Key findings included reports of ineffective communication between NH staff and pharmacy as well as other system failures within the medication distribution and bedside medication administration processes. In addition, the qualitative study provided insight into how the RN viewed measures of a successful medication pass (accuracy) when compared with that of the certified medication technician (timeliness).

SUMMARY OF THE CLINICAL LITERATURE

The review of the clinical literature did not provide direction to many changes in practice in terms of devices or procedures (Bates-Jensen, Alessi, et al., 2003; Geyer et al., 2001; Graumlich et al., 2003; Viamontes et al., 2003). One theme, critical to nursing practice, was consistent across the clinical topics: inconsistent assessment at critical points in the residents' care for prevention and timely treatment of potentially dangerous conditions despite evidence to suggest there were risk factors that should be closely monitored (Bates-Jensen, Cadogan, Jorge, et al., 2003; Bates-Jensen, Cadogan, Osterweil, et al., 2003; Gurwitz et al., 2000, 2005; Longo et al., 2004; Miceli et al., 2004; Wipke-Tevis et al., 2004).

It was clear that the risk factors associated with the development of pressure ulcers were clearly explicated (Barker et al., 2002; Barry et al., 2002; Baumgarten et al., 2004; Berlowitz, Brandies, Anderson, et al., 2001; Berlowitz, Brandies, Morris, et al., 2001; Horn et al., 2004). In addition, there was an effective assessment mechanism using the MDS skin risk assessment items validated for its predictive abilities (Bates-Jensen, Cadogan, Jorge, et al., 2003; Vap & Dunaye, 2000) and another tool, the Braden Scale, that, although frequently used, was found to be less consistent in its predictive abilities (Bergstorm & Braden, 2002). Although the risk factors associated with falls were not as clearly explicated (Avidan et al., 2005; Harrison et al., 2001; Ooi et al., 2000; van Doorn et al., 2003), recommendations indicated that both initial risk assessments for falling and post-fall assessments are critical. The review of both infections and medication safety also suggested that acute changes were going undetected, which lead to rapid deterioration related to infections (Barry et al., 2002; Longo et al., 2004) or undetected ADEs (Barker et al., 2002; Gurwitz et al., 2000, 2005).

GENERAL OBSERVATIONS ON THE STATE OF NURSING HOME SAFETY

Synthesizing the organizational and clinical safety literature for the NH setting has provided the opportunity to explore both organizational and clinical evidence to guide the next steps for nurses and nursing leadership in the NH setting. Although Longo and colleagues (2004) were focused on acute infections, their qualitative study provides insight into a great challenge for NHs in terms of illness or risk recognition and action. Building on the findings of other studies, which suggested assessment was inconsistent in this setting, they explored the barriers for getting treatment for residents. These barriers were closely related to gaps noted in the organizational review and included failed communication, inappropriate and inaccurate information, and a lack of teamwork among providers.

Timely communication of resident status changes and ongoing monitoring of residents for subtle changes is critical to abate deterioration and prevent unnecessary decline. Moseley and Jones (2003) did find an association with the proportion of RNs to LPNs and assessment deficiencies, and Harrington and colleagues (2000) did associate lower RN and NA staffing with increasing deficiencies. A basic understanding of clinical roles and education preparation suggest that the RN is critical to the assessment process. Recognizing that there is a serious lack of assessment in the NH setting, nurse leaders must evaluate the most effective and appropriate use of RNs and APNs in a fiscally constrained environment.

Providing safe care to residents in the NH requires a sound understanding of current clinical evidence, well designed clinical systems, mindful staff members, and an environment in which safety concerns can be discussed for ongoing improvement to occur. According to the review of the literature, there are both organizational and clinical lessons to be learned so that NHs can continue to develop a culture of safety to provide the best possible care to the residents that they serve. Open, accurate, and timely communication among staff members is essential for the communication of information about residents at risk. More effective use of RN and APN time must be explored to ensure that timely and appropriate assessment is occurring to detect risk factors and abate the consequences of acute changes.

Although the literature on staffing remains inconsistent, the value role of the RN in this setting is clear in the many assessment issues noted and the lack of adherence to recognized practice guidelines.

IMPLICATIONS OF THE STUDIES REVIEWED FOR FUTURE RESEARCH

The implications for future research are three-fold. First, the role of the RN in this setting must be more clearly explicated to ensure that residents are receiving timely and appropriate assessment and safe care according to recognized standards. To explicate the role of the RN, better outcome measures must be developed that are nurse sensitive. A second clear agenda for NH research is the explication of the role of leadership, particularly nursing leadership, to create an environment where open and accurate communication can be accomplished among all of the diverse NH roles so that opportunities to improve care can be identified by all members of the team. Finally, a new frontier for the NH setting is the use of technology and the need to harness the information that has set in the NH system for years. Information mastery for staff and leadership is a necessary aspect of the organization that must be developed to provide sound information for strategic and focused change to occur.

ACKNOWLEDGMENTS

The authors want to thank David Zellmer for his diligence in supporting the development of this chapter.

REFERENCES

Agency for Health Care Policy and Research. (1992). *Pressure ulcers in adults: Prediction and prevention.* Rockville, MD: U.S. Department of Health and Human Services. Publication No. 92-0047.

Agency for Health Care Policy and Research. (1994). *Treatment of pressure ulcers.* Rockville, MD: U.S. Department of Health and Human Services Publication No. 95-0652.

American Geriatric Society. (2001). Guidelines for the prevention of falls in older persons. *Journal of the American Geriatric Society, 49*(5), 664–672.

American Medical Directors Association. (2004). *Common infections in the long term care setting.* Columbia, MD: American Medical Directors Association.

Anderson, R. A., Corazzini, K. N., & McDaniel, R. R. (2004). Complexity science and the dynamics of climate and communication: Reducing nursing home turnover. *The Gerontologist, 44*(3), 378–388.

Anderson, R. A., Issel, L. M., & McDaniel, R. R. (2003). Nursing homes as complex adaptive systems: Relationship between management practice and resident outcomes. *Nursing Research, 52*(1), 12–21.

Association of Health Systems Pharmacists. (2005). *ASHP guidelines.* Retrieved August 11, 2005, from www.ashp.org/bestpractices/guidelines

Avidan, A. Y., Fries, B. E., James, M. L., Szafara, K. L., Wright, G. T., & Chervin, R. D. (2005). Insomnia and hypnotic use recorded in the minimum data set, as predictors of falls and hip fractures in Michigan nursing homes. *Journal of the American Geriatrics Society, 53*(6), 955–962.

Barker, K. N., Flynn, E. A., Pepper, G. A., Bates, D. W., & Mikeal, R. L. (2002). Medication errors observed in 36 health care facilities. *Archives of Internal Medicine, 162*(16), 1897–1903.

Barry, C. R., Brown, K., Esker, D., Denning, M. D., Kruse, R. L., & Binder, E. F. (2002). Nursing assessment of ill nursing home residents. *Journal of Gerontological Nursing, 28*(5), 4–7.

Bates, D., Cullen, D., Laird, N., Petersen, L., Small, S., Servi, R., et al. (1995). Incidence of adverse drug events and potential adverse drug events. *Journal of the American Medical Association, 274*(1), 29–34.

Bates-Jensen, B. M., Alessi, C. A., Al-Samarrai, N. R., & Schnelle, J. F. (2003). The effects of an exercise and incontinence intervention on skin health outcomes in nursing home residents. *Journal of the American Geriatrics Society, 51*(3), 348–355.

Bates-Jensen, B. M., Cadogan, M., Jorge, J., & Schnelle, J. F. (2003). Standardized quality-assessment system to evaluate pressure ulcer care in the nursing home. *Journal of the American Geriatrics Society, 51*(9), 1195–1202.

Bates-Jensen, B. M., Cadogan, M., Osterweil, D., Levy-Storms, L., Jorge, J., Al-Samarrai, N., et al. (2003). The minimum data set pressure ulcer indicator: Does it reflect differences in care processes related to pressure ulcer prevention and treatment in nursing homes? *Journal of the American Geriatrics Society, 51*(9), 1203–1212.

Bates-Jensen, B. M., Schnelle, J. F., Alessi, C. A., Al-Samarrai, N. R., & Levy-Storms, L. (2004). The effects of staffing on in-bed times of nursing home residents. *Journal of the American Geriatrics Society, 52*(6), 931–938.

Baumgarten, M., Margolis, D., van Doorn, C., Gruber-Baldini, A. L., Hebel, J. R., Zimmerman, S., et al. (2004). Black/white differences in pressure ulcer incidence in nursing home residents. *Journal of the American Geriatrics Society, 52*(8), 1293–1298.

Beers, M. (1997). Explicit criteria for determining potentially inappropriate medication use by the elderly. *Archives of Internal Medicine, 157*(14), 1531–1536.

Berg, K., Mor, V., Morris, J., Murphy, K., Moore, T., & Harris, Y. (2002). Identification and evaluation of existing nursing home quality indicators. *Health Care Financing Review, 23*(4), 19–36.

Bergstrom, N., & Braden, B. B. (2002). Predictive validity of the Braden Scale among black and white subjects. *Nursing Research, 51*(6), 398–403.

Berlowitz, D. R., Bezerra, H. Q., Brandeis, G. H., Kader, B., & Anderson, J. J. (2000). Are we improving the quality of nursing home care: The case of pressure ulcers. *Journal of the American Geriatrics Society, 48*(1), 59–62.

Berlowitz, D. R., Brandeis, G. H., Anderson, J. J, Ash, A. S., Kader, B., Morris, J. N., et al. (2001). Evaluation of a risk-adjustment model for pressure ulcer development using the minimum data set. *Journal of the American Geriatrics Society, 49*(7), 872–876.

Berlowitz, D. R., Brandeis, G. H., Morris, J. N., Ash, A. S., Anderson, J. J., Kader, B., et al. (2001). Deriving a risk-adjustment model for pressure ulcer development using the minimum data set. *Journal of the American Geriatrics Society, 49*(7), 866–871.

Boockvar, K., Fishman, E., Kyriacou, C. K., Monias, A., Gavi, S., & Cortes, T. (2004). Adverse events due to discontinuations in drug use and dose changes in patients transferred between acute and long term care facilities. *Archives of Internal Medicine, 164*(5), 545–550.

Boockvar, K. S., Gruber-Baldini, A. L., Burton, L., Zimmerman, S., May, C., & Magaziner, J. (2005). Outcomes of infection in nursing home residents with and without early hospital transfer. *Journal of the American Geriatrics Society, 53*(4), 590–596.

Bostick, J. E. (2004). Relationship of nursing personnel and nursing home care quality. *Journal of Nursing Care Quality, 19*(2), 130–136.

Bowers, B. J., Esmond, S., & Jacobson, N. (2003). Turnover reinterpreted: CNAs talk about why they leave. *Journal of Gerontological Nursing, 29*(3), 36–43.

Brannon, D., Zinn, J. S., Mor, V., & Davis, J. (2002). An exploration of job, organizational, and environmental factors associated with high and low nursing assistant turnover. *The Gerontologist, 42*(2), 159–168.

Briesacher, B., Limcango, R., Simoni-Wastila, L., Doshi, J., & Gurwitz, J. (2005). Evaluation of nationally mandated drug use reviews to improve patient safety in nursing homes: A natural experiment. *Journal of the American Geriatrics Society, 53*(6), 991–996.

Campbell, S. L. (2003). Empowering nursing staff and residents in long-term care. *Geriatric Nursing, 24*(3), 170–175.

Capezuti, E., Maislin, G., Strumpf, N., & Evans, L. K. (2002). Side rail use and bed-related fall outcomes among nursing home residents. *Journal of the American Geriatrics Society, 50*(1), 90–96.

Castle, N. G. (2000). Differences in nursing homes with increasing and decreasing use of physical restraints. *Medical Care, 38*(12), 1154–1163.

Castle, N. G. (2001). Administrator turnover and quality of care in nursing homes. *The Gerontologist, 41*(6), 757–767.

Castle, N. G. (2002). Nursing homes with persistent deficiency citations for physical restraint use. *Medical Care, 40*(10), 868–878.

Castle, N.G. (2003). Providing outcomes information to nursing homes: Can it improve quality of care? *The Gerontologist, 43*(4), 483–492.

Castle, N. G. (2005). Turnover begets turnover. *The Gerontologist, 45*(2), 186–195.

Castle, N. G., & Engberg, J. (2005). Staff turnover and quality of care in nursing homes. *Medical Care, 43*(6), 616–626.

Clever, K., Smith, G., Bowser, C., & Monroe, K. (2002). Evaluating the efficacy of a uniquely delivered skin protectant and its effect on the formation of sacral/buttock pressure ulcers. *Ostomy Wound Management, 48*(12), 60–67.

Coleman, E. A., Martua, J. M., Lin, M. K., & Kramer, A. M. (2002). Pressure ulcers prevalence in long term nursing home residents since the implementation of OBRA'87. *Journal of the American Geriatric Society, 50*(4), 728–732.

Curry, L., Porter, M., Michalski, M., & Gruman, C. (2000). Individualized care: Perceptions of certified nurse's aides. *Journal of Gerontological Nursing, 26*(7), 45–51.

Dellefield, M. E. (2004). Prevalence rate of pressure ulcers in California nursing homes: Using the OSCAR database to develop a risk-adjustment model. *Journal of Gerontological Nursing, 31*(11) 13–21.

Dorr, D. A., Horn, S. D., & Smout, R. J. (2005). Cost analysis of nursing home registered nurse staffing times. *Journal of the American Geriatrics Society, 53*(5), 840–845.

Dunn, K. S. (2001). The effect of physical restraints on fall rates in older adults who are institutionalized. *Journal of Gerontological Nursing, 27*(10), 41–48.

Geyer, M. J., Brienza, D. M., Karg, P., Trefler, E., & Kelsey, S. (2001). A randomized control trial to evaluate pressure-reducing seat cushions for elderly wheelchair users. *Advances in Skin & Wound Care, 14*(3), 120–129.

Graumlich, J. F., Blough, L. S., McLaughlin, R. G., Milbrandt., J. C., Claderon, C. L., Agha, S. A., et al. (2003). Healing pressure ulcers with collagen or hydrocolloid: A randomized clinical trail. *Journal of the American Geriatric Society, 51*(2), 147–154.

Gurwitz, J. H., Field, T. S., Avorn, J., McCormick, D., Jain, S., Eckler, M., et al. (2000). Incidence and preventability of adverse drug events in nursing homes. *The American Journal of Medicine, 109*, 87–94.

Gurwitz, J. H., Field, T. S., Judge, J., Rochon, P., Harrold, L. R., Cadoret, C., et al. (2005). The incidence of adverse drug events in two large academic long-term care facilities. *The American Journal of Medicine, 118*(3), 251–258.

Harrington, C. (2005a). Nurse staffing in nursing homes in the United States: Part 1. *Journal of Gerontological Nursing, 31*(2), 18–23.

Harrington, C. (2005b). Nurse staffing in nursing homes in the United States: Part 2. *Journal of Gerontological Nursing, 31*(3), 9–15.

Harrington, C., & Swan, J. H. (2003). Nursing home staffing, turnover, and case mix. *Medical Care Research and Review, 60*(3), 366–392.

Harrington, C., Zimmerman, D., Karon, S. L., Robinson, J., & Beutel, P. (2000). Nursing home staffing and its relationship to deficiencies. *Journal of Gerontology, 55B*(5), S278–S287.

Harrison, B., Booth, D., & Algase, D. (2001). Studying fall risk factors among nursing home residents who fell. *Journal of Gerontological Nursing, 27*(10), 26–34.

Horn, S. D., Bender, S. A., Ferguson, M. L., Smout, R. J., Bergstrom, N., Taler, G., et al. (2004). The national pressure ulcer long-term care study: Pressure ulcer development in long-term care residents. *Journal of the American Geriatrics Society, 52*(3), 259–367.

Hunter, S., Anderson, J., Hanson, D., Thompson, P., Langemo, D., & Klug, M. (2003). *Journal of Wound Ostomy Continence Nursing, 30*(5), 250–258.

Institute of Medicine. (1999). *To err is human: Building a safer health system.* Washington, DC: National Academy Press.

Kaushal, R., Bates, D. W., Landrigan, C., McKena, K. J., Clapp, M. D., Federico, F., et al. (2001). Medication errors and adverse events in pediatric inpatients. *Journal of the American Medical Association, 285*(16), 2114–2120.

Kerr, E. A., Smith, D. M., Hogan, M. M., Hofer, T. P., Krein, S. L., Bermann, M., et al. (2003). Building a better quality measure: Are some patients with poor quality actually getting good care? *Medical Care, 41*(10), 1173–1182.

Leape, L. L., & Berwick, D. M. (2005). Five years after to Err is Human: What have we learned? *Journal of the American Medical Association, 293*(19), 2384–2390.

Longo, D. R., Young, J., Mehr, D., Lindbloom, E., & Salerno, L. D. (2004). Barriers to timely care of acute infections in nursing homes: a preliminary qualitative study. *Journal of the American Medical Directors Association, 5*, S5–S10.

Lucas, J. A., Avi-Itzhak, T., Robinson, J. P., Morris, C. G., Koren, M. J., & Reinhard, S. C. (2005). Continuous quality improvement as an innovation: Which nursing facilities adopt it? *The Gerontologist, 45*(1), 68–77.

McCarty, E. F., & Drebing, C. (2002). Burden and professional caregivers: Tracking the impact. *Journal for Nurses in Staff Development, 18*(5), 250–257.

Miceli, D., Strumpf, N., Reinhard, S., Zanna, M., & Fritz, E. (2004). Current approaches to postfall assessment in nursing homes. *Journal of the American Medical Directors Association, 5*(6), 387–394.

Mor, V., Berg, K., Angelleli, J., Gifford, D., Morris, J., & Moore T. (2003). The quality of quality measurement in U.S. nursing homes. *Gerontologist, 43*(Suppl. 2), 37–46.

Moseley, C. B., & Jones, L. (2003). Registered nurse staffing and OBRA deficiencies in Nevada nursing facilities. *Journal of Gerontological Nursing, 29*(3), 44–50.

Mueller, C. & Karon, S. L. (2004). ANA nurse sensitive quality indicators for long-term care facilities. *Journal of Nursing Care Quality, 19*(1), 39–47.

Ochs, R. F., Horn, S. D., van Rijswijk, L., Pietsch, C., & Smout, R. J. (2005). Comparison of air-fluidized therapy with other support surfaces used to treat pressure ulcers in nursing home residents. *Ostomy Wound Management, 51*(2), 38–68.

Ooi, W. L., Hossain, M., & Lipsitz, L. A. (2000). The association between orthostatic hypotension and recurrent falls in nursing home residents. *The American Journal of Medicine, 108*, 106–111.

Parsons, S. K., Simmons, W. P., Penn, K., & Furlough, M. (2003). Determinants of satisfaction and turnover among nursing assistants: The results of a statewide survey. *Journal of Gerontological Nursing, 29*(3), 51–58.

Pennington, K., Scott, J., & Magilvy, K. (2003). The role of certified nursing assistants in nursing homes. *Journal of Nursing Administration, 33*(11), 578–584.

Perri, M., Menon, A. M., Deshpande, A. D., Shinde, S. B., Jiang, R., Cooper, J. W., et al. (2005). Adverse outcomes associated with inappropriate drug use in nursing homes. *The Annuals of Pharmacotherapy, 39*, 405–411.

Rantz, M. J., Hicks, L., Grando, V., Petroski, G. F., Madsen, R. W., Mehr, D. R., et al. (2004). Nursing home quality, cost, staffing, and staff mix. *The Gerontologist, 44*(1), 24–38.

Rantz, M. J., Popejoy, L., Petroski, G. F., Madsen, R. W., Mehr, D. R., Zwygart-Stauffacher, M., et al. (2001). Randomized clinical trial of a quality improvement intervention in nursing homes. *The Gerontologist, 41*(4), 525–538.

Ryden, M. B., Snyder, M., Gross, C. R., Savik, K., Pearson, V., Krichbaum, K., et al. (2000). Value-added outcomes: The use of advanced practice nurses in long-term care facilities. *The Gerontologist, 40*(6), 654–662.

Scott-Cawiezell, J. (2005). [Underlying causes of communication barriers and systems failures influencing nursing home medication safety practices]. Unpublished raw data.

Scott-Cawiezell, J., Main, D. S., Vojir, C. P., Jones, K., Moore L., Nutting, P. A., et al. (in press). Linking nursing home working conditions and organizational performance. *Healthcare Management Review.*

Smith, P., & Rusnak, P. (1997). APIC guidelines for infection prevention and control in long term care. *American Journal of Infection Control, 25*(6), 488–512.

Swagerty, D. L., Lee, R. H., Smith, B., & Taunton, R. L. (2005). The context for nursing home resident care: The role of leaders in developing strategies. *Journal of Gerontological Nursing, 31*(2), 40–48.

Trick, W. E., Weinstein, R. A., DeMarais, P. L., Tomaska, W., Nathan, C., McAllister, S. K., et al. (2004). Comparison of routine gloves use and contact-isolation precautions to prevent transmission of multi-drug resistant bacteria in a long-term care facility. *Journal of the American Geriatrics Society, 52*(12), 2003–2009.

van Doorn, C., Gruber-Baldini, A. L., Zimmerman, S., Hebel, J. R., Port, C. L., Baumgarten, M., et al. (2003). Dementia as a risk factor for falls and fall injuries among nursing home residents. *Journal of the American Geriatrics Society, 51*(9), 1213–1218.

Vap, P. W., & Dunaye, T. (2000). Pressure ulcer risk assessment in long-term care nursing. *Journal of Gerontological Nursing, 26*(6), 37–45.

Viamontes, L., Temple, D., Wytall, D., & Walker, A. (2003). An evaluation of an adhesive hydrocellular foam dressing and a self-adherent soft silicone foam dressing in a nursing home setting. *Ostomy Wound Management, 49*(8), 48–58.

Vogelsmeier, A., Scott-Cawiezell, J., & Zellmer, D. (in press). Barriers to safe medication administration in the nursing home. *Journal of Gerontological Nursing.*

Wipke-Tevis, D. D., Williams, D. A., Rantz, M. J., Popejoy, L. L., Madsen, R. W., Petroski, G. F., et al. (2004). Nursing home quality and pressure ulcer prevention and management practices. *Journal of the American Geriatrics Society, 52*(4), 583–588.

Winzelberg, G. S. (2003). The quest for nursing home quality: Learning history's lessons. *Archives of Internal Medicine, 163*(21), 2552–2556.

Zhang, X., & Grabowski, D. C. (2004). Nursing home staffing and quality under the nursing home reform act. *The Gerontologist, 44*(1), 13–23.

Zimmerman, S., Gruber-Baldini, A. L., Hebel, J. R., Sloane, P. D., & Magaziner, J. (2002). Nursing home facility risk factors for infection and hospitalization: Importance of registered nurse turnover, administration, and social factors. *Journal of the American Geriatrics Society, 50*(12), 1987–1995.

PART IV

Emerging Issues in Patient Safety

Chapter 9

Informatics for Patient Safety: A Nursing Research Perspective

Suzanne Bakken

ABSTRACT

In Crossing the Quality Chasm, *the Institute of Medicine (IOM) Committee on Quality of Health Care in America identified the critical role of information technology in designing a health system that produces care that is "safe, effective, patient-centered, timely, efficient, and equitable" (Committee on Quality of Health Care in America, 2001, p. 164). A subsequent IOM report contends that improved information systems are essential to a new health care delivery system that "both prevents errors and learns from them when they occur" (Committee on Data Standards for Patient Safety, 2004, p. 1). This review specifically highlights the role of informatics processes and information technology in promoting patient safety and summarizes relevant nursing research. First, the components of an informatics infrastructure for patient safety are described within the context of the national framework for delivering consumer-centric and information-rich health care and using the National Health Information Infrastructure (NHII) (Thompson & Brailer, 2004). Second, relevant nursing research is summarized; this includes research studies that contributed to the development of selected infrastructure components as well as studies specifically focused on patient safety. Third, knowledge gaps and opportunities for nursing research*

*are identified for each main topic. The health information technologies deployed as
part of the national framework must support nursing practice in a manner that enables prevention of medical errors and promotion of patient safety and contributes
to the development of practice-based nursing knowledge as well as best practices for
patient safety. The seminal work that has been completed to date is necessary, but
not sufficient, to achieve this objective.*

Keywords: patient safety, nursing, informatics

In *Crossing the Quality Chasm*, the Institute of Medicine (IOM) Committee on
Quality of Health Care in America identified the critical role of information technology (IT) in designing a health system that produces care that is "safe, effective, patient-centered, timely, efficient, and equitable" (Committee on Quality of
Health Care in America, 2001, p. 164). A subsequent IOM report contends that
improved information systems are essential to a new health care delivery system
that "both prevents errors and learns from them when they occur" (Committee
on Data Standards for Patient Safety, 2004, p. 1). This review specifically highlights the role of informatics processes and information technology in promoting
patient safety and summarizes relevant nursing research. First, the components of
an informatics infrastructure for patient safety are described within the context
of the national framework for delivering consumer-centric and information-rich
health care and using the National Health Information Infrastructure (NHII)
(Thompson & Brailer, 2004). Second, relevant nursing research is summarized;
this includes research studies that contributed to the development of selected infrastructure components as well as studies specifically focused on patient safety.
Third, knowledge gaps and opportunities for nursing research are identified for
each main topic.

Definitions for patient safety concepts vary. For the purpose of this review,
the following patient safety-related definitions from the Committee on Data Standards for Patient Safety (2004) apply:

- An error may be an act of commission or an act of omission.
- An adverse event results in unintended harm to the patient by an act of
  commission or omission rather than by the underlying disease or condition of the patient.
- A near miss is an act of commission or omission that could have harmed
  the patient, but did not cause harm as a result of chance, prevention, or
  mitigation.

The research studies in this review were retrieved through a variety of
methods. First, a series of Medline searches was conducted using the keywords

patient safety, decision support, computer-based provider order entry, shared decision making, self-care, self-management, personal health record, and patient portal combined with nurse or nursing and with computer or informatics. Second, the Agency for Healthcare Research and Quality (AHRQ) Patient Safety Resource Web site (www.psnet.ahrq.gov/) was searched for research articles pertaining to informatics and patient safety and to nursing and patient safety. Third, the *Proceedings of the 2005 American Medical Informatics Association* were manually searched. Fourth, the author's familiarity with NHII allowed identification of research studies relevant to various infrastructure components. Fifth, programs of nursing informatics research were reviewed for their relevance to patient safety. Because of the breadth of the perspective and the associated search strategies, the review includes patient safety–relevant studies not explicitly identified by their authors as informatics research, and papers from the nursing informatics literature not explicitly identified by their authors as patient safety research.

INFORMATICS INFRASTRUCTURE FOR PATIENT SAFETY

In 2004, Tommy Thompson, Secretary of Health and Human Resources, and David Brailer, National Coordinator for Health Information Technology, released a strategic action framework for delivering consumer-centric and information-rich health care. The framework has four goals, all relevant to patient safety: (1) inform clinical practice, (2) interconnect clinicians, (3) personalize care, and (4) improve population health (Thompson & Brailer, 2004). Strategies for each goal, along with patient safety examples, are summarized in Table 9.1.

NHII is central to the strategic action framework goals. It is enabled by technology, but, more important, it incorporates values, practices, relationships, laws, standards, systems, and applications that support all facets of three inter-related dimensions of health: individual (personal) health, health care (caregiver-oriented), and public (population) health (National Center for Vital and Health Statistics, 1998). The NHII aims to provide ubiquitous health care information and decision support. Components of an informatics infrastructure that supports patient safety across NHII dimensions include the following: (1) data acquisition methods and user interfaces, (2) standards that facilitate health care data exchange among heterogeneous systems, (3) data repositories and clinical event monitors, (4) data mining techniques, (5) digital sources of evidence or knowledge, (6) communication technologies, and (7) informatics competencies (Bakken, 2001; Committee on Data Standards for Patient Safety, 2004). Illustrative patient safety examples of informatics infrastructure components are shown in Table 9.2.

TABLE 9.1   Strategic Action Framework Goals and Strategies With Patient Safety–Related Examples

Goals and strategies	Patient safety examples
Inform clinical practice • Incentivize electronic health record (EHR) adoption • Reduce risk of EHR investment • Promote EHR diffusion in rural and underserved areas Interconnect clinicians through creation of interoperable systems • Foster regional collaboration • Develop a national health information network • Coordinate federal health information systems Personalize care through consumer-centric information to enable personalization of care, individual's management of health and illness, and assistance in personal health decisions • Encourage use of personal health records • Enhance informed consumer choice • Promote telehealth systems Improve population health through uses of aggregated data including quality improvement, patient safety, clinical trials and other types of research, and public health • Unify public health surveillance architectures • Streamline quality and health status monitoring • Accelerate research and dissemination of evidence	• EHRs • Computer-based provider order entry (CPOE) • Automated falls risk alert • Context-specific information retrieval • Data mining for adverse event detection • Data standards that support data sharing across organizations (e.g., Health Level 7 messaging, Clinical Document Architecture, and decision support standards; Continuity of Care Record standard) • Patient safety event taxonomy to support voluntary and mandatory reporting • Personal health records that contain data elements such as medication lists, allergies, major diagnoses, laboratory results • Self-management tools • Consumer decision aids • Telemonitoring of vital signs and laboratory values • Regional patient safety data warehouse • Electronic dissemination of patient safety-related evidence (e.g., Patient Safety Network [www.psnet.ahrq.gov]) • Integration of geographical information system (GIS) data with clinical data

TABLE 9.2   Components of National Health Information Infrastructure for Patient Safety

Component	Patient safety examples
Data acquisition methods and user interfaces	Data entry (keyboard, mouse, voice, touch screen, graffiti) or received from another computer system (e.g., hemodynamic monitor to clinical information system)
Data exchange standards	Health Level 7 Reference Information Model; Patient Safety Event Taxonomy
Data repositories and clinical event monitors	Automated alerts generated through clinical event monitor for abnormal laboratory value, drug–drug interaction, high risk for pressure ulcer
Data mining techniques	Machine learning algorithm or natural language processing for potential adverse event detection
Digital sources of evidence or knowledge	Practice guidelines, Micromedex, Cochrane Systematic Reviews
Communication technologies	Internet, mobile technologies (e.g., cellular telephone, personal digital assistant)
Informatics competencies	Use decision support systems, expert systems, and aids for clinical decision making or differential diagnosis; Identify, evaluate, and apply the most relevant information

NURSING RESEARCH

The goals of the strategic action framework help to organize the relevant nursing research. Following the review of research related to the four goals, research in the area of nursing informatics competencies—a prerequisite for efficient and effective use of informatics-based patient safety tools across all four goals-is summarized. Knowledge gaps and suggestions for future research are described following each section.

Inform Clinical Practice

Key informatics-based patient safety tools include electronic health records, clinical decision support systems such as computer-based provider order entry (CPOE) systems, and bar code administration systems (Committee on Data Standards for Patient Safety, 2004). Relevant nursing research in this area focuses on CPOE, clinical decision support systems for prevention and management of patient falls and pressure ulcers, and bar code administration systems for medications and blood products. These tools were identified by Ball, Weaver, and Abbott as "enabling technologies to revitalize the role of nursing in an era of patient safety" (2003, p. 29). In addition, the National Quality Forum (2003) identified CPOE systems, strategies for pressure ulcer risk assessment, and medication unit-dose systems as key patient safety practices for immediate implementation.

CPOE Systems

Although recently there have been several highly visible CPOE system failures (Koppel, Metlay, Cohen, Abaluck, Localio, Kimmel, et al., 2005), many studies document the positive effect of CPOE on aspects of patient safety, such as prevention of adverse drug events (ADEs) (Bates, Leape, Cullen, Laird, Peterson, Teich, et al., 1998; Bates, 1999; Galanter, Didomenico, & Polikaitis, 2005). Nursing research related to CPOE has primarily focused on processes rather than outcomes. For example, Snyder and Fields (2005) assessed organizational readiness for CPOE system innovation in a sample predominantly comprising registered nurses from 22 critical care, intermediate, and medical-surgical units across three community hospitals. The responses prior to CPOE implementation indicated moderate to strong agreement regarding innovation readiness in all innovation categories. Of note, in contrast to other health care organizations, respondents reported extensive experience with work-related IT innovation during the prior 12 months. Reynolds, Peres, and Tatham (2005) evaluated a CPOE work-around, hypothesized to affect patient safety, in which medication orders were written into the comment fields of Nursing Communication Orders as free text, consequently bypassing decision support such as drug–drug interaction. Their analysis revealed that (1) less than 25% of Nursing Communication Orders related to medications and (2) the high-volume users had a lower percentage (11%) of medication orders than low-volume users. Moreover, the comment field was sometimes used as a holding place for telephone orders until the official order was entered. This analysis provided the impetus for policy changes, educational efforts, and refinement of order sets.

Prevention and Management of Patient Falls

A systematic review focused on interventions to reduce falls in the elderly in the community or in institutional or hospital care identified the likely benefit of risk factor screening and intervention in community and residential care settings (Gillespie, Gillespie, Robertson, Lamb, Cumming, and Rowe, 2005). In this volume, Currie summarizes various approaches to falls prevention and management. Although the potential effect of automated falls risk assessment on fall rates has been noted, no randomized controlled trials (RCTs) were located for this review that specifically examined the effect of clinical decision support systems for prevention or management of patient falls in any setting. Two recent research reports described the development of computer-based approaches for falls prevention. Liaw, Sulaiman, Pearce, Sims, Hill, Grain, et al. (2003) identified the methodological, information model, and terminology issues associated with the Australian Falls Risk Assessment and Management System through iterative development and testing with clinicians and consumers. Currie, Mellino, Cimino, and Bakken (2004) addressed similar issues of representation of falls-related concepts within the context of introducing a fall and injury risk assessment tool integrated into a Web-based clinical information system. Common across these two studies was the identification of the need for standardized terminologies and information models to support automated falls risk assessment and management.

Pressure Ulcer Prevention and Management

Pressure ulcer prevention and management is a key patient safety concern for nursing, and relevant guidelines exist. Zielstorff and colleagues (Zielstorff, Barnett, Estey, Hamilton, Vickery, Welebob, et al., 1997; Zielstorff, Barnett, Fitzmaurice, Estey, Hamilton, Vickery, et al., 1996; Zielstorff, Estey, Vickery, Hamilton, Fitzmaurice, & Barnett, 1997) developed a pressure ulcer prevention and management system to assist clinicians with patient-specific decision making. End users were satisfied with the system; however, preliminary results in a volunteer sample of 15 nurses showed no effect on pressure ulcer knowledge or clinical decision making skills (Zielstorff, Estey et al.). Quaglini, Grandi, Baiardi, Mazzoleni, Fassino, Franchi, et al. (2000) evaluated a computer-based guideline for pressure ulcer prevention after nurses used it for 40 patients. The nurses reported satisfaction with the tool in terms of documentation improvement and increase in knowledge. Clarke, Bradley, Whytock, Handfield, van der Wal, and Gundry (2005) evaluated nurses' perceptions regarding the implementation of the Wound and Skin Intelligence System. Although the nurses found certain system aspects (e.g., risk assessment tools, plans of care, and wound care grid) useful, the time it took and the lack of competencies required to use the decision support system were significant barriers. No studies were located that evaluated the effect of decision support on pressure ulcer rates.

Bar Code Administration Systems

An AHRQ evidence report that critically analyzed patient safety practices identified four areas in which bar coding shows promise for improving patient safety: patient identification, medication dispensing and administration, specimen handling, and medical record keeping (University of California at San Francisco [UCSF]–Stanford University Evidence-Based Practice Center,

2001). Nurse researchers have evaluated two specific types of applications that integrate bar coding: bar code medication administration (BCMA) and transfusion administration. It is estimated that 5% of U.S. hospitals currently use BCMA (Wright & Katz, 2005). A number of studies have documented the positive effect of BCMA on medication administration errors in addition to nurse acceptance of the technology. Coyle and Heinen (2005) reported a 23% decrease in medication administration errors during the first year of BCMA in a single Veterans Affairs Medical Center and a 66% decrease after 5 years. Moreover, nurses accepted the BCMA and contributed to its evolutionary design. Anderson and Wittwer (2004) reported similar statistics of a 59% to 70% decrease in medication administration errors on a variety of nursing units and positive effect on nurse satisfaction. However, although these studies consistently report a positive impression of BCMA, others urge attention to the possible new paths to ADEs. For example, in an ethnographic, cross-sectional study of medication passes before and after BCMA implementation, Patterson, Cook, and Render (2002) identified five negative effects: (1) nurse confusion regarding automated removal of medications by BCMA, (2) degraded nurse-physician coordination, (3) nurses dropping activities (e.g., replacing wrist band scanning with typing in patient identification) to reduce workload during busy periods, (4) increased prioritization of timely medication administration during goal conflicts, and (5) decreased ability to deviate from routine sequences (e.g., tapering of medication doses). The authors highlighted the need to intervene through BCMA design, organizational policy, and training initiatives so that these negative effects are eliminated and new paths to ADEs can be prevented, and they have more recently proposed 15 best practices (Patterson, Rogers, & Render, 2004).

Several reports have documented unacceptable rates of transfusion errors in general, with ABO-incompatible transfusions ranging from 1 in 138,672 to 1 in 41,000 (Andreu, Morel, Forestier, Debeir, Rebibo, Janvier, et al., 2002; Linden, Wagner, Voytovich, & Sheehan, 2000). Also of note is the significant proportion of errors that are attributed to nurses. For example, in a study that used the medical event reporting system for transfusion medicine (MERS-TM) at three hospitals, high-severity events with potential for patient harm accounted for 5% of 4,670 events, with nursing-related events comprising 78% of high-severity events (Callum, Merkley, Coovadia, Lima, & Kaplan, 2004). In a nurse-led study, Porcella and Walker (2005) estimated the relative risk of finding a misidentification event in blood products administration before and after implementation of a tool that captures data related to sample collection, sample arrival in the blood bank, blood bank dispensing of blood product, and administration of blood product. The system compares the scanned patient wristband bar codes to bar codes on requisitions, samples, and products and indicates a match or error message. The relative risk of finding a misidentification event in any stage of the process increased 30-fold from the manual to the bar code process.

Knowledge Gaps and Future Research

Besides the few studies related to bar code administration systems, nursing research related to informatics use for patient safety toward the goal of informing clinical practice has primarily focused on process evaluations rather than examining the effectiveness of various informatics applications on patient outcomes such as ADEs, falls, and pressure ulcers. Although process evaluations are essential to understand technology-enhanced nursing practice (Casper, Karsh, Or, Carayon, Grenier, Sebern, et al., 2005), it is vital that the effect of such systems on nursing-sensitive outcomes also be examined through well-controlled study designs.

Interconnect Clinicians Through Creation of Interoperable Systems

Health care data exchange standards support the creation of interoperable systems (i.e., systems that receive and understand data from other systems) and data reuse for multiple purposes such as error and adverse event detection and prevention. The IOM Committee on Data Standards for Patient Safety specifically recommended the acceleration of development and adoption of standards in three key areas: terminologies, data interchange formats (e.g., reference terminology models, Health Level 7 Reference Information Model), and knowledge representation (e.g., guideline representation language, Arden Syntax for decision support rules). The primary foci of nursing research in this area have been the creation of nursing terminologies and development and testing of data interchange formats. There has been little nursing-specific work related to the development of a generic guideline representation model for representing clinical guidelines in a computer-executable format, an essential prerequisite for decision support tools.

Terminologies

Within the context of the Nursing Minimum Data Set (NMDS), decades of research have resulted in a set of core nursing terminologies that represent the practice of nursing, facilitate integration of nursing data into electronic health records, and can be used for patient safety purposes (e.g., decision support for prevention and detection of errors and adverse events) as well as aggregation for quality management, evidence-based practice, and clinical nursing research (Beyea, 2000; Johnson, Maas, & Moorhead, 2000; Martin, 2004; McCloskey & Bulechek, 2000; North American Nursing Diagnosis Association International, 2005; Saba, 2004). In addition, nurse researchers have demonstrated the utility of nonnursing terminologies for describing nursing practice (Bakken, Cimino, Haskell, Kukafka, Matsumoto, Chan, et al., 2000; Griffith & Robinson, 1992, 1993; Henry, Holzemer, Reilly, & Campbell, 1994) and have led efforts to integrate nursing concepts into health care terminologies, with broad coverage for the health care domain such as the Logical Observation Identifiers, Names, and Codes (LOINC) database and Systematized Nomenclature of Medicine (SNOMED) Clinical Terms (Bakken, Warren, Lundberg, Casey, Correia, Konicek, et al., 2002; Matney, Bakken, & Huff, 2003), which have been identified as required health care terminologies for federal use in the United States. The aspects of nursing care summarized by each terminology are summarized in Table 9.3.

Although many authors have described the potential role of standardized nursing terminologies in promoting patient safety, few studies have actually examined this issue. Recently, Keenan, and Yakel (2005) identified the role of the Hands-on Automated Nursing Data System (HANDS) tool, which incorporates the NANDA Taxonomy, Nursing Interventions Classification, and Nursing Outcomes Classification, in promoting safer nursing care. They found that the increased visibility of nursing care facilitated by HANDS promoted greater understanding of care (collective mind) and improved continuity of care, key aspects of patient safety.

Data Interchange Formats

Nurse researchers have conducted research in the areas of reference terminology models (RTMs) and the Health Level 7 Reference Information Model. In particular, investigators have conducted substantial research on transforming organized lists of nursing diagnoses and nursing interventions into formal structures such as RTMs (Choi, Jenkins, Cimino, White, & Bakken, 2005; Hardiker, Bakken, Casey, & Hoy, 2002; Hardiker & Rector, 1998, 2001; Ozbolt, 2000a, 2000b, 2003a). Less work has been conducted in the area of goals and outcomes (Bakken, Cimino et al., 2000; Bakken, Warren, Casey, Konicek, Lundberg, Pooke, et al., 2002; Ozbolt, 2003b). RTMs facilitate mapping among the various nursing terminologies and enable computer processing of terms for purposes such as decision support for error prevention. The culmination of this work was the development of an international standard that specifies RTMs for nursing diagnoses and nursing interventions (Bakken, Coenen, & Saba, 2004), and it has been tested in several studies. Bakken, Cashen, Mendonca, O'Brien, & Zieniewicz (2000) demonstrated the utility of the nursing intervention RTM to represent standardized interventions from the Omaha System and Home Health Care Classification. Moss, Coenen, and Mills (2003) confirmed the ubiquity of action and target concepts (required in RTM model) in a sample of 21,065 documented pain interventions. And other investigators provided evidence regarding the usefulness of the RTM for representing nursing diagnoses (Bakken, Warren, Lundberg et al., 2002; Hwang, Cimino, & Bakken, 2003) and its potential for natural language processing (NLP) of nursing narratives (i.e., free text) (Bakken, Hyun, Friedman, & Johnson, 2005).

TABLE 9.3 Standardized Terminologies With Utility for Nursing Care

Terminology	Contents	ANA[b]	UMLS[c]	HL7[d]	SNOMED[e]	Availability
Nursing-specific						
Clinical Care Classification[a]	Nursing diagnoses, interventions, outcomes, goals	x	x	x	x	Public domain
Omaha System	Problems, interventions, outcomes	x	x	x	x	Public domain
North American Nursing Diagnosis Association Taxonomy	Nursing diagnoses	x	x	x	x	License
Nursing Interventions Classification	Nursing interventions	x	x	x	x	License
Nursing Outcomes Classification	Patient/Client outcomes	x	x	x	x	License
Patient Care Data Set	Patient problems, care goals, care orders	x	x	x		Only at Vanderbilt University
Perioperative Nursing Data Set	Nursing diagnoses, interventions, patient outcomes	x	x	x	x	License
Others						
Current Procedural Terminology codes	Medical services		x			License
Logical Observation Identifiers, Names, and Codes (LOINC)	Vital signs, obstetric measurements, clinical assessment scales, research instruments	x	x	x	Laboratory LOINC only	Copyrighted, but free for use
SNOMED Clinical Terms	MD/RN diagnoses, health care interventions, procedures, findings, substances, organisms, events	x	x	x	x	5-year federal license

[a]Formerly, the Home Health Care Classification
[b]Recognized by the American Nurses Association
[c]Included in Unified Medical Language System
[d]Registered with Health Level 7
[e]Included in SNOMED Clinical Terms

In addition to the development and testing of RTMs, researchers have examined the utility of the Health Level 7 Reference Information Model, a standard that supports data exchange among heterogeneous information systems, to support nursing. Danko, Kennedy, Haskell, Androwich, Button, Correia, et al. (2003) documented the adequacy of the "Act" class in the Health Level 7 Reference Information Model for modeling breast cancer education interventions through a use case analysis approach. Goossen, Ozbold, Coenen, Park, Mead, Ehnfors, et al. (2004) focused their analysis on the Observation class of the Health Level 7 Reference Information Model. They developed a provisional domain model for the nursing process and conducted a small-scale evaluation, concluding that it was possible to map patient information from the nursing domain model to the Health Level 7 Reference Information Model. Both reports suggest the need for further testing to ensure adequate support for data exchange for the nursing domain.

Knowledge Representation

In terms of knowledge representation, although nurses are frequent users of clinical practice guidelines and many nurse investigators are in the process of developing decision support systems (e.g., the N-CODES Project) (O'Neill, Dluhy, Fortier, & Michel, 2004), there has been little nursing-specific work on guideline representation interchange formats. Roberts (2005) utilized a smoking cessation guideline represented in the Guideline Interchange Format as part of a study about clinical practice guideline–related knowledge representation models and comprehension-generated inferences of nurse practitioners and physicians at varying levels of expertise. This study identified similarities in content knowledge, but the differences in knowledge structures between nurses and physicians suggest the importance of nursing participation in translation of paper-based guidelines to computer-interpretable formats.

Another aspect of knowledge representation for guidelines is the terminology required to represent guideline concepts. Dykes, Currie, and Cimino (2003) examined the extent to which Health Insurance Portability and Accountability Act of 1996 (HIPAA)–mandated terminologies alone and in conjunction with SNOMED CT and LOINC represented concepts from a congestive heart failure evaluation and management guideline. SNOMED CT and LOINC represented 86.2% of the concepts, and overall 91.9% of the 260 unique concepts were represented by at least one terminology.

Knowledge Gaps and Future Research

The nursing research related to interconnecting clinicians through interoperable systems demonstrates a significant body of research related to terminology development and substantial efforts toward creation of computable representations of nursing diagnoses and interventions and testing of the Health Level 7 Reference Information Model. The current work related to representing goals and outcomes suggests that continued research is needed from the perspective of development of an RTM and testing of the Health Level 7 Reference Information Model. There is little nursing research in the area of clinical guideline interchange format. However, it is needed to ensure that computer-executable models support nurses' mental models and interpretations of clinical practice guidelines as well as those of physicians, so that nurses can optimally use the guideline-based decision support systems.

Personalize Care Through Consumer-Centric Information

A number of authors have identified the patient's role in promoting safety and preventing errors (Hibbard, Peters, Slovic, & Tusler, 2005; Vincent & Coulter, 2002; Weingart, Pagovich, Sands, Li, Aronson, Davis, et al., 2005). These include patient involvement in (1) helping to reach an accurate diagnosis; (2) deciding on an appropriate treatment or management strategy; (3) choosing a suitably experienced and safe provider; (4) ensuring that treatment is appropriately administered, monitored, and adhered to; and (5) identifying side effects or adverse events quickly and taking appropriate action (Vincent & Coulter). However, in a convenience sample of 195 participants, Hibbard et al. found that consumers may be reluctant to participate in some preventive actions even when they perceive them to be effective. In particular, consumers were less likely to take preventive action when it required questioning health professionals' actions or judgments (e.g., confirming right medication and dose or asking health care workers whether they have washed their hands). The study showed that reading about medical errors, education, self-efficacy, and perceived effectiveness were significant predictors of likelihood of taking preventive actions in a path analysis. Informatics tools have the potential to provide information and education and to improve self-efficacy for prevention of medical errors. As shown in Table 9.4, 13 of AHRQ's 20 tips (2000) to help patients prevent medical errors can be supported by one or more consumer-oriented informatics tools. These include tools that support shared decision making, self-care, interactive education, and support; patient portals that integrate results review and secure communication with providers; personal health records (PHRs); and electronic benchmarking reports. In the following paragraphs, nursing research related to these tools is summarized. This is followed by a discussion of health literacy as relevant to consumer-oriented informatics tools and selected nursing research studies.

Shared Decision-Making Tools

Ruland (2004) described the relevance of patient preferences and shared decision making to patient safety including emphasis on intended outcomes from the

TABLE 9.4 Informatics Tools of Relevance to AHRQ Patient Tips to Help Prevent Medical Errors

Patient tip	Shared decision making tools	Self-care tools	Interactive education & support tools	Health portals	Personal health record	Bench-marking tools
Become an active member of your health care team.	•	•	•	•	•	•
Make sure doctors know about everything you are taking, including prescriptions, over-the-counter medicines, and dietary supplements such as vitamins and herbs.					•	
Make sure your doctor knows about any allergies and adverse reactions you have had to medicines.					•	
Ask for information about your medicines in terms you can understand when your medicines are prescribed and when you receive them.	•	•	•	•	•	
If you have any questions about the directions on your medicine labels, ask.	•	•		•		
Ask for written information about the side effects your medicine could cause.	•	•	•	•	•	
If you have a choice, choose a hospital at which many patients have the procedure or surgery you need.						•
When you are being discharged from the hospital, ask your doctor to explain the treatment plan you will use at home.		•		•	•	
Speak up if you have questions or concerns	•		•	•	•	
Make sure that all health professionals involved in your care have important health information about you.	•	•	•	•	• •	
Know that more is not always better.						
If you have a test, don't assume that no news is good news.	•	•		•	•	
Learn about your condition and treatments by asking your doctor and nurse and by using other reliable sources.	•	•	•	• •	• •	

perspective of the patient and lack of relevant data, misinterpretation of data, and ineffective communication as major sources of error. She identified six types of informatics tools to support shared decision making and risk communication from the perspective of patient safety: (1) interactive education to improve risk comprehension; (2) multiple, individualized formats for conveying risk; (3) individualized risk calculations; (4) application of decision analysis methods to calculate options with the highest expected value; (5) automated updates of evidence to support shared decision making; and (6) utilization of different preference-elicitation techniques and formats.

Several nurse investigators have developed paper-based shared decision-making tools, including O'Connor's Ottawa Decision Support Framework (O'Connor, Fiset, DeGrasse, Graham, Evans, Stacy, et al., 1999; O'Connor, Tugwell, Wells, Elmslie, Jollie, Hollingsworth, et al., 1998). Ruland and associates (Ruland, 1999; Ruland, Kresevic, Brennan, & Lorensen, 1997; Ruland, Kresevic, & Lorensen, 1997; Ruland, White, Stevens, Fanciullo, & Khilani, 2003) have developed and tested Creating Better Health Outcomes by Improving Communication about Patients' Expectations (CHOICE), a computer-based decision support system for shared decision making, in a variety of patient populations. Ruland (2002) evaluated the use of CHOICE in assisting nurse elicitation of patients' preferences for functional performance during the admission interview. In the intervention group, preference information was added to patients' charts and used for subsequent care planning. Nursing care in the experimental group as compared to the two control groups was more consistent with patient preferences ($F = 11.4$; $P < 0.001$) and improved patients' preference achievement ($F = 4.9$; $P < 0.05$). Consistency between patients' preferences and nurses' care priorities was associated with higher-preference achievement ($r = 0.49$; $P < 0.001$). In an evaluation of CHOICE for symptom management in cancer, patients completed an assessment of symptoms and preferences prior to seeing their provider in the clinic (Ruland et al., 2003). Patients in the experimental group and their clinicians received a printout for use during the clinical encounter. In a sample of 52 patients, the experimental group demonstrated greater congruence between symptoms captured by CHOICE and symptoms addressed in the visit than did patients in the control group. There were no differences between the groups on patient satisfaction.

Self-Care Tools

Many nursing interventions are aimed at improving patient self-care or self-management. Several investigators have specifically focused on computer-based approaches to self-management of medications, a key patient safety issue. Neafsey, Strickler, Shellman, and Padula (2001) developed an interactive multimedia computer software program to increase older adults' knowledge about interactions between prescription and over-the-counter medications and alcohol and to in-crease their self-efficacy to avoid such interactions. The program, which was designed for the learning styles and psychomotor skills of older adults and imple-mented on a touchscreen notebook computer, was pilot tested on 60 older adults. Those in the experimental group had greater knowledge and self-efficacy scores than the controls. Moreover, they reported their intent to make specific changes in self-medication behaviors. Alegmagno, Niles, and Treiber (2004) also ad-dressed medication use in the elderly population. Community-based seniors ($n =$ 412) completed a computer-based screening for medication misuse and viewed video clips related to their own potential misuse. The intervention also included a medication reminder checklist and a 7-day pill-dispensing box. During a 2-month follow-up period, one-third of the participants reported visiting their physician to discuss medication misuse feedback.

Using a quasi-experimental, nonequivalent control group design, Yeh, Chen, and Liu (2005) addressed another aspect of patient safety: self-care ability. They examined the effect of a multimedia software program that included printed instructions as compared to standard care in patients hospitalized for hip replace-ment. Experimental subjects demonstrated higher self-efficacy, less assistance for functional activities, and shorter length of stay.

Interactive Education and Support Tools

A series of studies by Gustafson and associates (Gustafson, Hawkins, Boberg, McTavish, Owens, Wise, et al., 2002; Gustafson, Hawkins, Pingree, McTavish, Arora, Mendenhall, et al., 2001; Shaw, McTavish, Hawkins, Gustafson, & Pin-gree, 2000) has consistently documented the effect of the Comprehensive Health Enhancement Support System (CHESS), one of the earliest computer-based sys-tems for providing education, information, and support, on perceptions of quality of life and emotional support. CHESS is typically used in home or community settings and includes information, communication, journaling, and analysis (e.g., assessments, health tracking, treatment decisions, and action plan). Studies of CHESS in underserved populations (black, low socioeconomic status) demon-strated more use of information and analysis services rather than communication services, as compared to white participants, who tended to use communication services such as e-mail or bulletin boards most often.

In nursing, Brennan has conducted multiple RCTs of computer-based in-formational, support, and decision support services aimed at improving self-care, coping, and decision making in a variety of patient populations. An early field trial focused on family caregivers of persons with Alzheimer's disease found that even though decision support was the least-used function in the resource and there were no significant differences in decision-making skill, decision-making confidence was significantly increased (Brennan, Moore, & Smyth, 1995). There were no significant differences in social isolation. In a study of persons living with AIDS, Brennan and Ripich (1994) identified that communication services were used more often than information and support services. HeartCare, an Internet-based system for patient home recovery after coronary artery bypass graft surgery, provides health information and support that is tailored to patients' individual needs and stages of the recovery process (Brennan, Bjorndottir, Rogers, Jones, Moore, & Visovsky, 2000; Brennan, Moore, Bjorndottir, Jones, Visovsky, & Rogers, 2001; Brennan, Caldwell, Moore, Screenath, & Jones, 1998). The effect on clinical outcomes is under evaluation in an RCT.

The Women to Women Project tested the effect of a computer-based peer support and information intervention on chronically ill, rural women (Cudney, Winters, Weinert, & Anderson, 2005; Hill, Schillo, & Weinert, 2004; Hill & Weinert, 2004; Weinert, 2005; Weinert, Cudney, & Winters, 2005). Weinert et al. reported significant differences between the intervention and control groups in computer skills, computer comfort, and Internet knowledge. The authors suggest that the women in the intervention group will have a sustained ability to access Internet-based health information to assist with the management of their chronic illness. Preliminary data analysis regarding the effect of the intervention demonstrates that the intervention is helping to increase the women's ability to adapt to their chronic illnesses (Weinert) and to improve social support in a vulnerable sample with low social support and high psychosocial distress (Hill et al.).

Health Portals

Health portals are typically designed to meet the customized needs of a designated group of people. Such portals may serve a single purpose, such as provision of information from a variety of sources, or they may deliver a variety of patient-oriented services. For example, MedLinePlus (http://medlineplus.gov/) provides a single-service, consumer-oriented health information and education in both English and Spanish. In contrast, portals such as My Chart at the Cleveland Clinic (Harris, 2005), the Veteran's Affairs' My Healthevet (www.myhealth.va.gov/), and Palo Alto Medical Foundation's PAMFOnline (www.pamfonline.org) include services such as viewing of medical information, test results, health reminders, and schedules; appointment request; prescription renewal; and patient education. The latter has significant overlap with PHRs (described in the next section).

Moody (2005) described the importance of e-health Web portals as a tool for nurses to use to empower patients and caregivers, but no research studies were retrieved for this review that specifically addressed health portals from the perspective of nursing and patient safety. Health portals have the potential to contribute to patient safety through education and empowerment of patients, timeliness of communication, and prevention of errors of omission.

Personal Health Records

A PHR is

> *an electronic application through which individuals can access, manage, and share their health information in a secure and confidential environment. It allows people to access and coordinate their lifelong health information and make appropriate parts of it available to those who need it* (Working Group on Policies for Electronic Information Sharing Between Doctors and Patients, 2004, p. 13).

Tang and Lansky (2005) point out that a PHR contains not only provider-centric information such as that which patients can view through a health portal, but also information entered by the patient such as symptoms, over-the-counter medications, exercise and food diaries, and data from home monitoring devices. PHRs currently primarily exist in three forms: (1) patient view into an existing EHR through a patient portal (e.g., the Veteran's Affairs' My Healthevet [www.myhealth.va.gov/] and Palo Alto Medical Foundation's PAMFOnline [www.pamfonline.org]); (2) freestanding software application on the Internet (e.g., ihealthrecord [www.ihealthrecord.org/]); and (3) freestanding software application on a personal device (e.g., CapMed [www.capmed.com]).

Although there has been nursing input for efforts aimed at defining PHR components and functions, such as the 2004 NHII Summit, no studies were located that specifically addressed nursing and the PHR.

Electronic Benchmarking Reports

The need for consumer-oriented reports that guide individuals and families in the selection of health care services (e.g., Health Employers Data and Information Set) or evaluation of services received against a specific benchmark (e.g., www.compareyourcare.org/) is widely acknowledged. Nursing research in this area is limited and focuses on nursing indicators of quality in nursing homes. Harrington and colleagues (Harrington, Collier, O'Meara, Kitchener, Simon, & Schnell, 2003; Harrington, O'Meara, Collier, & Schnelle, 2003; Harrington, O'Meara, Kitchener, Simon, & Schnelle, 2003) led the design of a Web-based report card for nursing facilities in California. The authors contend that existing nursing home quality Web sites typically lacked data such as resident characteristics, staff turnover rates, and financial indicators. The Web-based system that was implemented included six key areas for information: facility characteristics and ownership; resident characteristics; staffing indicators (e.g., hours, turnover rates); clinical quality indicators; deficiencies, complaints, and enforcement actions; and financial indicators (e.g., direct care expenditures, wages, benefits).

Health Literacy

A recent IOM report noted that 90 million Americans have difficulty understanding and acting on health information (Committee on Health Literacy, 2004). Studies document that inadequate health literacy is associated with increased risk of hospitalization, patient report of worse health status, and inadequate understanding of condition and treatment (Ad Hoc Committee on Health Literacy for the Council on Scientific Affairs, American Medical Association, 1999). For example, Williams, Baker, Parker, and Nurss (1998) demonstrated significant differences in patients' knowledge of their chronic disease among diabetic and hypertensive patients with inadequate, marginal, or adequate health literacy. In addition, Davis, Williams, Marin, Parker, and Glass (2002) conducted an extensive literature review on the topic of health literacy and cancer communication. Their analysis provides evidence that low literacy adversely affects stage of diagnosis, impairs communication and discussion about risks and benefits of treatment options, and limits understanding of informed consent. The findings of these studies suggest that many adults possess inadequate health literacy, which presents a barrier to understanding their conditions and managing their treatment plans.

Several authors have identified health literacy as a barrier to using consumer-oriented informatics tools across the lifespan (Chang, Bakken, Brown, Houston, Kreps, Kukafka, et al., 2004; Gerber, Brodsky, Lawless, Smolin, Arozullah, Smith, et al., 2005; Gray, Klein, Noyce, Sesselberg, & Cantrill, 2005). McCray (2005) specifically points out that "the literacy demands of these personalized, targeted, and tailored information interventions have not been seriously studied" (p. 157). Somewhat conversely, the potential power of such tools, when developed with consideration to readability issues as a strategy for information and education for persons with varying levels of health literacy, has also been noted. For example, computer-based methods for health education is one of four significant research issues identified by the Ad Hoc Committee on Health Literacy for the Council on Scientific Affairs, American Medical Association (Ad Hoc Committee on Health Literacy for the Council on Scientific Affairs, American Medical Association, 1999). In a white paper from the American Medical Informatics Association, Chang et al. (2004) proposed recommendations related to informatics use in underserved populations and specified the need to develop content and formats for health information for varying literacy levels. Of national significance, Thompson and Brailer's (2004) strategic action framework notes the importance of adapting personalized care information for reading levels, as well as for other aspects, such as cultural traditions.

Only a small number of researchers have investigated the effect of computer-based low literacy interventions on patient outcomes. For example, Gerber and colleagues (2005) evaluated a clinic-based multimedia intervention for diabetes education targeted to individuals with low health-literacy levels. There were no significant differences between the intervention and control group in hemoglobin A1c, body mass index, blood pressure, knowledge, self-efficacy, or self-reported medical care. There was an increase in perceived susceptibility to diabetes complications in the intervention group that was greatest among those with lower health literacy. In addition, there was relatively less use of the multimedia intervention among those with low literacy. Few nurse investigators have reported the development of informatics-based tools specifically tailored or targeted to level of literacy. Choi (2005) developed a suite of Web-based educational resources for families of babies in the neonatal intensive care unit with Patent *Ductus Arteriosus* to improve family understanding of their neonate's condition and, ultimately, to facilitate family-centered decision making. Literacy is measured using the Short Test of Functional Health Literacy in Adults (S-TOFLA), and tailored informational and educational content is provided based on literacy score. Wydra (2001) conducted an RCT to test a prototype interactive multimedia module to assist adults receiving cancer treatment and with limited literacy and computer skills to manage fatigue and improve self-care ability. As compared to usual care, those in the experimental group significantly improved self-care ability.

Knowledge Gaps and Future Research

Additional nursing research is needed in regard to the use and effect of the various informatics tools within the context of patient safety for shared decision making, self-care, interactive education and support, health portals, PHRs, and electronic benchmarking reports. Although extensive work on shared decision making exists, few nursing research studies explicitly use computer-based shared decision making tools in the context of patient safety. Further research is required for the development and evaluation of the six types of tools identified by Ruland.

Due to the essential role that informed patients and caregivers play in preventing and detecting medical errors, self-care tools, interactive information and support systems, and health information portals, particularly those tailored to individual needs, have the potential to empower consumers to play this role. Additional studies are needed in a variety of populations to determine how to best use such electronic nursing intervention strategies to improve the quality and safety of care.

Given the phenomena studied by nurse investigators, nursing research has the potential to significantly contribute to the development and evaluation of 10 of the 64 proposed core functions of the PHR proposed by the Working Group on Policies for Electronic Information Sharing Between Doctors and Patients (2004): (1) manage list of other therapeutic modalities (e.g., counseling, occupational therapy, alternative); (2) case management; (3) patient diaries; (4) easy to use terminology; (5) standardized code sets and nomenclature; (6) patient education, self-care content, and consensus guidelines; (7) clinician-directed links to patient education self-care content and consensus guidelines; (8) adherence messaging for specific medications; (9) adherence messaging for specific conditions; and (10) patient-specific instructions. All are relevant to patient safety. In addition, studies are needed that evaluate the effect of PHRs on patient knowledge, empowerment, decision making, adherence to therapeutic regimens and health promotion guidelines, perceptions of engagement with health care clinicians, and clinical outcomes such as hemoglobin A1c and viral load.

Studies are also needed that evaluate the best approaches for presentation of patient safety data to consumers and that examine the effect of patient safety–related information on consumer decision making and satisfaction with services received. Moreover, it is vital that report cards in other care settings incorporate nursing-sensitive patient safety indicators such as those specified by the American Nurses Association (ANA) for acute care (1995).

Resources that are well matched to the health literacy of consumers have the potential to decrease misinformation and promote communication between patients, their families, and providers—key aspects of preventing medical errors and improving patient safety. Qualitative studies are needed to evaluate how the information is understood and used. Moreover, quantitative studies are needed to evaluate the influence of computer-based systems tailored to health literacy level on patient safety indicators such as medication errors and patient falls.

Improve Population Health Through Uses of Aggregated Data

This section focuses primarily on efforts that support the Thompson and Brailer (2004) strategy to streamline quality and health status monitoring as one of three strategies (Table 9.1) to improve population health through uses of aggregated data. Strategies that support the unification of public health surveillance architectures and acceleration of research and dissemination of evidence are viewed as outside the scope of this review. Beyond the requirements to interconnect clinicians, two aspects of the NHII are particularly important to enable the goal of improving population health through uses of aggregated data: data repositories and data mining techniques. Computational modeling techniques also have a potential role for developing and testing hypotheses related to patient safety interventions.

Patient Safety Databases

Data repositories include local clinical repositories that are typically optimized for patient care and data warehouses that are optimized for data analysis for a variety of purposes, including quality improvement and patient safety. The IOM

TABLE 9.5   Examples of Patient Safety Databases

Database	Organization	Reporting
National Nosocomial Infections Surveillance System	CDC[a]	Voluntary
Dialysis Surveillance Network	CDC	Voluntary
Vaccine Adverse Event Report System	CDC, FDA[b]	Mandatory
Medicare Patient Safety Monitoring System	CMS[c]	Voluntary
Patient Safety Reporting System	VHA/NASA[d]	Voluntary
New York Patient Occurrence Reporting and Tracking System	New York State	Mandatory
Medical Event Reporting System for Transfusion Medicine	Columbia University	Voluntary
MedMARx	USP[e]	Voluntary
Sentinel Event	JCAHO[f]	Voluntary
National Database of Nursing Quality Indicators	ANA[g]	Voluntary

[a]Centers for Disease Control and Prevention
[b]Food and Drug Administration
[c]Center for Medicare & Medicaid Services
[d]Veterans Health Administration/National Aeronautical and Space Agency
[e]United States Pharmacopeia
[f]Joint Commission on Accreditation of Healthcare Organizations
[g]American Nurses Association

Committee on Data Standards for Patient Safety recommended the creation of a common safety reporting format to populate regulatory and voluntary patient safety databases at the regional and national level to support learning across organization. Such databases (Table 9.5) facilitate learning across organizations and enable analysis of events that rarely occur in a single institution.

The ANA initiated the development of the National Database of Nursing Quality Indicators (NDNQI), a database of nursing-sensitive quality indicators collected at the unit level. Contributors to NDNQI include 767 hospitals in 50 states and the District of Columbia. The indicators include three areas of key relevance to patient safety: pressure ulcers, falls with and without injury, and nurse staffing (e.g., nursing hours per patient day, staff mix, and agency staff utilization). A number of studies have demonstrated the utility of NDNQI for examining the relationship between staffing variables and patient outcomes (Dunton, Gajewski, Taunton, & Moore, 2004). And the California Nursing Outcomes Coalition (CalNOC) database extends NDNQI (Aydin, Bolton, Donaldson, Brown, Buffum, Elashoff, et al., 2004; Brown, Donaldson, Aydin, & Carlson, 2001).

Donaldson, Brown, Aydin, Bolton, and Rutledge (2005) illustrated the use of two nurse-related quality indicators from CalNOC—patient falls incidence and hospital-acquired pressure ulcer prevalence—as benchmarks in operational quality dashboards.

Data Mining

Data mining techniques, also known as knowledge discovery in databases, encompass traditional statistical approaches, artificial intelligence methods, and NLP. Within the health care context, data mining typically focuses on reusing information collected during the course of care for other purposes such as quality assurance, clinical research, and patient safety. Researchers have demonstrated the promise of automated adverse event detection using data mining techniques (Bates, Evans, Murff, Stetson, Pizziferri, & Hripcsak, 2003a, 2003b; Murff, Forster, Peterson, Fiskio, Heiman, & Bates, 2003; Murff, Patel, Hripcsak, & Bates, 2003). For instance, Melton and Hripcsak (2005) applied NLP techniques to detect 45 New York Patient Occurrence Reporting and Tracking System event types in hospital discharge summaries. The NLP adverse event detection system outperformed traditional detection methods, with an average specificity of 0.9996 per event type for detecting cases with events.

There has been little nursing research related to data mining for patient safety purposes. One exception is Goodwin, who directs a program of research utilizing a variety of data mining techniques (e.g., logistic regression, neural networks, classification and regression trees, inductive algorithms, and fuzzy logic) to predict preterm birth as part of a strategy for prevention of preterm birth(Goodwin, VanDyne, Lin, & Talbert, 2003). Such risk identification strategies are consistent with the IOM Committee on Data Standards for Patient Safety recommendation that the federal government pursue a robust applied patient safety agenda that includes identification of patients at risk for high-risk events. Goodwin, Innacchione, and Hammond's (2000) recent results using data mining techniques show that seven demographic variables result in 0.72 area under the receiver operating characteristic (ROC) curve and that the addition of more than a thousand additional variables adds only 0.03 area under the curve. Another application of data mining for patient safety purposes in nursing is the work of Abbott, Quirolgico, Manchand, Canfield, and Adya (1998), who examined the potential of the Minimum Data Set (MDS), a resident assessment tool for long-term care facilities, to predict admission to acute care from long-term care.

Computational Modeling

Only one series of related reports was retrieved that applied computational modeling techniques to patient safety in the context of nursing care. Effken et al.

(Effken, Brewer, Patil, Lamb, Verran, & Carley, 2003a, 2003b; Effken, Brewer, Patil, Lamb, Verran, & Carley, 2004; Effken, Brewer, Patil, Lamb, Verran, & Carley, 2005) used a computational modeling program, OrgAhead, to model patient care units' achievement of patient safety (regarding medication errors and falls) and quality outcomes. Validation studies were conducted to verify the correspondence between actual and virtual units. Hypotheses for innovations were generated and tested with the modeling program. For all but the highest-performing unit, the investigators were able to generate practical strategies that improved performance of the virtual units by 6% to 8% (Effken et al., 2003b).

Knowledge Gaps and Future Research

Nursing research has resulted in major progress toward the creation of databases that contain nursing-sensitive quality indicators; however, there remains the need for additional research to broaden the scope of the indicators across care settings and levels of nursing practice (i.e., advanced practice nursing as well as basic nursing practice). Further investigation of the applicability and utility of data mining and computational modeling techniques for nursing-relevant patient safety research is also required.

Informatics Competencies

Although research related to informatics competencies in nursing has been conducted for more than a decade, because of increasing emphasis on patient safety and consideration of the role that technology can play in addressing the nursing shortage, there is now heightened interest in ensuring that graduates of nursing programs and practicing nurses have sufficient informatics competencies to meet the demands of various health care practice settings (Carty & Rosenfeld, 1998; Grobe, 1989; Peterson & Gerdin-Jelger, 1988; Staggers, Gassert, & Curran, 2001; 2002).

The most substantial work on informatics competency definitions for nursing has been led by Staggers et al. (2001, 2002), who published a set of informatics competencies for nurses at four levels of practice: beginning nurse, experienced nurse, informatics specialist, and informatics innovator. Investigators developed and initially validated the competencies through literature review and expert consensus. Building on this work and others, the ANA (American Nurses Association, 2001) published the *Scope and Standards of Nursing Informatics Practice*. The document not only delineates informatics nurse specialist practice, but also describes informatics competencies for beginning and experienced nurses.

Several researchers have examined informatics content and related competencies in nursing curricula. McNeil, Elfrink, and Pierce (2004) recently reported the results of an online survey of deans/directors from 266 baccalaureate and higher nursing education programs in the United States to determine the extent of informatics content in the curriculum and faculty expertise. The most frequently taught aspects of informatics content in the undergraduate curriculum were how to access electronic resources, ethical use of information systems and the computer-based patient record, and evidence-based practice. Data and information system standards were the least visible content areas. Among the respondents, only two programs rated their faculty as experts in teaching and using information technology.

Desjardins, Cook, Jenkins, and Bakken (2005) described the effect of an innovative informatics for evidence-based practice (IEBP) curriculum that combined didactic course work and personal digital assistant-based documentation of clinical encounters on nursing informatics competencies in three student cohorts at the Columbia University School of Nursing. A repeated-measures, nonequivalent comparison group design was used to determine differences in self-rated informatics competencies pre- and post-IEBP and between cohorts at graduation. The types of computer skill competencies on which the students rated themselves as competent on at admission were generic in nature and reflective of basic computer literacy. Informatics competencies increased significantly from admission to graduation in all areas for the class of 2002 and in almost all areas for the class of 2003. None of the three cohorts achieved competence in the area of computer skills: education despite curricular revisions. There were no differences among the cohorts at graduation, suggesting that the various curricular innovations were equally successful in promoting informatics competency.

Other researchers (Tanner, Pierce, & Pravikoff, 2004) have focused on information literacy, a component of informatics competency based on a set of knowledge and skills related to information retrieval that was proposed by the library community in 1989 (American Library Association, 1989), updated in 1998 (National Forum on Information Literacy, 1998), and closely tied to evidence-based practice (Sackett, Richardson, Rosenberg, & Haynes, 1998). Information literacy includes knowing when a need for information exists, identifying information needed to address a given problem or issue, finding needed information and evaluating the information; organizing the information, and using the information effectively to address the problem or issue at hand (American Library Association, 1989). The findings of Tanner et al.'s (2004) national survey of nurses are congruent with the American Library Association's 1998 progress report (National Forum on Information Literacy). The investigators found that although the majority (64.5%) of nurses had information needs on a regular basis, more than half of the respondents never searched electronic databases. Moreover, two-thirds reported "never" to frequency of evaluating research reports, and 52% reported "never" to frequency of using research in practice.

In a related study, Pravikoff, Tanner, and Pierce (2005) reported that the nurses felt more confident asking colleagues or peers and searching the Internet and World Wide Web than using bibliographic databases such as PubMed or Cumulative Index to Nursing and Allied Health Literature to find specific information. Their findings suggest that nurses are inadequately trained in the use of tools that would help them find evidence on which to base their practice.

Knowledge Gaps and Future Research

Literature suggests that although there is heightened awareness of the importance of informatics competencies (Saranto & Hovenga, 2004), practicing nurses do not possess the necessary informatics competencies to fully utilize informatics tools. In addition, integration of informatics competencies into nursing curriculum is limited. Lack of informatics competencies can result in suboptimal use of informatics tools designed to enhance patient safety.

CONCLUSIONS

In a recent paper entitled *Strategic Action in Health Information Technology: Why the Obvious Has Taken So Long*, Shortliffe (2005) notes that "Today the United States is poised to achieve what has been sought and anticipated for at least three decades"(p. 1222) and highlights recent governmental and nongovernmental activities that support this proposition. The health information technologies deployed as part of the strategic action framework must support nursing practice in a manner that enables prevention of medical errors and promotion of patient safety and contributes to the development of practice-based nursing knowledge as well as best practices for patient safety. The seminal work that has been completed to date is necessary, but not sufficient, to achieve this objective. Recommendations for progressing toward this objective, in addition to those specified at the end of each section, include the following:

- Nursing research focused on the use of informatics for patient safety needs to move from formative or process evaluations to outcome evaluations
- Nursing informatics researchers should explicitly assess their research for potential contributions to error prevention and promotion of patient safety
- Nurse researchers should increase their participation and leadership in interdisciplinary patient safety–oriented informatics research
- The phenomenon of near misses should be explicitly explored from the perspective of nurses' work and informatics support for prevention of near misses
- Doctoral programs in nursing informatics should evaluate their curricula from the perspective of patient safety and make revisions as necessary

- Doctoral programs with an emphasis on patient safety should evaluate their curricula from the perspective of informatics and make revisions as necessary
- Nurse leaders should work in relevant policy arenas to ensure that the policies that are developed in regard to health information technologies are inclusive of nurses and advanced practice nurses (e.g., incentives for EHR adoption must not be limited to physicians)
- Increased mechanisms for funding research at the intersection of patient safety, nursing, and informatics should be developed

REFERENCES

Abbott, P. A., Quirolgico, S., Manchand, R., Canfield, K., & Adya, M. (1998). *Can the US Minimum Data Set be used for predicting admissions to acute care facilities?* Proceedings of MedInfo98; (pp. 1318–1321). Amsterdam: IOS Press.

Ad Hoc Committee on Health Literacy for the Council on Scientific Affairs, American Medical Association (1999). Health literacy: Report of the Council on Scientific Affairs. *Journal of the American Medical Association, 281*(6), 552–557.

Agency for Healthcare Research and Quality (2000). *Patient fact sheet: 20 tips to help prevent medical errors.* Retrieved November 1, 2005, from www.ahrq.gov/consumer/20tips.htm

Alemagno, S. A., Niles, S. A., & Treiber, E. A. (2004). Using computers to reduce medication misuse of community-based seniors: Results of a pilot intervention program. *Geriatric Nursing, 25*(5), 281–285.

American Library Association (1989). *Presidential Committee on Information Literacy. Final report.* Chicago.

American Nurses Association (2004). *National Database of Nursing Quality Indicators.* Retrieved 2005, from www.nursingworld.org/quality/database.htm

American Nurses Association (1995). *Nursing report card for acute care.* Washington, DC: American Nurses Publishing.

American Nurses Association (2001). *Scope and Standards of Nursing Informatics Practice.* Washington, DC: American Nurses Publishing.

Anderson, S., & Wittwer, W. (2004). Using bar-code point-of-care technology for patient safety. *Journal of Healthcare Quality, 26*(6), 5–11.

Andreu, G., Morel, P., Forestier, F., Debeir, J., Rebibo, D., Janvier, G., et al. (2002). Hemovigilance network in France: Organization and analysis of immediate transfusion incident reports from 1994 to 1998. *Transfusion, 42*(10), 1356–1364.

Aydin, C. E., Bolton, L. B., Donaldson, N., Brown, D. S., Buffum, M., Elashoff, J. D., et al. (2004). Creating and analyzing a statewide nursing quality measurement database. *Journal of Nursing Scholarship, 36*(4), 371–378.

Bakken, S. (2001). An informatics infrastructure is essential for evidence-based practice. *Journal of the American Medical Informatics Association, 8*(3), 199–201.

Bakken, S., Cashen, M. S., Mendonca, E. A., O'Brien, A., & Zieniewicz, J. (2000). Representing nursing activities within a concept-oriented terminological system: Evaluation of a type definition. *Journal of the American Medical Informatics Association, 7*(1), 81–90.

Bakken, S., Cimino, J. J., Haskell, R., Kukafka, R., Matsumoto, C., Chan, G. K., et al. (2000). Evaluation of the clinical LOINC (Logical Observation Identifiers, Names, and Codes) semantic structure as a terminology model for standardized assessment measures. *Journal of the American Medical Informatics Association, 7*(6), 529–538.

Bakken, S., Coenen, A., & Saba, V. (2004). ISO reference technology model: nursing diagnosis and action models look to testing for practical application. *Healthcare Informatics, 21*(9), 52.

Bakken, S., Hyun, S., Friedman, C., & Johnson, S. B. (2005). ISO reference terminology models for nursing: Applicability for natural language processing of nursing narratives. *International Journal of Medical Informatics, 74*(7–8), 615–622.

Bakken, S., Warren, J. J., Casey, A., Konicek, D., Lundberg, C., & Pooke, M. (2002). Information model and terminology model issues related to goals. *American Medical Informatics Association Annual Symposium Proceedings* (pp. 17–21). Bethesda, MD: American Medical Informatics Association.

Bakken, S., Warren, J. J., Lundberg, C., Casey, A., Correia, C., Konicek, D., et al. (2002). An evaluation of the usefulness of two terminology models for integrating nursing diagnosis concepts into SNOMED Clinical Terms. *International Journal of Medical Informatics, 68*(1–3), 71–77.

Ball, M. J., Weaver, C., & Abbott, P. A. (2003). Enabling technologies promise to revitalize the role of nursing in an era of patient safety. *International Journal of Medical Informatics, 69*(1), 29–38.

Bates, D., Leape, L., Cullen, D., Laird, N., Peterson, L., Teich, J., et al. (1998). Effect of computerized physician order entry and a team intervention on prevention of serious medication errors. *Journal of the American Medical Association, 280*, 1311–1316.

Bates, D. W. (1999). The impact of computerized physician order entry on medication error prevention. *Journal of the American Medical Informatics Association, 6*(4), 313–321.

Bates, D. W., Evans, R. S., Murff, H., Stetson, P. D., Pizziferri, L., & Hripcsak, G. (2003a). Detecting adverse events using information technology. *Journal of the American Medical Informatics Association, 10*(2), 115–128.

Bates, D. W., Evans, R. S., Murff, H., Stetson, P. D., Pizziferri, L., & Hripcsak, G. (2003b). Policy and the future of adverse event detection using information technology. *Journal of the American Medical Informatics Association, 10*(2), 226–228.

Beyea, S. (2000). Perioperative data elements: Interventions and outcomes. *Association of Operating Room Nurses Journal, 71*(2), 344–353.

Brennan, P. (1997). The ComputerLink projects: A decade of experience. *Studies in Health Technology and Informatics, 46*, 521–526.

Brennan, P., Bjorndottir, G., Rogers, M., Jones, J., Moore, S., & Visovsky, C. (2000). Launching HeartCare. In V. Saba, R. Carr, W. Sermeus & P. Rocha (Eds.), *Nursing informatics 2000. One step beyond: The evolution of technology and nursing. Proceedings of the 7th IMIA International Conference on Nursing Use of Computers and Information Science* (pp. 438–445). Auckland, New Zealand: Adis International.

Brennan, P., Moore, S., Bjornsdottir, G., Jones, J., Visovsky, C., & Rogers, M. (2001). HeartCare: An Internet-based information and support system for patient home recovery after coronary artery bypass graft (CABG) surgery. *Journal of Advanced Nursing*, 35(5), 699–708.

Brennan, P. F., Caldwell, B., Moore, S. M., Screenath, N., & Jones, J. (1998). Designing HeartCare: Custom computerized home care for patients recovering from CABG surgery. In C. G. Chute (Ed.), *American Medical Informatics Association Annual Fall Symposium Proceedings* (pp. 381–385). Orlando, FL: Hanley & Belfus.

Brennan, P. F., Moore, S. M., & Smyth, K. A. (1995). The effects of a special computer network on caregivers of persons with Alzheimer's disease. *Nursing Research, 44*(3), 166–172.

Brennan, P. F., & Ripich, S. (1994). Use of a home-care computer network by persons with AIDS. *International Journal of Technology Assessment in Health Care, 10*(2), 258–272.

Brown, D. S., Donaldson, N., Aydin, C. E., & Carlson, N. (2001). Hospital nursing benchmarks: The California Nursing Outcomes Coalition project. *Journal of Healthcare Quality, 23*(4), 22–27.

Callum, J. L., Merkley, L. L., Coovadia, A. S., Lima, A. P., & Kaplan, H. S. (2004). Experience with the medical event reporting system for transfusion medicine (MERS-TM) at three hospitals. *Transfusion and Apheresis Science, 31*(2), 133–143.

Carty, B., & Rosenfeld, P. (1998). From computer technology to information technology: Findings from a national study of nursing education. *Computers in Nursing, 16*, 259–265.

Casper, G. R., Karsh, B. T., Or, C. K. L., Carayon, P., Grenier, A. S., Sebern, M., et al. (2005). Designing a technology enhanced practice for home nursing care of patients with congestive heart failure. *American Medical Informatics Association Annual Symposium Proceedings*, (pp. 116–120). Bethesda, MD: American Medical Informatics Association.

Chang, B. L., Bakken, S., Brown, S. S., Houston, T. K., Kreps, G. L., Kukafka, R., et al. (2004). Bridging the digital divide: Reaching vulnerable populations. *Journal of the American Medical Informatics Association, 11*(6), 448–457.

Choi, J. (2005). Web-based educational resources for low literacy families in the NICU. *American Medical Informatics Association Annual Symposium Proceedings*, (p. 922). Bethesda, MD: American Medical Informatics Association.

Choi, J., Jenkins, M. L., Cimino, J. J., White, T. M., & Bakken, S. (2005). Toward semantic interoperability in home health care: Formally representing OASIS items for integration into a concept-oriented terminology. *Journal of the American Medical Informatics Association, 12*(4), 410–417.

Clarke, H. F., Bradley, C., Whytock, S., Handfield, S., van der Wal, R., & Gundry, S. (2005). Pressure ulcers: Implementation of evidence-based nursing practice. *Journal of Advanced Nursing, 49*(6), 578–590.

Committee on Data Standards for Patient Safety. (2004). *Patient Safety: Achieving a New Standard for Care*. Washington, DC: Board on Health Care Services, Institute of Medicine.

Committee on Health Literacy. (2004). *Health Literacy: A Prescription to End Confusion*. Washington, DC: Institute of Medicine of the National Academies.

Committee on Quality of Health Care in America. (2001). *Crossing the Quality Chasm: A New Health System for the 21st Century.* Washington, DC: Institute of Medicine, National Academy of Sciences.

Coyle, G. A., & Heinen, M. (2005). Evolution of BCMA within the Department of Veterans Affairs. *Nursing Administration Quarterly, 29*(1), 32–38.

Cudney, S., Winters, C., Weinert, C., & Anderson, K. (2005). Social support in cyberspace: Lessons learned. *Rehabilitation Nursing, 30*(1), 25–28; discussion 29.

Currie, L. M., Mellino, L. V., Cimino, J. J., & Bakken, S. (2004). Development and representation of a fall-injury risk assessment instrument in a clinical information system. *Medinfo, 11*(Pt. 1), (pp. 721–725), Bethesda, MD: American Medical Informatics Association.

Danko, A., Kennedy, R., Haskell, R., Androwich, I. M., Button, P., Correia, C. M., et al. (2003). Modeling nursing interventions in the act class of HL7 RIM Version 3. *Journal of Biomedical Informatics, 36*(4–5), 294–303.

Davis, T., Williams, M., Marin, E., Parker, R., & Glass, J. (2002). Health literacy and cancer communication. *CA: A Cancer Journal for Clinicians, 52*(3), 134–149.

Desjardins, K. S., Cook, S. S., Jenkins, M., & Bakken, S. (2005). Effect of an informatics for Evidence-based Practice Curriculum on nursing informatics competencies. *International Journal of Medical Informatics, 74*(11–12):1012–1020.

Donaldson, N., Brown, D. S., Aydin, C. E., Bolton, M. L., & Rutledge, D. N. (2005). Leveraging nurse-related dashboard benchmarks to expedite performance improvement and document excellence. *Journal of Nursing Administration, 35*(4), 163–172.

Dunton, N., Gajewski, B., Taunton, R. L., & Moore, J. (2004). Nurse staffing and patient falls on acute care hospital units. *Nursing Outlook, 52*(1), 53–59.

Dykes, P. C., Currie, L. M., & Cimino, J. J. (2003). Adequacy of evolving national standardized terminologies for interdisciplinary coded concepts in an automated clinical pathway. *Journal of Biomedical Informatics, 36*(4–5), 313–325.

Effken, J. A., Brewer, B. B., Patil, A., Lamb, G. S., Verran, J. A., & Carley, K. (2003a). Using computational modeling to study the impact of workplace characteristics on patient safety outcomes. *American Medical Informatics Association Annual Symposium Proceedings,* (p. 837). Bethesda, MD: American Medical Informatics Association.

Effken, J. A., Brewer, B. B., Patil, A., Lamb, G. S., Verran, J. A., & Carley, K. (2004). Using computational modeling to improve patient care unit safety and quality outcomes. *Medinfo, 11*(Pt. 1), (pp. 726–730), Bethesda, MD: American Medical Informatics Association.

Effken, J. A., Brewer, B. B., Patil, A., Lamb, G. S., Verran, J. A., & Carley, K. (2005). Using OrgAhead, a computational modeling program, to improve patient care unit safety and quality outcomes. *International Journal of Medical Informatics, 74*(7–8), 605–613.

Effken, J. A., Brewer, B. B., Patil, A., Lamb, G. S., Verran, J. A., & Carley, K. (2003b). Using computational modeling to transform nursing data into actionable information. *Journal of Biomedical Informatics, 36*(4–5), 351–361.

Galanter, W. L., Didomenico, R. J., & Polikaitis, A. (2005). A trial of automated decision support alerts for contraindicated medications using computerized physician order entry. *Journal of the American Medical Informatics Association, 12*(3), 269–274.

Gerber, B. S., Brodsky, I. G., Lawless, K. A., Smolin, L. I., Arozullah, A. M., Smith, E. V., et al. (2005). Implementation and evaluation of a low-literacy diabetes education computer multimedia application. *Diabetes Care*, 28(7), 1574–1580.

Gillespie, L. D., Gillespie, W. J., Robertson, M. C., Lamb, S. E., Cumming, R. G., & Rowe, B. H. (2005). Interventions for preventing falls in elderly people. *Cochrane Database of Systematic Reviews* (4).

Goodwin, L., VanDyne, M., Lin, S., & Talbert, S. (2003). Data mining issues and opportunities for building nursing knowledge. *Journal of Biomedical Informatics*, 36(4–5), 379–388.

Goodwin, L. K., Innacchione, M. A., & Hammond, W. E. (2000). Data mining methodology for outcomes analysis in complex clinical problems. In V. Saba, R. Carr, W. Sermeus & P. Rocha (Eds.), *Nursing Informatics 2000. One Step Beyond: The Evolution of Technology and Nursing. Proceedings of the 7th IMIA International Conference on Nursing Use of Computers and Information Science* (pp. 66–72). Auckland, New Zealand: Adis International.

Goossen, W. T., Ozbolt, J. G., Coenen, A., Park, H. A., Mead, C., Ehnfors, M., et al. (2004). Development of a provisional domain model for the nursing process for use within the Health Level 7 reference information model. *Journal of the American Medical Informatics Association*, 11(3), 186–194.

Gray, N. J., Klein, J. D., Noyce, P. R., Sesselberg, T. S., & Cantrill, J. A. (2005). The Internet: A window on adolescent health literacy. *Journal of Adolescent Health*, 37(3), 243.

Griffith, H. M., & Robinson, K. R. (1992). Survey of the degree to which critical care nurses are performing Current Procedural Terminology-coded services. *American Journal of Critical Care*, 1, 91–98.

Griffith, H. M., & Robinson, K. R. (1993). Current Procedural Terminology (CPT) coded services provided by nurse specialists. *Image: Journal of Nursing Scholarship*, 25, 178–186.

Grobe, S. (1989). Nursing informatics competencies. *Methods of Information in Medicine*, 28, 267–269.

Gustafson, D., Hawkins, R., Boberg, E., McTavish, F., Owens, B., Wise, M., et al. (2002). CHESS: 10 years of research and development in consumer health informatics for broad populations, including the underserved. *International Journal of Medical Informatics*, 65(3), 169–177.

Gustafson, D., Hawkins, R., Pingree, S., McTavish, F., Arora, N., Mendenhall, J., et al. (2001). Effect of computer support on younger women with breast cancer. *Journal of General Internal Medicine*, 16(7), 435–445.

Hardiker, N. R., Bakken, S., Casey, A., & Hoy, D. (2002). Formal nursing terminology systems: A means to an end. *Journal of Biomedical Informatics*, 35(5–6), 298–305.

Hardiker, N. R., & Rector, A. L. (1998). Modeling nursing terminology using the GRAIL representation language. *Journal of the American Medical Informatics Association*, 5(1), 120–128.

Hardiker, N. R., & Rector, A. L. (2001). Structural validation of nursing terminologies. *Journal of the American Medical Informatics Association*, 8, 212–221.

Harrington, C., Collier, E., O'Meara, J., Kitchener, M., Simon, L. P., & Schnelle, J. F. (2003). Federal and state nursing facility websites: Just what the consumer needs? *American Journal of Medical Quality*, 18(1), 21–37.

Harrington, C., O'Meara, J., Collier, E., & Schnelle, J. F. (2003). Nursing indicators of quality in nursing homes. A Web-based approach. *Journal of Gerontology Nursing, 29*(10), 5–11.

Harrington, C., O'Meara, J., Kitchener, M., Simon, L. P., & Schnelle, J. F. (2003). Designing a report card for nursing facilities: What information is needed and why. *Gerontologist, 43*(2), 47–57.

Harris, C. M. (2005). *My chart: Your personal health connection.* Paper presented at the Connecting Americans to Their Health Care Conference, Washington, DC.

Henry, S. B., Holzemer, W. L., Reilly, C. A., & Campbell, K. E. (1994). Terms used by nurses to describe patient problems: can SNOMED III represent nursing concepts in the patient record? *Journal of the American Medical Informatics Association, 1*(1), 61–74.

Hibbard, J. H., Peters, E., Slovic, P., & Tusler, M. (2005). Can patients be part of the solution? Views on their role in preventing medical errors. *Medical Care Research Review, 62*(5), 601–616.

Hill, W., Schillo, L., & Weinert, C. (2004). Effect of a computer-based intervention on social support for chronically ill rural women. *Rehabilitation Nursing, 29*(5), 169–173.

Hill, W. G., & Weinert, C. (2004). An evaluation of an online intervention to provide social support and health education. *Computes, Informatics, Nursing, 22*(5), 282–288.

Hwang, J. I., Cimino, J. J., & Bakken, S. (2003). Integrating nursing diagnostic concepts into the Medical Entities Dictionary using the ISO Reference Terminology Model for Nursing Diagnosis. *Journal of the American Medical Informatics Association, 10*(4), 382–388.

Johnson, M., Maas, M., & Moorhead, S. (Eds.) (2000). *Nursing Outcomes Classification (NOC)* (2nd ed.). St. Louis: C. V. Mosby.

Keenan, G., & Yakel, E. (2005). Promoting safe nursing care by bringing visibility to the disciplinary aspects of interdisciplinary care. *American Medical Informatics Association Annual Symposium Proceedings* (pp. 385–389). Bethesda, MD: American Medical Informatics Association.

Koppel, R., Metlay, J. P., Cohen, A., Abaluck, B., Localio, A. R., Kimmel, S. E., et al. (2005). Role of computerized physician order entry systems in facilitating medication errors. *Journal of the American Medical Association, 293*(10), 1197–1203.

Liaw, S. T., Sulaiman, N., Pearce, C., Sims, J., Hill, K., Grain, H., et al. (2003). Falls prevention within the Australian general practice data model: Methodology, information model, and terminology issues. *Journal of the American Medical Informatics Association, 10*(5), 425–432.

Linden, J. V., Wagner, K., Voytovich, A. E., & Sheehan, J. (2000). Transfusion errors in New York State: An analysis of 10 years' experience. *Transfusion, 40*(10), 1207–1213.

Martin, K. S. (2004). *The Omaha System—A Key to Practice, Documentation, and Information Management* (2nd ed.): Elsevier.

Matney, S., Bakken, S., & Huff, S. M. (2003). Representing nursing assessments in clinical information systems using the logical observation identifiers, names, and codes database. *Journal of Biomedical Informatics, 36*(4–5), 287–293.

McCloskey, J. C., & Bulechek, G. M. (2000). *Nursing interventions classification* (3rd ed.). St. Louis: C. V. Mosby.

McCray, A. T. (2005). Promoting health literacy. *Journal of the American Medical Informatics Association, 12*(2), 152–163.

McNeil, B., Elfrink, V., & Pierce, S. (2004). Preparing student nurses, faculty and clinicians for 21st century informatics practice: Findings from a national survey of nursing education programs in the United States. *Medinfo*, (pp. 903–907), Bethesda, MD: American Medical Informatics Association.

Melton, G. B., & Hripcsak, G. (2005). Automated detection of adverse events using natural language processing of discharge summaries. *Journal of the American Medical Informatics Association*, 12(4), 448–457.

Moody, L. E. (2005). E-health web portals: Delivering holistic healthcare and making home the point of care. *Holistic Nursing Practice*, 19(4), 156–160.

Moss, J., Coenen, A., & Mills, M. (2003). Evaluation of the draft international standard for a reference terminology model for nursing actions. *Journal of Biomedical Informatics*, 36(4–5), 271–278.

Murff, H. J., Forster, A. J., Peterson, J. F., Fiskio, J. M., Heiman, H. L., & Bates, D. W. (2003). Electronically screening discharge summaries for adverse medical events. *Journal of the American Medical Informatics Association*, 10(4), 339–350.

Murff, H. J., Patel, V. L., Hripcsak, G., & Bates, D. W. (2003). Detecting adverse events for patient safety research: A review of current methodologies. *Journal of Biomedical Informatics*, 36(1–2), 131–143.

National Forum on Information Literacy. (1998). *A progress report on information literacy: An update on the American Library Association Presidential Committee on Information Literacy: Final report*. San Jose, CA.

National Quality Forum. (2003). *Safe Practices for Better Health Care*. Washington, DC.

Neafsey, P. J., Strickler, Z., Shellman, J., & Padula, A. T. (2001). Delivering health information about self-medication to older adults: Use of touchscreen-equipped notebook computers. *Journal of Gerontology Nursing*, 27(11), 19–27.

North American Nursing Diagnosis Association (NANDA) International. (2005). *Nursing diagnoses: Definitions and classification 2005–2006*. Philadelphia, PA: NANDA International.

O'Connor, A., Fiset, V., DeGrasse, C., Graham, I., Evans, W., Stacy, D., et al. (1999). Decision aids for patients considering options affecting cancer outcomes: Evidence of efficacy and policy implications. *Journal of the National Cancer Institute Monographs*, 25, 67–79.

O'Connor, A., Tugwell, P., Wells, G., Elmslie, T., Jollie, E., Hollingworth, G., et al. (1998). A decision aid for women considering hormone therapy after menopause: Decision support framework and evaluation. *Patient Education and Counseling*, 33, 267–279.

O'Neill, E. S., Dluhy, N. M., Fortier, P. J., & Michel, H. (2004). The N-CODES project: The first year. *Computers, Informatics, Nursing*, 22(6), 345–350.

Ozbolt, J. (2000a). Terminology standards for nursing: Collaboration at the summit. *Journal of the American Medical Informatics Association*, 7(6), 517–522.

Ozbolt, J. (2000b). Toward a reference terminology model for nursing: The 1999 Nursing Vocabulary Summit Conference. In V. Saba, R. Carr, W. Sermeus & P. Rocha (Eds.), *7th International Congress Nursing Informatics. One Step Beyond: The Evolution of Technology and Nursing* (pp. 267–276). Auckland, New Zealand: Adis International.

Ozbolt, J. (2003a). The Nursing Terminology Summit Conferences: A case study of successful collaboration for change. *Journal of Biomedical Informatics*, 36(4–5), 362–374.

Ozbolt, J. (2003b). Reference terminology for therapeutic goals: A new approach. *American Medical Informatics Association Annual Symposium Proceedings* (pp. 504–508). Bethesda, MD: American Medical Informatics Association.

Patterson, E. S., Cook, R. I., & Render, M. L. (2002). Improving patient safety by identifying side effects from introducing bar coding in medication administration. *Journal of the American Medical Informatics Association, 9*(5), 540–553.

Patterson, E. S., Rogers, M. L., & Render, M. L. (2004). Fifteen best practice recommendations for bar-code medication administration in the Veterans Health Administration. *Joint Commission Journal of Quality and Safety, 30*(7), 355–365.

Peterson, H., & Gerdin-Jelger, U. (1988). *Preparing nurses for using information systems: Recommended informatics competencies.* New York: NLN Publications.

Porcella, A., & Walker, K. (2005). Patient safety with blood products administration using wireless and bar-code technology. *American Medical Informatics Association Annual Symposium Proceedings* (pp. 614–618). Bethesda, MD: American Medical Informatics Association.

Pravikoff, D. S., Tanner, A. B., & Pierce, S. T. (2005). Readiness of U.S. nurses for evidence-based practice. *American Journal of Nursing, 105*(9), 40–51; quiz 52.

Quaglini, S., Grandi, M., Baiardi, P., Mazzoleni, M. C., Fassino, C., Franchi, G., et al. (2000). A computerized guideline for pressure ulcer prevention. *International Journal of Medical Informatics, 58–59,* 207–217.

Reynolds, K., Peres, A., & Tatham, J. M. (2005). The impact on patient safety of free-text entry of nursing orders into an electronic medical record in an integrated delivery system. *American Medical Informatics Association Annual Symposium Proceedings* (p. 1095). Bethesda, MD: American Medical Informatics Association.

Roberts, W. D. (2005). *Clinical practice guideline-related knowledge representation models and comprehension-generated inferences of nurse practitioners and physicians at varying levels of expertise.* New York: Columbia University.

Ruland, C. (1999). Decision support for patient preference-based care planning: Effects on nursing care and patient outcomes. *Journal of the American Medical Informatics Association, 6*(4), 304–312.

Ruland, C. M. (2002). Handheld technology to improve patient care: Evaluating a support system for preference-based care planning at the bedside. *Journal of the American Medical Informatics Association, 9*(2), 192–201.

Ruland, C. M. (2004). Improving patient safety through informatics tools for shared decision making and risk communication. *International Journal of Medical Informatics, 73* (7–8), 551–557.

Ruland, C. M., Kresevic, D., Brennan, P. F., & Lorensen, M. (1997). Decision support for assessing patient preferences for geriatric care. *Studies in Health Technologies and Informatics, 46,* 296–299.

Ruland, C. M., Kresevic, D., & Lorensen, M. (1997). Including patient preferences in nurses' assessment of older patients. *Journal of Clinical Nursing, 6*(6), 495–504.

Ruland, C. M., White, T., Stevens, M., Fanciullo, G., & Khilani, S. M. (2003). Effects of a computerized system to support shared decision making in symptom management of cancer patients: Preliminary results. *Journal of the American Medical Informatics Association, 10*(6), 573–579.

Saba, V. (2004). *Clinical Care Classification*. Retrieved October 14, 2004, from http://www.sabacare.com

Sackett, D. L., Richardson, W. S., Rosenberg, W., & Haynes, R. B. (1998). *Evidenced-based medicine: How to practice and teach EBM*. Edinburgh: Churchill Livingstone.

Saranto, K., & Hovenga, E. (2004). Information literacy-what is it about? Literature review of the concept and the context. *International Journal of Medical Informatics, 73*, 503–513.

Shaw, B. R., McTavish, F., Hawkins, R., Gustafson, D. H., & Pingree, S. (2000). Experiences of women with breast cancer: Exchanging social support over the CHESS computer network. *Journal of Health Communication, 5*(2), 135–159.

Shortliffe, E. H. (2005). Strategic action in health information technology: Why the obvious has taken so long. *Health Affairs (Millwood), 24*(5), 1222–1233.

Snyder, R., & Fields, W. (2005). Assessing hospital readiness for Computerized Provider Order Entry (CPOE) innovation. *American Medical Informatics Association Annual Symposium Proceedings*, (p. 1118). Bethesda, MD: American Medical Informatics Association.

Staggers, N., Gassert, C. A., & Curran, C. (2001). Informatics competencies for nurses at four levels of practice. *Journal of Nursing Education, 40*(7), 303–316.

Staggers, N., Gassert, C. A., & Curran, C. (2002). A Delphi study to determine informatics competencies for nurses at four levels of practice. *Nursing Research, 51*(6), 383–390.

Tang, P. C., & Lansky, D. (2005). The missing link: Bridging the patient-provider health information gap. *Health Affairs (Millwood), 24*(5), 1290–1295.

Tanner, A., Pierce, S., & Pravikoff, D. (2004). Readiness for evidence-based practice: Information literacy needs of nurses in the United States. *Medinfo*, (pp. 936–940). Bethesda, MD: American Medical Informatics Association.

Thompson, T., & Brailer, D. (2004). *The decade of health information technology: Delivering consumer-centric and information-rich health care. Framework for strategic action*. Washington, DC: Office of the National Coordinator for Health Information Technology. U.S. Department of Health and Human Services.

University of California at San Francisco (UCSF)—Stanford University Evidence-based Practice Center. (2001). *Making health care safer: A critical analysis of patient safety practices* (Publication No. 01-E058). Rockville, MD: Agency for Healthcare Research and Quality.

Vincent, C. A., & Coulter, A. (2002). Patient safety: What about the patient? *Quality and Safe Health Care, 11*(1), 76–80.

Weinert, C. (2005). Social support in cyberspace: The next generation. *Computers, Informatics, Nursing, 23*(1), 7–15.

Weinert, C., Cudney, S., & Winters, C. (2005). Social support in cyberspace: The next generation. *Computers, Informatics, Nursing, 23*(1), 7–15.

Weingart, S. N., Pagovich, O., Sands, D. Z., Li, J. M., Aronson, M. D., Davis, R. B., et al. (2005). What can hospitalized patients tell us about adverse events? Learning from patient-reported incidents. *Journal of General Internal Medicine, 20*(9), 830–836.

Williams, M., Baker, D., Parker, R., & Nurss, J. (1998). Relationship of functional health literacy to patients' knowledge of their chronic disease. A study of patients with hypertension and diabetes. *Archives of Internal Medicine, 158*(2), 166–172.

Working Group on Policies for Electronic Information Sharing Between Doctors and Patients. (2004). *Connecting Americans to their healthcare: Final report*. New York, NY: Connecting for Health, Markle Foundation.

Wright, A. A., & Katz, I. T. (2005). Bar coding for patient safety. *New England Journal of Medicine, 353*(4), 329–331.

Wydra, E. W. (2001). The effectiveness of a self-care management interactive multimedia module. *Oncology Nursing Forum, 28*(9), 1399–1407.

Yeh, M. L., Chen, H. H., & Liu, P. H. (2005). Effects of multimedia with printed nursing guide in education on self-efficacy and functional activity and hospitalization in patients with hip replacement. *Patient Education and Counseling, 57*(2), 217–224.

Zielstorff, R. D., Barnett, G. O., Estey, G., Hamilton, G., Vickery, A., Welebob, E., et al. (1997). A knowledge-based decision support system for prevention and treatment of pressure ulcers. *Studies in Health Technology and Informatics, 46*, 291–295.

Zielstorff, R. D., Barnett, G. O., Fitzmaurice, J. B., Estey, G., Hamilton, G., Vickery, A., et al. (1996). A decision support system for prevention and treatment of pressure ulcers based on AHCPR guidelines. *American Medical Informatics Association Annual Symposium Proceedings*, (pp. 562–566), Bethesda, MD: American Medical Informatics Association.

Zielstorff, R. D., Estey, G., Vickery, A., Hamilton, G., Fitzmaurice, J. B., & Barnett, G. O. (1997). Evaluation of a decision support system for pressure ulcer prevention and management: Preliminary findings. *American Medical Informatics Association Annual Symposium Proceedings*, (pp. 248–252), Bethesda, MD: American Medical Informatics Association.

Chapter 10

Organizational Climate and Culture Factors

Sean P. Clarke

ABSTRACT

Nurses and others have expressed a great deal of interest in the potential for incorporating notions about organizational culture and climate in research and practice aiming to improve health care safety. In this review, definitions and measures of these terms are explored, the state of the research literature connecting culture and climate with safety is reviewed, and directions for future research and leadership practice are outlined.

Keywords: patient safety, nursing, organizational climate

The current era of patient safety research and practice that began with publication of the Institute of Medicine's landmark report *To Err Is Human* is now entering its seventh year. And although health professionals and leaders have long been conscious of safety concerns, the intense attention paid to safety issues in the recent past has been characterized by several new lines of thinking. One such development has been focused public and professional concern regarding poor patient outcomes as indicators of problems in care. Another has been a recognition that there has been relatively limited use of information technologies at the point of care. And yet another has been attention to enormous variation in the uptake of basic evidence–based practices by health care providers and organizations. Arguably, however, the most important development has been a sustained move toward thinking of safety problems in terms of systems issues. Root-cause analysis has supplanted a tendency to automatically attribute bad outcomes to the last pair of hands to touch the patient before an accident or error.

Clinicians and managers have long noted differences in the atmospheres or environments of health care organizations and subunits within those organizations (nursing units, specialty areas, etc.). Although they are not always able to articulate exactly what these differences are beyond general impressions (cold, friendly, disorganized, tense), they insist that the distinctions are real and that these factors influence both work lives and the process and outcomes of care. Contrasts can be especially striking across hospitals and other providers in the same geographical area that serve the same types of patients or have the same basic structural characteristics. Some of these variations appear to reflect the clienteles the organization or its subunit serves and historical forces, particularly the conditions under which it was founded, its most influential leaders over time, and how it has responded (or failed to respond) to social, technological, and economic shifts. In other situations, more immediate operating conditions and circumstances seem to affect the atmosphere or environment, for example, budget cuts, high turnover rates, or a lack of stable frontline or top-level leadership. In many ways, it is not surprising that as the search for improvements in patient safety continues, talk of environment and atmosphere (researched and defined in a more refined way) have entered into safety discussions.

Safety has become a pressing concern for nurses and others in health care because of the growing sophistication and technological intensity of patient care services in health care organizations. Tolerance for potentially avoidable poor outcomes in health care is also waning. Obviously, having as many factors in place in health care settings that favor safe practice and good outcomes is crucial. A high-reliability organization has consistently excellent outcomes in providing complex services and generally has a strong safety record (usually manifested as a low rate of accidents). Many believe that high-reliability organizations not only ensure that the correct raw materials of personnel and equipment are in place, but also commit to employee development and quality management strategies that make safety the primary goal of the organization (Page, 2004). Certainly, many hope that the notion of high-reliability organizations applies beyond industrial settings and aeronautics to health care facilities (Gaba, Singer, Sinaiko, Brown, & Ciavarelli, 2003).

There has been considerable emphasis on the application of technology, especially computerized provider order entry, dispensing technologies, and bar coding technology as a means of improving patient safety. Others have pressed for reforms in product labeling. Still others have emphasized the need for policies and procedures designed to ensure better flow of communication or decrease the odds that patients will be exposed to risky conditions. Attention to specific safety problems and ensuring near-universal application of best practices are certainly valid approaches. However, the number of technological and procedural solutions that are affordable and can be feasibly implemented across a range of institutions is limited, and it is also highly improbable that there will ever be sufficient time or resources to eliminate every potential safety hazard.

Many hope that some overarching organizational properties exist that support innovations, favor adoption of best practices, and decrease the need for senior management to be involved in micro-level practice decisions. Thus, leadership approaches that address systemic problems organizationwide will clearly be needed as well—a bundle of factors can be thought of either as ingredients, or the products, of positive organizational culture and climate.

The purpose of this review is not to duplicate published reviews of instruments (e.g., Ashkanasy, Broadfoot, & Falkus, 2000; Gershon, Stone, Bakken, & Larsen, 2004; Scott, Mannion, Davies, & Marshall, 2003; Tregunno, 2005) used in climate and culture research in health care or earlier overviews of the literature (e.g., Hickam, Severance, Feldstein, Ray, Gorman, Schuldheis et al., 2003; Page, 2004; Scott, Mannion, Marshall, & Davies, 2003; Tregunno). Rather, it is to provide an overview of points of agreement and controversy in definitions and measurement of climate and culture, outline the state of findings in the area, and make suggestions for practice and future research.

DEFINITIONS

Organizational Culture

Definitions of organizational culture abound (Martin, 2002). Most characterize it as the accumulation of invisible, often unspoken ideas, values, and approaches that permeate organizational life. The term culture and the notion that it can be studied systematically have roots in anthropology. Most have tried to characterize the culture of a specific organization or subunit of that organization. However, it is possible to think about the culture of a profession in general or of a profession in a particular country (e.g., the culture of American nursing). When examining organizations, particularly in an international context, it is also possible to consider the culture of business or work in a sector of a society in terms of what is valued and prioritized (Hofstede & Peterson, 2000).

The phrase "the way we do things around here" arises frequently when organizational culture is mentioned. Culture typically begins with what an organization perceives as its purpose and priorities and what types of activities are valued and which are less valued. Organizational culture is typically discussed in terms of a deeply engrained set of ideas and experiences that serve as a frame for actions and experiences in workplaces. It is possible to view culture as at least partially reflecting the cumulation or totality of leadership decisions in organizations over time. Such decisions in a health care organization might relate to a focus on patient needs, quality monitoring, training, and employee involvement in decision making. Those decisions directly and indirectly influence employee outcomes, including satisfaction and perceptions of the work environment, as well as organizational outcomes (such as quality of work, financial performance, and reputation). The performance of health care organizations on all of these levels can, over time, themselves influence culture.

Schein (1992) describes three levels or types of manifestations of culture: artifacts (readily observed, often physical traces in physical layout and design), espoused values (what insiders tell us are the strategies, goals, and policies of an organization), and basic underlying assumptions (unspoken ideas at the heart of the organization's success). Not surprisingly, organizational culture is typically considered to evolve over years. Few would say that it changes over weeks.

Many scholars conceptualize culture as a shared experience in organizations, and most quantitative researchers proceed with the assumption that it is shared, and that each organization has a unique configuration of cultural properties. However, each of these contentions is debatable and all have been discussed extensively by organizational behavior scholars (Martin, 2002). In addition to enumerating and lucidly explaining differences across various definitions and conceptualizations of organizational culture, Martin outlines three distinct approaches to the study of culture in organizations: integration (highlighting common experiences and perspectives across the organization), differentiation (describing unity within subunits or subgroups of employees but also important contrasts across these groups that may serve functional purposes), and fragmentation (an approach that resembles differentiation but takes the stance that the various different cultures are in fundamental conflict with each other). The integration approach has dominated much of the literature about culture in health care organizations; however, its critics argue that researchers and leaders who adopt it are often expressing a tacit preference for a degree of unity among workers that may not be possible or desirable in modern organizations.

Climate

As at least one group of authors has commented, the notion of organizational climate is an allusion to meteorology and enduring weather patterns (Scott, Mannion, Davies, et al., 2003). Organizational climate refers to an atmosphere, a moveable set of perceptions related to working and practice conditions, many of which are influenced by managers. It tends to be more grounded in the psychological experience of organizational life than culture.

Stone, Harrison, Geldman, Linzer, Peng, Roblin et al.'s (2005) integration and secondary analysis of six major studies of organizational climate in different health care settings identified two key domains of employee climate perceptions. The first was "core climate," including opinions about leaders' values and strategies and structural characteristics of the organization (e.g., communication, governance, and information technology use). The second was "process climate domains," encompassing perceptions about working conditions (e.g., aspects of supervision, work design, group process, and commitment to quality).

Climate is often thought of as subject to change within months, if not weeks, in the face of events and decisions in an organization. Some see climate factors as the most obvious or immediate reflections or results of culture. However, the exact distinction between culture and climate remains a matter of debate in the organizational studies literature (Ashkanasy, Wilderom, & Peterson, 2000).

Related Terms

Work Environments and Human Resource Practices

Tregunno (2005), among other authors, has stated that inconsistent use of terminology in results not only from difficulties in defining and distinguishing culture and climate, but also from writers' tendencies to use these two concepts and a number of related or cognate terms, such as *work environments* and *human resources management* (HRM), interchangeably. Confusion is exacerbated by the extensive interconnections between these ideas. For example, HRM practices (e.g., hiring, staff development, compensation, and participatory approaches) (Buchan, 2004) can be a reflection of underlying organizational culture or climate and can certainly contribute to climate.

Environment and *climate* might appear to be synonymous, but environments tend to encompass a broader range of factors. *Work environment* tends to refer to the perceptions of workers (in this case, nurses) regarding elements of the organization that relate to activities on the job (Tregunno, 2005). *Practice environment* refers more specifically to the presence of organizational elements emphasized as key to high-quality nursing care by educators, as well as leaders in the profession and advocacy groups (Estabrooks, Tourangeau, Humphrey, Hesketh, Giovannetti, & Thomson, 2002). These attributes include bedside clinician involvement in decision making related to clinical practice and organizational decisions affecting their work, evidence of respect for the professional nurse throughout the organization, quality monitoring and improvement activities, and opportunities and respect for continuing and higher education for nurses in the facility.

Some health care organizations that demonstrate all of these environmental elements have been designated Magnet health care facilities (McClure & Hinshaw, 2002). Research to identify objective outcomes in these organizations is ongoing. Whether some, most, or all Magnet facilities have distinct, desirable organizational climate or culture traits is not clear, conceptually or empirically, although some writers see the Magnet organizations as embodying a specific type of organizational culture (Miller & Brunell, 2004). Hickam and colleagues' (2003) review did not consider Magnet research to deal with cultural factors, but placed it instead in a broader category of research on outcomes related to organizational factors.

Safety Culture and Climate

Uniform use of terminology is further complicated by appearance of yet another pair of terms: *safety climate* and *safety culture*. Clinicians, managers, and researchers commonly use these terms in reference to the tendency of workers in a health care organization to question each other, adopt an active versus passive attitude about rooting out and resolving problems, and take a proactive (rather than fatalistic) stance toward safety problems.

The definition of *safety culture* adopted by a workgroup commissioned by the Agency for Healthcare Research and Quality (AHRQ) to develop the major tool now being used in the United States was as follows: "[G]roup values, attitudes, perceptions, competencies and behavior" influencing performance of organizations with respect to safety. "Organizations with a positive safety culture are characterized by . . . mutual trust . . . shared perceptions of the importance of safety, and confidence in the efficacy of preventive measures." ("Organizing for Safety," as cited by Sorra & Nieva, 2004, p. 1).

Safety climate has been described as the manifestations or indications of safety culture in terms of perceptions and attitudes at a particular point in time (Gaba et al., 2003). Specifically, receptiveness to and adoption of technologies; uptake of lower-tech best practices intended to enhance safety, including sound communication and collaboration; and a nonpunitive and open approach to reporting and analyzing errors and near misses are commonly included under the umbrella of safety climate. But some definitions have been even more specifically tied to a particular safety concern. DeJoy, Gershon, Murphy, and Wilson (1996) and Gershon, Karkashian, Vlanov, Kummer, Kasting, and Green-McKenzie (1999) have done extensive research on a triad of elements of climate they believe are related to sharps safety, including perceptions of management commitment to safety, job hindrances, and feedback and training on safety. A later version of the tool includes cleanliness and orderliness, minimal conflict, and availability of personal protective equipment and engineering controls (e.g., safety-engineered equipment to prevent bloodborne pathogen exposures) (Gershon, Karkashian, Grosch, Murphy, Escamilla-Cejudo, Flanagan et al., 2000).

Other related terms, even narrower in scope, have also appeared. These include *error-reporting culture* and *error-reporting climate*. Several authors have made general statements that punitive cultures interfere with the reporting of errors and corrective actions (Page, 2004), and many survey researchers (e.g. Connelly & Powers, 2005) have found that perceptions of strong disincentives for reporting errors are among the most and severe climate problems in health care settings. Because silence interferes with short- and long-term responses to errors and safety-related events, many authors have urged managers to work toward a culture of trust to optimize both reporting and, ultimately, safety (Firth-Cozens, 2004).

Measurement of Organizational Culture and Climate

Although quantitative research has been done in the broader field of culture, it is safe to say that much culture research uses qualitative fieldwork techniques. Organizational climate research has been more closely aligned with the positivist (i.e., measurement-oriented and hypothesis-testing) approach in organizational studies, and climate researchers tend to believe that key climate elements can and should be measured using surveys. Attempts to reconcile the qualitative and quantitative traditions in organizational culture research, particularly through the use of survey instruments, has met with mixed reviews and represents a major area of contention within the field (Martin, 2002).

Two groups of authors have recently enumerated available tools to measure climate and culture, both narrowly and broadly conceptualized. Scott, Mannion, Davies, et al. (2003) reviewed literature dealing with organizational culture published up until June 2001 and identified nine distinct instruments from health care studies, and four used in education and industry research believed to show potential for health care research. They contrasted tools that attempted to categorize facilities into cultural types with those that evaluated how strongly one or more cultural elements operate in organizations. The number of items in the tools ranged from 13–135. Gershon and colleagues (2004), using somewhat broader criteria (by including organizational climate tools) and slightly different search approaches and screening criteria, arrived at 10 instruments. Overlap between their list and that of Scott et al. was minimal. This could reflect the outcomes and safety screen that Gershon's group used, in contrast to the broader focus on articles dealing with health care management adopted by Scott's team.

Since the reviews reported by Scott, Mannion, Davies, et al. (2003) and Gershon et al. (2004), the AHRQ commissioned and distributed a safety culture survey tool through its Web site (www.ahrq.gov) that is intended for wide use in quality assurance and research efforts (Nieva & Sorra, 2003; Sorra & Nieva, 2004). The tool measures perceptions of workers in organizational subunits regarding manager behaviors, continuous improvement, teamwork, communication, feedback, nonpunitive responses to error and, staffing. It examines organizationwide support for patient safety efforts as well as teamwork and communication across subunits in the organization. It also measures several summary perceptions, specifically, ratings of safety of care and of the frequency of and completeness of error reporting. Pilot work provides good evidence for factor structure and reliability and preliminary evidence of validity. Dissemination of the tool has been extensive, and findings of various kinds should be forthcoming in the literature shortly.

ISSUES IN RESEARCH ON CLIMATE, CULTURE, AND SAFETY

Linking Climate and Culture With Outcomes

Individual clinicians' judgments and actions affect patient outcomes most directly, but it is important not to forget the myriad environmental conditions that affect the quality of practice of individual workers as well as the health care team as a whole. If climate and culture do affect quality of care and patient outcomes, it is surely principally through their indirect influences on the process of clinical care.

Many of the same issues that confront researchers who attempt to connect staffing levels in hospitals and other health care organizations with patient outcomes (Clarke, 2003, 2005, in press; Clarke & Aiken, 2003) also challenge researchers interested in connecting climate and culture with safety outcomes. The key to nearly any correlational research, quantitative or qualitative, is a range of observed values on both the independent (explanatory) variable and the dependent (outcomes) measures across the study sample. This means that the sampling strategy must result in a pool of hospitals, nursing units, or time periods for the same hospitals or units where variation on culture or climate measures is seen. Examining a group of settings believed or known to have a limited range of climate or cultural factors (uniformly positive organizational characteristics or particularly negative ones) makes it doubtful that associations between climate and culture or outcomes will be detected.

Staffing researchers can use changes in staffing levels (their independent variable) over time within the same organizations or subunits thereof as the source of variation in their studies. Even so, the reason for temporal variation in staffing must be thought through, as do the possibilities that weekly, monthly, and seasonal variations and changes over the course of years in treatment approaches and clienteles will affect types of patients seen by an organization or its subunit. Any changes in patient characteristics or background variables that occur alongside organizational changes will confound any associations with outcomes that might be observed, even with sound risk-adjustment methods. However, the slow nature of change in climate (and especially in culture) means that there are major limitations in using natural shifts over time in organizations to conduct research. The alternative, therefore, is to compare institutions or nursing units and their outcomes against each other at a common point in time. This can be expensive and labor-intensive, unless nurses or other workers can be surveyed across many institutions in a cost-effective manner. For an early description of an approach that generated institution-specific organizational data about facilities across entire states and countries, see Aiken, Sochalski, and Lake (1997).

Collecting sound outcomes data is critical and often problematic. The rarer the outcomes or the more subtle the differences in climate/culture or outcomes that are of interest, the larger the number of institutions or units that must be studied to stand a reasonable chance of identifying any associations that might exist. High-quality information about nursing-sensitive patient safety outcomes across large numbers of organizations has been difficult to obtain. However, various initiatives, such as the American Nurses Association National Database of Nursing Quality Indicators (www.nursingquality.org), special statewide databases (Aydin, Bolton, Donaldson, Brown, Buffum, Elashoff et al., 2004), as well as data warehousing efforts in the U.S. military and Veterans Affairs systems and by the Centers for Disease Control and Prevention through the National Healthcare Safety Network, are also opening new possibilities for data linkages for research in this area.

The selection of specific outcome variables represents yet another major challenge. Ensuring that the dependent variables studied are not merely alternate ways of observing the organizational properties in question is critical. For example, questionnaires may reveal that employees believe that particular institutions value continuing education. Having a high proportion of individuals involved in continuing education programs on safety issues in these institutions would not be particularly meaningful (except for demonstrating convergent validity of measures). Searching for outcomes that are distinct from climate and culture themselves are important to avoid study designs that lead to circular conclusions (for example, that workers in organizations with positive safety climates perceive them to be safer [Hoff, Jameson, Hannan, & Flink, 2004]).

It is also vital to ensure in studies of culture and climate that the outcomes selected are not principally influenced by factors outside the control of nurses and their managers. Under such circumstances, any statistical associations of outcomes with climate and culture can be nearly impossible to plausibly relate to nurses and nursing care. Outcomes could show minimal sensitivity to the conditions under which nurses practice when underlying illnesses or adverse social conditions in the patient populations treated are particularly severe, or the outcome in question is almost completely determined on the interventions of a health care discipline other than nursing. As a result, whether mortality or certain complications are valid indicators of the quality of nursing care in an institution and are truly "nursing sensitive" is still being debated.

Options for reliably measuring safety outcomes, whether safe processes in health care, positive outcomes, or both, are decidedly limited (Clarke, in press). Measuring health care errors is especially difficult. Incident reports, intended to serve a quality-monitoring function in health care organizations, are not consistently filled out by nurses and other clinicians. Multiple decision points, from recognizing an error to judging it worthy of reporting to seeing the benefits of reporting against any risks or drawbacks to having the resources (particularly time) to complete the report are all influenced by conditions in an organization (including climate and culture) as well as personal characteristics and social psychological processes. Retrospective survey reports of errors and adverse events will be affected by recall biases and a variety of other cognitive factors, some of which may vary from respondent to respondent. Rates of reported errors are not necessarily meaningless and may serve as general indicators of safety, but extreme caution should be exercised before considering them to be reliable indicators of the specific phenomena in question—actual medication errors, for example.

The types of outcomes data relating to safety that can be collected in a cost-effective manner on a sufficient scale to allow outcomes research are limited. Direct observation of patients and their care is expensive, intrusive, and raises both methodological and ethical challenges. Although patient care records can be useful in many types of research, wide variations in charting practices across clinicians and organizations are common. In the case of safety research, unless these variations in recording practices are of specific interest, they limit the usefulness of chart review (also an expensive data collection method) as a technique in outcomes research on organizational factors. The major remaining approach, therefore, is to use indirect or unobtrusive measures of accidents or errors gathered from databases that hold other primary purposes. Hospital discharge abstracts, a byproduct of the billing process, provide extensive (albeit imperfect) information about reasons for admission, important demographic characteristics, clinical services received, complications, and inpatient mortality. Creative uses could be made of readings archived from monitoring equipment, as well as databases from specific departments within organizations, such as pharmacy, laboratory, central supply, and telecommunications.

Difficulties in drawing sound conclusions regarding causal sequencing from cross-sectional research (i.e. recognizing that correlation is not equivalent to causation) are also a concern in health outcomes research on organizational factors. Climate and culture research is certainly no exception. Differential outcomes across organizations may be the result of positive organizational conditions, outcomes may cause culture and climate shifts, or mechanisms may operate in both directions. For instance, positive climate/culture could favor better outcomes, but good outcomes may also improve morale and influence managers in staying the course with respect to certain supervisory styles or resource allocation decisions. In the specific context of safety work, interactions between patients and staff and various events and accidents shape perceptions of institutions over time (Scott, Mannion, Marshall et al., 2003). This results in unavoidable confounding of outcomes with climate/culture measures. Researchers should explore options for measuring objective indicators of safety in addition to survey reports. Future research must adopt a mix of designs and measures to ensure that interpretation of results is not always plagued by the limitations of correlational methods and measures whose interpretation is ambiguous.

Study Design in Assessing Organizational Change and Its Effects

Empirical research on whether culture and climate can be changed (and if so, how) and what improvements in outcomes can be expected alongside movement on these dimensions has been limited, despite the relevance of these issues to practice on the front lines. Perhaps this is not surprising, given the challenges researchers face in measuring aspects of climate and culture and studying the associations between the organizational properties and safety even at single points in time.

There are many design and analysis challenges in organizational change research. What types of score increases or decreases assessed by quantitative instruments constitute meaningful shifts in organizational conditions? If climate or culture appear to shift over time, are the changes in question real (i.e., has there been true movement in working conditions or values), or rather do they reflect a change in employees' perceptions (i.e., the organization is really not different, but the employees' satisfaction with it has changed or there is some sort of halo effect)? Further, unless exactly the same employees are surveyed repeatedly, alternate explanations for change over time include the possibility that such shifts really result from different people being surveyed. In examining effects of changes in climate/culture with less-than-optimal design controls (e.g., in single institutions over time), there is always the possibility that other factors have changed in institutions concurrently and are responsible for any differential outcomes that might be identified.

Once interventions can be empirically shown to improve climate and culture, it will then presumably be possible to track whether these changes are actually related to superior clinical care and better outcomes. Martin (2002) notes that true longitudinal research on organizational culture change is rare because of the enormous efforts involved and the high odds of disappointing results. She further comments, however, that well-conducted research along such lines could have a tremendous effect in helping managers and others choose the most effective strategies for achieving realistic organizational goals (in this case, optimal safety outcomes).

SUMMARIZING THE LITERATURE

Safety-Related Culture and Climate Elements in Healthcare Settings

The wide uptake of the AHRQ-sponsored Hospital Survey on Patient Safety Culture (Nieva & Sorra, 2003; Sorra & Nieva, 2004) is destined to lead to nationally representative survey benchmarks and dramatically enhance the ability of hospitals and other health care facilities (as well as researchers) to compare facilities to each other. Awaiting this, there have been recent indications of the state of organizational climate and culture in U.S. health care. Careful stratified surveys of 15 hospitals in California carried out in 2001 revealed several patterns (Singer, Gaba, Geppert, Sinaiko, Howard, & Park, 2003). Responses to 30 questions regarding safety climate across their organizations, in their departments, in daily operations, in communicating with other health care workers, as well as shame and fatigue as barriers to good care were analyzed. Overall, 8% to 70% of workers surveyed gave answers suggesting either clearly problematic or neutral (and therefore less than ideal) conditions. Managers were considerably more positive about the state of their institutions than nonmanagerial health care workers; clinicians in general and nurses in particular were distinct from other groups of hospital workers in voicing greater concerns regarding safety climate. Clear differences were seen across the hospitals themselves, suggesting that safety climate varies across health care workplaces.

Gaba and colleagues (2003) contrasted these results with those from similar surveys (with question wording tailored to their particular work scenarios) of naval aviators. They found that response patterns suggestive of climate problems were anywhere from nearly twice to nearly 12 times as common in hospitals as in naval squadrons. Specifically, far more hospital workers than aviators disagreed that senior leaders demonstrated a commitment to safety concerns, that attention to standard operating procedures was consistent, that quality management was consistent and proactive, that resources were adequate, and that communication across the organization and about errors and problems was frequent and candid. They concluded that problems may be engrained in the health care sector itself and that changing the safety climate in hospitals and other facilities may require major investments over time.

Culture and Climate Relations to Outcomes

Recent reviews of climate and culture literature have been consistent in their conclusions. Tregunno's (2005) review, concentrating particularly on studies in nursing, found "striking" variability in measures of climate and culture used and outcomes studied and noted that many researchers have failed to find evidence of an effect of climate or culture on outcomes. Scott, Mannion, Marshall et al. (2003) similarly concluded that although the findings of the literature as a whole are suggestive of a role of culture in outcomes, neither the slim body of results nor methodological quality of the studies used to generate them are supportive of a simple relationship between culture and organizational performance in health care.

The state of research on climate and culture as predictors of safety outcomes mirrors that of the broader literature about organizational or organization-level variables in health care safety. The review of research articles published from the 1980s through early 2002 by Hickam et al. (2003) examined evidence linking safety outcomes with organizational factors (in addition to staffing, work design, and environmental factors). They observed that organizational culture studies predominated (13 of 19 papers cited examined it), but found little evidence consistent with an effect of culture on safety-related patient outcomes, medical errors, or their detection. They concluded that organizational culture appeared to be tied (albeit inconclusively) to error reporting. Taking the body of evidence as a whole, they concluded that research results inside and outside of health care settings were encouraging and provided guidance for future research, but were insufficient to draw conclusions about the effect of organizational factors. Hoff et al. (2004) also reviewed research articles that linked organizational factors with medical errors and safety. They found that this literature was published mostly in management and quality assurance journals, rather than research-oriented publications dealing with clinical care. Other organizational elements studied in the various papers included team factors and interventions, feedback on performance, initiation of the use of practice guidelines, education, and various forms of technology. Medication errors were the major outcome studied. With few exceptions, they found little clustering of the evidence in the same journals and few series of articles written by the same lead authors. Only 9 of the 42 articles they identified after screening contained sufficient detail in methods and findings to support claims of linkages between organization factors and safety. None of the three articles identified as dealing with culture was deemed to meet this criterion.

One body of literature that ties climate with safety outcomes relevant to nursing is rarely cited in reviews, perhaps because its operationalizations of climate fall outside the boundaries of literature searches. Nonetheless, considerable evidence suggests that organizational climate is associated with percutaneous injuries with used sharps (needlesticks) and other forms of bloodborne pathogen exposures among health care workers and as well as behavioral risk factors for these injuries and exposures. Compliance with universal precautions (UP) was linked to the three climate elements (management support, hindrances, and feedback/training) in nurses in 177 urban hospital nurses; actual injuries were linked to hindrances alone (Grosch, Gershon, Murphy, & DeJoy, 1999). Connections between climate and compliance with UP were particularly strong among 225 correctional health workers (Gershon et al., 1999). Clarke and colleagues (Clarke, Rockett, Sloane, & Aiken, 2002; Clarke, Sloane, & Aiken, 2002) similarly reported that low perceptions of resource adequacy and managerial support aggregated to the unit and hospital level were associated with high risks for needlesticks and near-miss incidents in two independent samples of hospitals and hospital nurses.

Despite limited empirical data to support an association between climate and cultural factors and safety, many believe that attention to climate and culture factors hold considerable promise for improving health care. And one of the four major recommendations of the Institute of Medicine's panel on transforming work environments for nurses to promote safety (Page, 2004) was the creation and maintenance of cultures of safety (others recommendations involved management issues, the design of work processes, and staffing). However, the review of literature that accompanied the panel's detailed recommendations on this point included anecdotal evidence and scholarly analyses and commentaries, rather than empirical evidence of either an association of culture and climate or of changes in these parameters with safety outcomes.

CONCLUSIONS

As it evolves, literature about organizational climate and culture increasingly resembles another body of research and scholarship familiar to many nurses—that relating to social support. Both the connection of social support to health and health-related behaviors and the association of organizational culture and climate with institutional outcomes are intuitively appealing and are congruent with values in nursing. Despite limited empirical evidence for causal links, social support and social integration have been assumed to be precursors of health outcomes. Similarly, positive organizational climate and culture have been linked with safer health care in the minds of many. However, the state of the science in both cases is not always as strong as one might hope. There are major definitional inconsistencies, loose use of terms, and large numbers of instruments that force readers of either of these literatures to first consider how the concepts in question were measured in each study. On the whole, the implications for clinical practice (in the case of social support research) and for administrative/leadership practice (in the case of culture and climate research) remain unclear.

Opportunities still exist to improve the state of affairs in research linking organizational culture and climate to safety. Given the limited success in linking health organization performance (let alone safety) to organizational culture to date, Scott, Mannion, Marshall et al. (2003) advocate methodological innovation, closer attention to theoretical considerations, and multidisciplinary and multimethod approaches. However, after careful reflection, some scholars have concluded that the search for connections between culture, climate, and outcomes could be an unattainable quest (Martin, 2002) and that other research questions in these areas should be more vigorously investigated. Research will undoubtedly continue to search for these connections, but will certainly be constrained by theoretical and methodological challenges.

Several caveats should be borne in mind by nurse managers seeking insights from the culture and climate literatures, beyond recognizing that there is scant empirical evidence connecting culture and climate to safety outcomes. Organizational cultural change, especially because it is so complex and slow-moving, may be a dubious goal for a managers or executives expected to show concrete outcomes quickly, especially when they may not be in their roles long enough to follow through on such initiatives. Also, Schein (2002) emphasizes that making value judgments regarding cultures (bad versus good) may be unproductive, because all cultures at least partially reflect decisions and ways of being that have influenced an organization's survival over time. Finding leverage points from various aspects of a culture to change practices in an institution or on a unit is often a far more feasible approach than aggressive attempts at changing the culture itself, especially over the short term. Because resources in general (and resources for change, in particular) are scarce in health care, deciding which safety improvement strategies work best for organizations with different culture and climate characteristics deserves empirical examination. Such data are not yet available.

Culture and climate should not be used to avoid hard questions about leader effectiveness by blaming poor safety on demotivated or recalcitrant employees. Caution should also be exercised to ensure that climate and culture do not become pat excuses for high levels of errors or adverse events, low compliance with policies and procedures, or reluctance to adopt technologies. Culture and climate should not be used to sidestep questions of basic resource adequacy in health care settings, either. Scarce resources, an ongoing feature of life in nearly all health care organizations, raise many practical issues that touch on organizational culture. Cook and Rasmussen (2005) outline an intriguing model of system dynamics and patient care in which they liken situations of fully tapped health care resources to the nuclear power plant concept of "going solid" (derived from the image of a boiler completely full of liquid with nowhere for steam to go). They offer an intriguing notion about where research on culture and safety might proceed when they write that "shared, accurate and precise knowledge of the dynamics and location of the current operating point and boundary locations is a necessary component of safety culture" (p. 133). Perhaps future studies of safety culture should consider how resource allocation decisions are made, from the executive suite to the bedside, and aim toward better definitions of the boundaries of safe health care settings for patients and nurses.

In conclusion, pending further evidence, climate and culture are perhaps best thought of by safety researchers and leaders in clinical settings as modifying and moderating factors in influencing the safety of certain staffing and resource levels, and as offering levers and constraints in implementing of change and innovation, rather than as variables to be studied in isolation from other organizational and safety issues. Whether in research arenas or in practice, clearly articulating definitions and distinguishing empirical fact from intuition will undoubtedly increase meaningful applications of climate and culture to the challenging and crucial work of improving patient safety.

ACKNOWLEDGMENT

Preparation of this chapter was assisted in part by K01 NR07895 Organizational Climate and Hospital Patient/Nurse Safety from the National Institute of Nursing Research (Sean P. Clarke, PhD, CRNP, Principal Investigator).

REFERENCES

Aiken, L. H., Sochalski, J., & Lake, E. T. (1997). Studying outcomes of organizational change in health services. *Medical Care, 35*(Suppl. 11), NS6–NS18.

Ashkanasy, N. M., Broadfoot, L. E., & Falkus, S. (2000). Questionnaire measures of organizational culture. In N. M. Ashkanasy, C. P. M. Wilderom, & M. F. Peterson (Eds.). *Handbook of organizational culture and climate* (pp. 131–145). Thousand Oaks, CA: Sage.

Ashkanasy, N. M., Wilderom, C. P. M., & Peterson, M. F. (Eds.) (2000). *Handbook of organizational culture and climate*. Thousand Oaks, CA: Sage.

Aydin C. E., Bolton, L. B., Donaldson, N., Brown, D. S., Buffum, M., Elashoff, J. D., et al. (2004). Creating and analyzing a statewide nursing quality measurement database. *Journal of Nursing Scholarship, 36*(4), 371–378.

Buchan, J. (2004). What difference does ("good") HRM make? *Human Resources for Health,* 2. Retrieved April 6, 2006, from www.human-resources-health.com/content/2/1/6

Clarke, S. P. (2003). Balancing staffing and safety. *Nursing Management, 34*(6), 44–48.

Clarke, S. P. (2005). The policy implications of staffing-outcomes research. *Journal of Nursing Administration, 35*(1), 17–19.

Clarke, S. P. (In press). Research on nurse staffing and its outcomes: Challenges and risks. In S. Nelson & S. Gordon (Eds.), *Confronting caring.* Ithaca, NY: Cornell University Press.

Clarke, S. P., & Aiken, L. H. (2003). Registered nurse staffing and patient and nurse outcomes in hospitals: A commentary. *Policy, Politics and Nursing Practice, 4*(2), 104–111.

Clarke, S. P., Sloane, D. M., & Aiken, L. H. (2002). The effects of hospital staffing and organizational climate on needlestick injuries to nurses. *American Journal of Public Health, 92,* 1115–1119.

Clarke, S. P., Rockett, J., Sloane, D. M., & Aiken, L. H. (2002). Organizational climate, staffing, and safety equipment as predictors of needlestick injuries and near-misses in hospital nurses. *American Journal of Infection Control, 30,* 207–216.

Connelly, L. M., & Powers, J. L. (2005). On-line patient safety climate survey: Tool development and lessons learned. Organizational climate of staff working conditions and safety—An integrative model. *Advances in patient safety: From research to implementation, Volume 4: Programs, tools and products* (Agency for Healthcare Research and Quality Publication No. 050024) (pp. 415–428). Rockville, MD: Agency for Healthcare Research and Quality. Retrieved October, 21, 2005, from www.ahrq.gov/qual/advances

Cook, R., & Rasmussen, J. (2005). "Going solid": A model of system dynamics and consequences for patient safety. *Quality and Safety in Health Care, 14,* 130–134.

DeJoy, D. M., Gershon, R. R. M., Murphy, L. R., & Wilson, M. G. (1996). A work-systems analysis of compliance with universal precautions among health care workers. *Health Education Quarterly, 23*(2), 159–174.

Estabrooks, C. A., Tourangeau, A. E., Humphrey, C. K., Hesketh, K. L., Giovannetti, P., & Thomson, D. (2002). Measuring the hospital practice environment: A Canadian context. *Research in Nursing and Health, 25*(4), 256–268.

Firth-Cozens, J. (2004). Organizational trust: The keystone to patient safety. *Quality and Safety in Health Care, 13,* 56–61.

Gaba, D. M., Singer, S. J., Sinaiko, A. D., Brown, J. B., & Ciavarelli, A. P. (2003). Differences in safety climate between hospital personnel and naval aviators. *Human Factors, 45,* 173–185.

Gershon, R. R., Stone, P. W., Bakken, S., & Larson, E. (2004). Measurement of organizational culture and climate in healthcare. *Journal of Nursing Administration, 34*(1), 33–40.

Gershon, R. R. M., Karkashian, C. D., Grosch, J. W., Murphy, L. R., Escamilla-Cejudo, A., Flanagan, P. A., et al. (2000). Hospital safety climate and its relationship with safe work practices and workplace exposure incidents. *American Journal of Infection Control, 28*(3), 211–221.

Gershon, R. R. M., Karkashian, C. D., Vlanov, D., Kummer, L., Kasting, C., Green-McKenzie, J., et al. (1999). Compliance with universal precautions in correctional health facilities. *Journal of Occupational and Environmental Medicine, 41*(3), 181–189.

Grosch, J. W., Gershon, R. R. M., Murphy, L. R., & DeJoy, D. M. (1999). Safety climate dimensions associated with occupational exposure to bloodborne pathogens in nurses. *American Journal of Industrial Medicine,* (Suppl. 1), 122–124.

Hickam, D. H., Severance, S., Feldstein, A., Ray, L., Gorman, P., Schuldheis, S., et al. (2003). Organizational factors. In *The effect of health care working conditions on patient safety.* (Evidence report/Technology assessment No. 74. pp. 50–54). Rockville, MD: Agency for Healthcare Research and Quality. Retrieved April 6, 2006, from www.ahrq.gov/downloads/pub/evidence/pdf/work/work.pdf

Hoff, T., Jameson, L., Hannan, E., & Flink, E. (2004). A review of the literature examining linkages between organizational factors, medical errors, and patient safety. *Medical Care Research and Review, 61*(6), 3–37.

Hofstede, G., & Peterson, M. F. (2000). Culture: National values and organizational practices. In N. M. Ashkanasy, C. P. M. Wilderom, & M. F. Peterson (Eds.) *Handbook of organizational culture and climate* (pp. 401–415). Thousand Oaks, CA: Sage.

McClure M. L., & Hinshaw A. S. (Eds.). (2002). *Magnet hospitals revisited: Attraction and retention of professional nurses.* Kansas City, MO: American Nurses Association.

Miller, J. A., & Brunell, M. L. (2004). Improving the nursing work culture. In J. F. Byers, & S. V. White (Eds.), *Patient safety: Principles and practice* (pp. 232–255).

Martin, J. (2002). *Organizational culture: Mapping the terrain.* Thousand Oaks, CA: Sage.

Nieva, V. F., & Sorra, J. (2003). Safety culture assessment: A tool for improving patient safety in health care organizations. *Quality and Safety in Health Care, 12,* 17–23.

Page A. (Ed.). (2004). *Keeping patients safe: Transforming the work environments of nurses.* Washington, DC: National Academies Press.

Schein, E. H. (1992). *Organizational culture and leadership* (2nd ed.). San Francisco: Jossey-Bass.

Scott, T., Mannion, R., Davies, H., & Marshall, M. (2003). The quantitative measurement of organizational culture in health care: A review of the available instruments. *Health Services Research, 38,* 923–945.

Scott, T., Mannion, R., Marshall, M., & Davies, H. (2003). Does organizational culture influence health care performance? A review of the evidence. *Journal of Health Services Research and Policy, 8*(2), 105–117.

Singer, S. J., Gaba, D. M., Geppert, J. J., Sinaiko, A. D., Howard, S. K., & Park, K. C. (2003). The culture of safety: Results of an organization-wide survey in 15 California hospitals. *Quality and Safety in Health Care, 12,* 112–118.

Sorra, J. S., & Nieva, V. F. (2004). *Hospital survey on patient safety culture.* (Agency for Healthcare Research and Quality Publication No. 04-0041). Rockville, MD: Agency for Healthcare Research and Quality.

Stone, P. W., Harrison, M. L., Feldman, P., Linzer, M., Peng, T., Roblin, D., et al. (2005). Organizational climate of staff working conditions and safety—An integrative model. *Advances in patient safety: From research to implementation, Volume 2: Concepts and Methodology* (Agency for Healthcare Research and Quality Publication No. 050022, pp. 467–481). Rockville, MD: Agency for Healthcare Research and Quality. Retrieved October, 21, 2005, from www.ahrq.gov/qual/advances

Tregunno, D. (2005). Organizational climate and culture. In L. McGillis Hall (Ed.), *Quality work environments for nurse and patient safety* (pp. 67–91). Sudbury, MA: Jones & Bartlett.

Chapter 11

Methodologies Used in Nursing Research Designed to Improve Patient Safety

Elizabeth Merwin and Deirdre Thornlow

ABSTRACT

Nursing research studies of patient safety for 2002–2005 were reviewed to determine methods used and methodological challenges within this field of research. Methods used in traditional clinical research and in health services research were often combined or adapted in innovative research designs to advance knowledge regarding nursing care and patient safety outcomes. This relatively new focus of complex research posed methodological challenges in areas such as measurement and the availability and analysis of data. The most frequent methods used included survey research, analysis of secondary data, and observational studies. This review points to the need to increase the incorporation of complex methodological training, including health services research, the analysis of secondary data and complex survey design in our doctoral programs, and to provide opportunities for researchers to gain further methodological training. Increased use of multi-site and multi-level studies is also needed.

Keywords: patient safety, nursing, methods

This review will identify the types and breadth of research methods used in patient safety nursing research. Approaches range from qualitative and quantitative methods to the incorporation of research methodologies from other disciplines. The challenges of conducting patient safety research go beyond the typical methodological concerns. Patient safety research faces the dual challenges of conducting not only clinical research, but also health services research. Some studies reviewed for this paper focused on health care systems, while others analyzed processes of care to identify solutions for clinical patient safety issues. The complex methodological challenges faced within health services research, that of conducting research in an ever-changing, multifaceted health care system, are made more difficult by the realities posed by the recent emergence of patient safety as a specific research focus. Most administrative data systems were not designed to incorporate needed data elements and ready-to-use variables that would facilitate rapid and targeted analysis for patient safety research.

Additionally, the abrupt focus on patient safety research has necessitated the retraining of many in the research work force. The labor-intensive efforts needed to develop new research methods, coupled with the time restraints required for retraining, has made the initiation of this research focus more difficult. Realization of this limitation, however, has promoted the creative development of research teams from different disciplines and innovative thinking in approaches to patient safety research. This review shows the variety of methods and the inventive approaches used to advance the field. It offers guidance for needed methodological training within our doctoral, postdoctoral, and continuing education programs. No area of nursing research offers greater opportunity to provide solutions for these methodological challenges or greater opportunity to move the field forward through the incorporation of advanced methodological approaches. The potential contribution of nursing research to improving the patient safety of our citizens is evident in the innovative approaches that have been documented in the literature. Providing further training and encouraging nurses to coordinate and conduct interdisciplinary research to improve patient safety will amplify this contribution.

BACKGROUND

Patient safety has achieved prominence in the context of today's troubled health care environment. The Institute of Medicine (IOM) series of reports about patient safety stimulated public debate on medical errors and health care quality and spawned national and regional efforts to measure and address the issue. The Agency for Health Care Research and Quality (AHRQ) was designated by Congress to provide leadership in implementing the country's research response to the 1999 IOM report on medical errors (www.ahrq.gov/qual/pscongrpt/

psinisum.htm). A patient safety research agenda has since been launched and funded by AHRQ. Governments, foundations, health plans, purchasing coalitions, and provider systems all initiated programs and joint ventures to better protect patients (Bullen, 2002). For example, beyond revising its accreditation standards so that more than 50% now focus on patient safety, the Joint Commission on Accreditation of Healthcare Organizations (JCAHO) (2003) also mandated patient safety goals; each goal includes expert and evidence-based recommendations to help health care organizations reduce specific types of health care errors. In the private sector, the Leapfrog Group, a conglomerate of private business executives, pressures hospitals to adopt patient safety practices such as physician order entry. In the hopes of eventually reducing health care costs, the Leapfrog Group posts health care organization report cards on its Web site to inform consumers of hospitals' attempts to improve efficiency and safety.

Not to be outdone, in 2001 AHRQ awarded $50 million in grants, contracts, and other activities to reduce medical errors and improve patient safety. This represented the single largest investment the federal government had made to combat the estimated 44,000–98,000 medical error–related patient deaths nationwide each year. In each of the succeeding fiscal years since the initial grant, AHRQ continued to devote millions of dollars of its budget to patient safety research, although since 2004, the majority of funds have been earmarked for information technology implementation and research. AHRQ also established a Center for Quality Improvement and Safety and, as a result, has become the leader of patient safety education, dissemination of best practices, and development of standards and measures (Leape & Berwick, 2005).

Typically, patient safety is conceptualized as the avoidance, prevention, and amelioration of adverse outcomes or injuries stemming from the processes of health care (Cooper, Gaba, Liang, Woods, & Blum, 2000). Investigators and providers alike search for ways to improve the delivery and safety of patient care. Many are intent on embedding patient safety practices into health care; however, evidence for the incorporation of various safety practices—including incident reporting, root-cause analysis, and promoting a culture of safety—comes from domains outside of medicine and possesses a weak evidentiary base in the health care literature (Shojana, Duncan, McDonald & Wachter, 2001). When evidence does exist, organizations have made attempts to translate such evidence into practice. In 2002, the National Quality Foundation published a list of 30 evidence-based practices deemed ready for implementation (Leape, Berwick, & Bates, 2002; Shojania, Duncan, McDonald, & Wachter, 2002); JCAHO has since required at least 10 of these practices be implemented in its accredited hospitals. Recognizing that no single action on its own can keep patients safe, the IOM is calling for "bundles of changes" in leadership and management, work force, work processes, and organizational culture (Institute of Medicine, 2004). Thus, when examining patient safety, it is essential to explore the extent to which differences in patient outcomes, including adverse events, are reflective of differences in organizational processes.

The purpose of this review is to critique the methods used in patient safety research related to nursing. This information is necessary to inform the needs for methodological training for nursing research and to guide methods development in this field of research.

METHODS

An electronic search of Medline and Cumulative Index to Nursing and Allied Health Literature (CINAHL) for 2000–2005 using the key words patient safety, nursing, and research, restricted to English, resulted in 323 articles. Articles were selected for full review if they appeared to report a full research study and if available to the authors through a health science library, over the Internet, or through AHRQ's Patient Safety Network. Articles that appeared to be conceptual, policy-oriented, highlighted case examples, or focused on improving practice or quality of care with only an indirect relationship to patient safety were not selected for further review. Initially it was difficult to identify research articles, and several searches were conducted with different combinations of key words: patient safety, nursing, research, and statistical methods. Of the 323 articles identified, 55 were selected for further review. Articles were further limited to 2002–2005, as there were only seven articles identified from 2000–2001 and in general they were less focused on patient safety than on quality outcomes. Seven were eliminated due to being too peripheral to the topic, two were duplicates, and 10 were unavailable for review. Five were dissertation abstracts related to patient safety that were not included in the review. The remaining 24 articles were contributed to the review from the search of MEDLINE and CINAHL data bases using key words patient safety, nursing, and research, with the stipulation that articles be in English. Two additional articles were added based on the author's prior knowledge of their relevance despite their absence from the literature search.

Two supplemental searches were conducted to locate additional relevant research studies. First, an electronic search of AHRQ's four-volume report *Advances in Patient Safety: From Research to Implementation* resulted in the identification of 100 documents containing the word nursing. These documents were reviewed to identify research studies specific to nursing practice. In general, if the study was predominately focused on nursing practice or on nursing personnel, the article was selected for review. This process resulted in 11 additional articles included in this review. Many articles were excluded from further review because nursing was included to a lesser degree or discussed only within more general studies of patient safety.

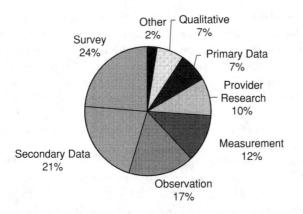

FIGURE 11.1   Types of Patient Safety Nursing Research 2002–2005.

Next, the authors searched the AHRQ online PSNet Patient Safety Network (www.psnet.ahrq.gov/), which includes a section about nursing-related articles and materials. This site was searched, and an additional five articles were identified for inclusion in this review. The methods described above resulted in a total of 42 research studies that were reviewed and that served as the basis to determine the methods used in patient safety nursing research. These articles were categorized by the predominant method used within the study. As Figure 11.1 shows, diverse methods were used in the patient safety research reviewed, with some of the studies incorporating multiple methods. The pie chart shows the percentages of the different types of methods used in this body of research. The most frequent methods used included survey research, analysis of secondary data, and observational studies. Studies also focused on improving measures of patient safety, provider research that included quality improvement types of initiatives, research studies that collected primary data, and studies that used qualitative methods such as focus groups. Although many studies used multiple methods, studies that used the most similar predominant method are discussed within sections of this review on each of these method types. This facilitates a presentation of the range of research topics and methods within each overall heading.

MEASUREMENT

With the increased focus on patient safety research, many recognized the need to establish new measures, choose appropriate measures, and standardize measures in order to ease integration into the new field. For example, Hodge, Asch, Olson, Kravitz, and Sauve (2002) used a modified Delphi approach with an expert panel to identify nursing-sensitive outcomes. Specifically, the investigators focused on outcomes relevant to patients, employers, and institutions that were perceived to be affected by changes in staffing ratios. The findings of this study offered direction to follow-up investigators in choosing nursing-relevant outcomes. However, following a comprehensive analysis of published literature from 1997–2004, Savitz, Jones, and Bernard (2005) observed that a prior focus on quality indicators was shifting toward patient safety. But the investigators noted the continued lack of agreement on measures, standardization of measures, and data availability for certain measures.

The lack of consistency in the selection of instruments and the perceived need to continue to develop instruments relevant to the topic is seen in the measurement studies reviewed. This is also seen in the choices and modification of instruments in the survey research reviewed. Stone, Harrison, Feldman, Linzer, Peng, Roblin, et al. (2005) proposed an integrated model of organizational climate to synthesize findings from AHRQ studies using different measures of organizational climate and to move the field toward establishing a standardized approach for this measure. Tailoring the measure of organizational climate to specific settings may be an important underlying issue to resolve in progressing toward standardization of this and other patient safety measures. For example, although Blegen, Pepper, and Rosse (2005) were aware of previously developed organizational and safety culture measures, this team used an instrument development approach to design the Hospital Unit Safety Climate measure for use in studies of acute care hospital inpatient units. Finalizing this tool required a literature review, item development by the research team, expert panel evaluation to generate a pilot tool, administration and evaluation of the pilot version including evaluation for reliability of subscales, and the use of factor analysis to establish the structural components of the tool.

Unveiled in 2001, AHRQ's patient safety indicators (www.qualityindicators. ahrq.gov/psi_overview.htm) motivated Simpson (2005) to operationalize a potential extension of the failure to rescue measure developed for use in general hospital/surgical patients to the obstetrical patient. The author documented the conceptual basis and application to the obstetrical patient and used practice guidelines to propose a data collection tool to facilitate the use of the new measure. This thoughtful application is a practical example of merging expert clinical knowledge with the adaptation of an existing measure for use with a different patient population. The same type of application could be helpful to guide the adaptation of measures developed for one setting to the needs of clients in another.

Throughout the literature reviewed for this review, issues regarding the choice of measures, the limited availability of measures, and the quest for better measures were common concerns. Although most of the investigators utilized previously developed measures in their studies, some also evaluated the reliability and validity of measures. Such research is needed to build the evidence base for those indicators that accurately measure patient safety.

QUALITATIVE APPROACHES

Focus Groups/Interviews

Several types of qualitative approaches have been used to advance patient safety research, including data collection through individual interviews and the use of focus groups. In one study, qualitative observations emerged from the implementation of a large quantitative study. Ebright, Urden, Patterson, and Chalko (2004) developed a study within a human performance framework using a cognitive task analysis technique to interview eight new registered nurses (RNs) regarding adverse events or near misses. An interdisciplinary approach was apparent in the design of the study, and themes were identified from the interviews. In another study following the completion of a large study of adverse drug events within a highly computerized health care system, Weir, Hoffman, Nebeker, & Hurdle (2005) identified unexpected qualitative observations regarding problems with the fit between the computerized system and processes of nursing care. And yet another study targeted an improved understanding of issues related to the reporting of errors within hospitals. Physicians and nurses from a health care system in one metropolitan area and its surrounding counties participated in nine focus groups. Investigators employed qualitative data approaches including content analysis and identification of themes (Jeffe, Dunagan, Garbutt, Burroughs, Gallagher, Hill, et al., 2004).

Ethnographic Studies/Observational Studies

Ethnography and human factors engineering have emerged as useful methodologies for patient safety research. Both approaches consider observation an important component. Ethnography has been used as a methodology in studies of communication and decision-making. Lingard, Espin, Whyte, Regehr, Baker, Reznick, et al. (2004) used ethnography to conduct observations of operating room team members, including 31 nursing staff. Communication events were identified and analyzed using data collected as field notes. Patterson, Cook, and Render (2002) used ethnographic observation to study the introduction of a new bar coding system for medication administration in three hospitals. A pre- and post-implementation design was used to identify unintended side effects resulting from the new system. Data collection methods identified cases, and investigators analyzed interruptions and other problems that surfaced when using the system.

Human factors engineering has been used to better understand technology (Carayon, Wetterneck, Hundt, Ozkaynak, Ram, DeSilvey, et al., 2005) and the process of work activities within medication administration (Harder, Bloomfield, Sendelbach, Shepherd, Rush, Sinclair, et al., 2005). An informative description of human factors engineering is available on the Food and Drug Administration Web site (www.fda.gov/cdrh/humfac/doit.html). Carayon and investigators used this method to study bar coding and intravascular (IV) pumps. Observational data were analyzed to formulate flow carts, determine variations and failures, and suggest solutions. Harder and colleagues used a human factors process analysis to guide the revision of a procedure for heparin administration to reduce errors. Following observations and interviews, a revised procedure was developed and implemented.

To better understand clinical decision-making, Potter, Wolf, Boxerman, Grayson, Sledge, Dunagan, et al. (2005) merged a human factors approach with a qualitative approach, thus effectively combining observation with a cognitive methodology. This study shows the value of uniting the expertise of a human factors observational study with expertise regarding clinical decisions. Ebright, Patterson, Chalks, and Render (2003) used both qualitative and quantitative methods to study the complex work of acute care RNs. Observations were made of eight nurses within two facilities from which specific decision cases (Sandelowski's concept) were identified. Nurses were interviewed using a critical decision method, which focused on the patterns of the work and the cognitive components of decision-making. Greengold et al. (2003) used observation to evaluate medication administration within an intervention study. The use of a medication nurse with responsibility only for administering medications for 15–18 patients was compared to a medication system whereby nurses caring for six patients were responsible for individual medication administration. Following direct observation, medication and process errors were determined. Descriptive information as well as differences in rates were also determined. This study offers an example of employing mixed methods in patient safety research.

QUANTITATIVE APPROACHES

Primary Data Collection

Several studies used primary collection methods to collect nurse- and patient-specific data. The data were collected either through structured interviews or the completion of specific data collection tools. Grayson, Boxerman, Potter, Wolf, Dunagan, Sorock, et al. (2005) conducted a case cross-over study to determine the odds for differences in conditions in the hospital working environment when a medical error occurred compared to other time periods. Nurses were interviewed after reporting an error and were questioned regarding conditions during the 30 minutes prior to the error, the work shift of the error, and the prior work shift. Structured interviews were also conducted by Evanoff, Potter, Wolf, Grayson, Dunagan, and Boxerman (2005), in a study of provider communications and priorities. The investigators selected patients randomly from one hospital and interviewed the resident, an RN, and a patient technician to determine whether they knew the name of the other providers caring for the patient and whether they knew of priorities for the patient's care. Descriptive data regarding agreements and inter-rater reliabilities for priorities were reported.

Mark, Salyer, and Wan (2003) evaluated a causal model of the relationships among unit context, professional practice, and nurse and patient outcomes using primary data collected from 64 hospitals, 124 units, 1,326 patients, and 1,682 RNs. Using structural equations modeling with the Mplus computer program, a measurement model was developed to represent a multilevel confirmatory factor analytic model. Hospital- and unit-level results were presented for several outcomes, including patient falls. Although data on medication errors were collected, this variable was not explained well by the model and was, therefore, excluded from the final multilevel causal model. This study offers a methodological example for conducting a multisite study using multilevel data and a complex statistical approach. Although primary data collection served as the source of data, this approach offers potential for conducting other multisite, multilevel data studies using secondary data.

Interventions/Practice Research

Examples of system and patient interventions exist within the literature, but often the interventions were practice-based changes initiated in pre-existing clinical settings for the purpose of improving patient safety. This is in contrast with clinical interventions that are typically developed with classical approaches to clinical research. Nevertheless, two research examples evaluating changes made to improve the safety of direct patient care were identified in this review. Olson, Cheek, and Morgenlander (2004) conducted a quality improvement project in a neurocritical care unit to determine whether the implementation of the Bispectral Index monitoring tool would influence the level of sedation medication administered by nurses. A student t-test was used to calculate means, standard deviations, and confidence intervals and to test for differences. Ho and French (2002) used a quasi-experimental design to evaluate a new method of administering oxygen to patients undergoing eye surgery with the specified goal of reducing the risk of fire due to high concentrations of oxygen within the area draped for surgery. Alternating weeks of use of the new method with the traditional method facilitated data collection. Different measures of both patient oxygenation levels and of gases in the draped area were compared using t tests. The motivation for the study was to determine whether to change to the new method.

Two systems interventions targeted toward improving patient safety were also identified. Thomas, Sexton, Neilands, Frankel, and Helmreich (2005) evaluated the effect of executive walking rounds. The authors point out that although walking rounds are often used, they had not been previously evaluated. Units within one hospital were randomly selected to receive walking rounds from a supervising executive once every 4 weeks for three visits (or not depending on assigned condition). The rounds were structured to focus on patient safety and promote dialogue with staff. A cumulative odds logistic regression model was developed based on a survey with a safety climate scale administered before and after the system intervention (Thomas et al., p. 7). In another quasi-experimental, pre- and post-test design, Ginsburg, Norton, Casebeer, and Lewis (2005) implemented an educational intervention in which nurse leaders from the experimental hospital were invited to participate in two patient safety workshops. Nurse leaders were surveyed before and after the intervention using an adapted tool for patient safety culture and a specific leadership tool. Repeated-measures analyses of variance with post hoc analysis were used to evaluate differences. Finally, hierarchical regression models were developed to explain the influence of study variables on the post-evaluation perception of patient safety culture using three safety factors as dependent variables.

SURVEY RESEARCH

Surveys were frequently used in patient safety research, but for varying purposes. For example, surveys were used to guide patient care procedures, nurses were surveyed as part of overall multidisciplinary evaluations, and statewide and national surveys were undertaken to better understand aspects of quality of care or the work environment. Gall and Bull (2004) performed a telephone survey to follow-up on clients discharged to home after a gastrointestinal procedure; the goal was to generate descriptive information useful in facilitating improved discharge care. St. Clair (2005) conducted an informal survey of practice patterns related to tracheostomy care to motivate a performance improvement initiative. Subsequent initiatives included a review of the literature and the development of a revised procedure. Perceptions of nurses regarding medication errors have been surveyed (Wakefield, Uden-Holman, & Wakefield, 2005; Mayo & Duncan, 2004). Wakefield et al. validated their survey instrument via factor analysis. Stratton, Blegen, Pepper, & Vaughn (2004) surveyed a convenience sample of pediatric and adult nurses to further understand differences in errors for pediatric clients versus adults;

actual differences in rates of reported medication errors for the two groups were also reported.

Response rates are always a challenge in survey research. Nurses in 25 randomly selected hospitals across the United States were surveyed regarding error rates for adverse events (Blegan, Vaughn, Pepper, Vojir, Stratton, Boyd, et al., 2004). The sampling procedures included distribution of the tools by hospital representatives resulting in a 30% response rate. Mayo and Duncan (2004) achieved a 20% response rate when surveying a random sample of nurses within one union. Sochalski (2004) conducted a secondary analysis of a one-state survey of a random sample of nurses regarding the relationship of nurse staffing and quality of care. The original survey investigators achieved a 52% response rate. Generally, in the studies analyzed for this review, the investigators used traditional survey methods requiring one-time completion of a survey tool. In contrast, Rogers, Hwang, Scott, Aiken, and Dinges (2004) conducted a more complex survey of a random sample of American Nurses Association (ANA) members. To facilitate a detailed evaluation of the relationship between the hours worked by nurses and errors, the author conducted a survey that required the completion of log books for a 2-week period, including daily recording of items. Of the 4,320 individuals sampled, 1,725 indicated interest in participating, 891 were eligible to participate and 40% did so. This innovative approach demonstrates the usefulness of survey research in studying more complex nursing research topics that require longitudinal data analysis.

The work environment and safety climate were also foci for studies. Nurses were included in a multidisciplinary survey using the Safety Climate Scale and Strategies for Leadership tool conducted by Pronovost, Weast, Holzmueller, Rosenstein, Kidwell, and Haller (2003). Ulrich, Buerhaus, Donelan, Norman, and Dittus (2005) conducted a follow-up survey regarding the work environment of nurses using a random sample of all RNs in the nation. Responses were weighted to represent the age and geographical distribution of nurses as identified in a prior survey. However, without relative standard errors presented for the estimates, it was difficult to evaluate the usefulness of this approach, because the sample size of 3,500 was small in relation to the country and offered the possibility of unstable estimates.

Secondary Data Analysis

Some of the more complex methodological studies were conducted by investigators using administrative datasets. These data often included discharge abstracts such as those collected through state health departments and available through national agencies such as AHRQ (retrieved December 13, 2005, from www.ahrq.gov/data/hcup/). These studies typically enlisted more than one administrative data source by merging datasets together, thus providing a more comprehensive dataset than is typically available within a single source. As discharge abstract data contain limited clinical information, investigators used existing data elements, including diagnoses and procedure codes, to create new variables to denote the patient's condition or represent outcomes of care. Typically the investigators recognized the importance of controlling for comorbidity in patient level studies, or the case mix of clients served by health care organizations for organizational level studies, and applied different mechanisms to measure either as appropriate. One such example of comorbidity software is provided by AHRQ, (retrieved December 13, 2005, from www.hcup-us.ahrq.gov/toolssoftware/comorbidity/comorbidity.jsp). In some studies, patient outcomes were derived from information available within administrative data using pre-established algorithms such as AHRQ's Patient Safety Indicators (retrieved December 13, 2005, from www.qualityindicators.ahrq.gov/psi_download.htm).

Often, combining administrative data sets alone were inadequate to study the research question posed, and authors combined the administrative data with data collected through primary research methods. In general, the investigators recognized the complex methodological issues posed by the clustering of patients who are treated on units within hospitals, or by the same doctor, or in other settings where similar nesting within different organizational subgroups occurs. Understanding that these observations are no longer independent, the investigators accounted for the clustering of observations within centers by using different types of hierarchical models.

Several studies were conducted using single- and multistate data. For example, Bernard and Ecinosa (2005) used Healthcare Cost and Utilization Project (HCUP) discharge abstract data from one state, combined it with data from cost reports, controlled for comorbidity, and then used logistical regression and hierarchical methods to model nursing-related patient safety indicators. In the same state, Encinosa and Bernard (2005) used 5 years of HCUP discharge abstract data and cost reports to study the relationship between hospital financial performance and nursing-sensitive patient safety indicators, controlling for time and using fixed effects for the 176 hospitals in their study to account for unobservable hospital characteristics. Needleman, Buerhaus, Mattke, Stewart, and Zelevinsky (2002) used data from 11 states and 799 hospitals to study the relationship between nurse staffing and patient outcomes. Patient outcomes were derived from discharge abstract data, and hospital-level staffing data were obtained; data were analyzed at the hospital level. To account for the influence of case mix on the hospital-level patient outcomes, the authors developed logistic regression models for the probability of risk for each patient for specific adverse outcomes and then used this information about the case mix of each hospital to adjust for the influence of case mix on outcomes.

Researchers also employed other types of secondary data. Dunton (2004) used ANA's National Database of Nurse Quality Indicators to study nurse staffing and patient falls. Dunton not only used linear models that accounted for the nesting of data, but also incorporated an innovative method to recognize that the data may become nonlinear at higher numbers of falls and accounted for this possibility using a knot (p. 56) to capture this nonlinear trend. This method offers promise, as studies seek to model both linear and nonlinear relationships. Hall, Doran, and Pink (2004) combined patient administrative data with staffing data collected directly from nurse managers to study nurse staffing and patient safety outcomes in 77 units at 17 hospitals. Using the organization's own measures to reflect the case mix of clients, multilevel hierarchical modeling was used to examine cost outcomes at the patient level, while patient outcomes were analyzed at the unit level with stepwise regression (due to the absence of patient safety outcomes at the patient level). Effken, Brewer, Patil, Lamb, Verran, and Carley (2004) used a computational modeling program called Orgahead to simulate changes within virtual units by combining data and data elements identified through a causal modeling study that reflected patient, unit, and organizational characteristics with quality and safety indicators collected from existing units. This mathematical modeling demonstrated the effect of changing specific data elements or groups of variables on specific outcomes. This innovation brings to the nursing literature an approach that combines the potential for tapping information within complex data systems with an ability to identify potential areas for improvement.

Aiken, Clarke, Sloane, Sochalski, and Silber (2002) combined secondary organizational and discharge abstract data from hospitals in one state with survey data collected from RNs in the same state. The investigators then merged the hospital discharge abstracts with vital statistics data to create a variable that identified deaths of clients following discharge. This innovative approach of combining different data sets with measures of patient conditions that allowed for differentiating complications of treatment from prior comorbidities enabled the investigators to estimate risk-adjusted patient outcomes while accounting for the clustering of data. Results highlighted the effect of different nurse-staffing ratios on patient mortality. Aiken and colleagues evaluated the effect of RN education levels on risk-adjusted outcomes using similar methods. Rothberg, Abraham, Lindenauer, and Rose (2005) evaluated the incremental cost-effectiveness of nurse staffing to mortality ratios discussed in Aiken, et al. (2002). Rothberg and co-investigators identified the cost effectiveness of different staffing ratios by estimating the costs per life saved in each of the ratios, using sensitivity analyses to explore the effect of the assumptions used in the models. This study demonstrates the need to incorporate cost-effectiveness analysis into patient safety studies. Such studies provide an effective mechanism for determining the actual costs incurred to achieve a certain level of patient safety outcome. Without this information, recommendations often are not perceived as credible, feasible, or ready for implementation by health policy and organizational decision makers. And finally, this series of investigations showcases studies building on one another to offer maximum results to the field. By so doing, the researchers provide an exemplar for responding to a current challenge within the field, which is the lack of integration of study designs and a collective building of a knowledge base.

OTHER METHODS

Other methods have been used in patient safety nursing research. One paper reported the use of a multimethod approach to studying patient safety in 29 rural hospitals. This paper is important in that the *American Journal of Nursing* offered continuing education credits to its readers following their review and test-taking. Cook Hoas, Guttmannova, and Joyner (2004) integrated findings from numerous patient safety–related studies and activities undertaken as a part of an R01 study with small, mainly nonaccredited hospitals. Data collection methods included a culture survey, a tool for reporting errors, a patient safety survey for staff, analysis of text from data collected in quarterly interviews, e-mail questionnaires, and analysis of responses to case studies presented for feedback. It was difficult to determine the specific methods used for the various components of the study, as they were not presented separately or in detail. Results from the studies and activities were integrated, and results were presented in an overall manner. The use of multimethods in areas where there is little prior research to inform the development of a study may be warranted. A rich, descriptive picture of the perspectives regarding patient safety and the patient safety activities occurring in small rural hospitals has the potential for offering direction for the development of a more structured research study for these understudied facilities. However, the lack of detail on the methods used in this review precludes evaluation, and the integration of findings from so many activities makes it difficult to discern the relevant findings.

DISCUSSION/LIMITATIONS

Using multiple search methods to locate published research represents a comprehensive approach to selecting articles that reflect the types of methods being used in patient safety nursing research. None of the selection modes for identifying research articles was completely objective—all required subjective decisions regarding the inclusion or exclusion of manuscripts. This is largely because the scope of patient safety nursing research, which is relevant to all clinical subspecialties and settings within the health system, resulted in many studies and professional papers that discuss the importance of patient safety or the relevance of their study to patient safety even when the study was not predominately focused on patient safety, as defined earlier.

The lack of consistent conceptual frameworks and definitions of patient safety outcomes made it difficult to determine boundaries for manuscript selection for this review. For example, any particular negative outcome (e.g., patient falls, medication errors) would require a full literature review to address the question of relevant methods used to study that particular outcome. Any study of a nursing intervention that aims to improve quality of care could be expected to affect patient safety. Because the term patient safety revealed many articles that were only peripherally related to the overall concept, decisions were made to select only those articles most relevant to the broadest concept of patient safety. This selection was made more difficult by the fact that nursing is a component of almost all patient safety studies; even those studies that did not focus primarily on nursing still had some relationship to nursing care. Despite these limitations, this review demonstrates the variety of methods and the inventive approaches being used to advance the field of patient safety nursing research.

CONCLUSION

Implications for the Use of Methodologies in Patient Safety Focused Nursing Research

This review demonstrates the variety of methods and the inventive approaches used to advance the field of patient safety nursing research. The field could be more quickly advanced through improved planning and coordination of ongoing and future research. Increased opportunities for collaborative research and for multisite studies need to be identified, and federal agencies need to fund the implementation of such strategies.

Additional work is needed regarding the development of measures to be used in patient safety nursing research. Most administrative data systems were not initially designed to incorporate data elements that would facilitate rapid or targeted analysis for patient safety research. Although measures have since been developed by governmental or regulatory agencies, or by individual investigators for personal use, further evaluation of the reliability and validity of the measures developed and deployed in patient safety research, and the subsequent dissemination of these results, would be a substantial contribution of nurse researchers. Creating an online database of patient safety measurement instruments that would include information regarding the use of each instrument in nursing research, current expert opinion regarding the use of the instrument, and reliability and validity findings, would be helpful in guiding researchers to appropriately select instruments. This warehouse may lead to more consistent use of instruments and measures over time. Perhaps this additional repository could be incorporated into AHRQ's National Quality Measures Clearinghouse (www.qualitymeasures.ahrq.gov/).

To enhance the contribution of patient safety nursing research it will be necessary to increase both multisite and longitudinal studies that capitalize on the strength of administrative data bases. Multimethod studies and clearly linked studies that build on previous findings are especially necessary. To do so, means must be established to provide opportunities to train investigators in the complex research methodologies and statistical analyses that are critical for this line of research, but may not have been included in prior educational programs. Although dissertations were not analyzed for this review, it is promising that five recent nursing dissertations focused on patient safety research. It will be important to increase training for new nurse researchers in this growing area. Doctoral programs in nursing must incorporate health services research methods, including the analysis of large data sets and the analysis of multilevel data, to facilitate the ability of nurse researchers to use advanced methodological approaches for patient safety research. Likewise, our finding that survey research emerged as a major research method should prompt increased attention to the design, implementation, and analysis of complex survey research designs. The innovative cognitive interviewing approaches, computational modeling, and human factors engineering approaches also suggest areas for further methodological training and development.

As noted, patient safety research is faced with the dual challenges of conducting not only clinical research, but also health services research. Who better to address these challenges than nurse researchers? The overall field of patient safety research benefits from the merging of the clinical knowledge of nurses with their understanding of the health care system and their research abilities. The contribution of nursing research to improving patient safety is evident in the documented literature. As this field grows, so will the contributions of nursing researchers to patient safety and health care delivery. Providing further training and encouraging nurses to coordinate and conduct interdisciplinary research to improve patient safety will amplify this contribution.

ACKNOWLEDGMENTS

This work was supported in part by the National Institute of Mental Health, R01 MH066293 Shortage of Health Professionals in Rural Areas (Elizabeth Merwin, principal investigator) and by 5F31NR009320 Relationship of Patient Safety to Patient Outcomes (Deirdre Thornlow, principal investigator).

REFERENCES

Aiken, L., Clarke, S., Sloane, D., Sochalski, J., & Silber, J. (2002). Hospital nurse staffing and patient mortality, nurse burnout, and job dissatisfaction. *Journal of the American Medical Association, 288*(16), 1987–1993.

Bernard, D., & Encinosa, W. E. (2005). Financial and demographic influences on medicare patient safety events. In *Advances in patient safety: From research to implementation* (Agency for Healthcare Research and Quality Publication No. 05-0021). Rockville, MD: Agency for Healthcare Research and Quality.

Blegen, M. A., Vaughn, T., Pepper, G., Vojir, C., Stratton, K., Boyd, M., & Armstrong, G. (2004). Patient and staff safety: Voluntary reporting. *American Journal of Medical Quality, 19,* 67–74.

Blegen, M. A., Pepper, G. A., & Rosse, J. (2005). Safety climate on hospital units: A new measure. In *Advances in patient safety: From research to implementation* (Agency for Healthcare Research and Quality Publication No. 05-0021). Rockville, MD: Agency for Healthcare Research and Quality.

Bullen, B. (2002). The way across the chasm. IOM reports help providers, government navigate toward higher-quality care. *Modern Healthcare, 32*(46), 30.

Carayon, P., Wetterneck, T. B., Hundt, A. S., Ozkaynak, M., Ram, P., DeSilvey, J., et al. (2005). Observing nurse interaction with infusion pump technologies. In *Advances in patient safety: From research to implementation* (Agency for Healthcare Research and Quality Publication No. 05-0021). Rockville, MD: Agency for Healthcare Research and Quality.

Cook, A. F., Hoas, H., Guttmannova, K., & Joyner, J. C. (2004). An error by any other name. *American Journal of Nursing, 104*(6), 32–44.

Cooper, J. B., Gaba, D. M., Liang, B., Woods, D., & Blum, L. N. (2000). National Patient Safety Foundation agenda for research and development in patient safety [Electronic version]. *Medscape General Medicine, 2*(4), 14. Retrieved April 13, 2006 from www. medscape.com/viewarticle/408064

Dunton, N., Gajewski, B., Taunton, R.L., and Moore, J. (2004). Nurse staffing and patient falls on acute care hospital units. *Nursing Outlook, 52*(1), 53–59.

Ebright, P. R., Patterson, E. S., Chalko, B. A., & Render, M. L. (2003). Understanding the complexity of registered nurse work in acute care settings. *Journal of Nursing Administration, 33*(12), 630–638.

Ebright, P. R., Urden, L., Patterson, E., & Chalko, B. (2004). Themes surrounding novice nurse near-miss and adverse-event situations. *Journal of Nursing Administration, 34*(11), 531–538.

Effken, J. A., Brewer, B. B., Patil, A., Lamb, G. S., Verran, J. A., & Carley, K. (2004). Using computational modeling to improve patient care unit safety and quality outcomes. *Medinfo, 11*(Pt. 1), 726–730.

Encinosa, W. E., & Bernard, D. M. (2005). Hospital finances and patient safety outcomes. *Inquiry, 42*(1), 60–72.

Evanoff, B., Potter, P., Wolf, L., Grayson, D., Dunagan, C. & Boxerman, S. (2005). Can we talk? Priorities for patient care differed among health care providers. In *Advances in patient safety: From research to implementation* (Agency for Healthcare Research and

Quality Publication No. 05-0021). Rockville, MD: Agency for Healthcare Research and Quality.

Gall, S., & Bull, J. (2004). Clinical risk: Discharging patients with no-one at home. *Gastroenterology Nursing, 27*(3), 111–114.

Ginsburg, L., Norton, P. G., Casebeer, A., & Lewis, S. (2005). An educational intervention to enhance nurse leaders' perceptions of patient safety culture. *Health Services Research, 40*(4), 997–1020.

Grayson, D., Boxerman, S., Potter, P., Wolf, L., Dunagan, C., Sorock, G., et al. (2005). Do transient working conditions trigger medical errors? In *Advances in patient safety: From research to implementation* (Agency for Healthcare Research and Quality Publication No. 05-0021). Rockville, MD: Agency for Healthcare Research and Quality.

Greengold, N. L., Shane, R., Schneider, P., Flynn, E., Elashoff, J., & Hoying, C. L. (2003). The impact of dedicated medication nurses on the medication administration error rate: A randomized controlled trial. *Archives of Internal Medicine, 163*(19), 2359–2367.

Hall, L. M., Doran, D., & Pink, G. H. (2004). Nurse staffing models, nursing hours, and patient safety outcomes. *Journal of Nursing Administration, 34*(1), 41–45.

Harder, K. A., Bloomfield, J. R., Sendelbach, S. E., Shepherd, M. F., Rush, P. S., Sinclair, J. S., Kirshbaum, M., Burns, D. E. (2005). Improving the safety of heparin administration by implementing a human factors process analysis. In *Advances in Patient Safety: From Research to Implementation* (Agency for Healthcare Research and Quality Publication No. 05-0021, vol. 3). Rockville, MD: Agency for Healthcare Research and Quality.

Ho, S., & French, P. (2002). Minimizing fire risk during eye surgery. *Clinical Nursing Research, 11*(4), 387–402.

Hodge, M. B., Asch, S. M., Olson, V. A., Kravitz, R. L., & Sauve, M. J. (2002). Developing indicators of nursing quality to evaluate nurse staffing ratios. *Journal of Nursing Administration, 32*(6), 338–345.

Institute of Medicine (2004). Creating and sustaining a culture of safety. In *Keeping patients safe: Transforming the work environment of nurses*. Washington, DC: The National Academies of Science.

Jeffe, D. B., Dunagan, W. C., Garbutt, J., Burroughs, T. E., Gallagher, T. H., & Hill, P. R. (2004). Using focus groups to understand physicians' and nurses' perspectives on error reporting in hospitals. *Joint Commission Journal on Quality & Safety, 30*(9), 471–479.

Joint Commission on Accreditation of Healthcare Organizations (2003). Facts about patient safety. Retrieved from http://www.JCAHO.org. Accessed 5/31/06.

Leape, L., Berwick, D., & Bates, D. (2002). What practices will most improve safety? *Journal of the American Medical Association, 288*(4), 501–507.

Leape, L.L. & Berwick, D.M. (2005). Five years after *To Err is Human*: What have we learned? *Journal of the American Medical Association, 293*(19), 2384–2390.

Lingard, L., Espin, S., Whyte, S., Regehr, G., Baker, G. R., Reznick, R., et al. (2004). Communication failures in the operating room: An observational classification of recurrent types and effects. *Quality & Safety in Health Care, 13*(5), 330–334.

Mark, B. A., Salyer, J., & Wan, T. (2003). Professional nursing practice: Impact on organizational and patient outcomes. *Journal of Nursing Administration, 33*(4), 224–234.

Mayo, A. M., & Duncan, D. (2004). Nurse perceptions of medication errors: What we need to know for patient safety. *Journal of Nursing Care Quality, 19*(3), 209–217.

Needleman, J., Buerhaus, P., Mattke, S., Stewart, M., & Zelevinsky, K. (2002). Nurse-staffing levels and the quality of care in hospitals. *New England Journal of Medicine, 346,* 1715–1722.

Olson, D. M., Cheek, D. J., & Morgenlander, J. C. (2004). The impact of bispectral index monitoring on rates of propofol administration. *AACN Clinical Issues, 15*(1), 63–73.

Patterson, E. S., Cook, R. I., & Render, M. L. (2002). Improving patient safety by identifying side effects from introducing bar coding in medication administration. *Journal of the American Medical Informatics Association, 9,* 540–553.

Potter, P., Wolf, L., Boxerman, S., Grayson, D., Sledge, J., Dunagan, C. et al. (2005). An analysis of nurses' cognitive work: A new perspective for understanding medical errors. In *Advances in patient safety: From research to implementation* (Agency for Healthcare Research Quality Publication No. 05-0021). Rockville, MD: Agency for Healthcare Research and Quality.

Pronovost, P. J., Weast, B., Holzmueller, C. G., Rosenstein, B. J., Kidwell, R. P., Haller, K. B., et al. (2003). Evaluation of the culture of safety: Survey of clinicians and managers in an academic medical center. *Quality & Safety in Health Care, 12*(6), 405–410.

Rogers, A. E., Hwang, W. T., Scott, L. D., Aiken, L. H., & Dinges, D. F. (2004). The working hours of hospital staff nurses and patient safety. *Health Affairs, 23*(4), 202–212.

Rothberg, M. B., Abraham, I., Lindenauer, P. K., & Rose, D. N. (2005). Improving nurse-to-patient staffing ratios as a cost-effective safety intervention. *Medical Care, 43*(8), 785–791.

Savitz, L. A., Jones, C. B., & Bernard, S. (2005). Quality indicators sensitive to nurse staffing in acute care settings. In *Advances in patient safety: From research to implementation* (Agency for Healthcare Research Quality Publication No. 05-0021). Rockville, MD: Agency for Healthcare Research and Quality.

Shojania, K., Duncan, B., McDonald, K., & Wachter, R. (2002). Safe but sound: Patient safety meets evidence-based medicine. *Journal of the American Medical Association, 288*(4), 508–513.

Shojania, K., Duncan, B., McDonald, K., & Wachter, R. (Eds.). (2001). Making health care safer: A critical analysis of patient safety practices. Evidence Report/Technology Assessment No. 43 (No. 01-E058). Rockville, MD: Agency for Healthcare Research and Quality.

Simpson, K. R. (2005). Failure to rescue: Implications for evaluating quality of care during labor and birth. *Journal of Perinatal & Neonatal Nursing, 19*(1), 24–34.

Sochalski, J. (2004). Is more better?: The relationship between nurse staffing and the quality of nursing care in hospitals. *Medical Care, 42*(Suppl. 2), 67–73.

St. Clair, J. (2005). A new model of tracheostomy care: Closing the research-practice gap. In, *Advances in Patient Safety: From Research to Implementation.* Agency for Healthcare Research and Quality. Agency for Healthcare Research Quality Publication No. 05-0021-CD, pp. 521–527.

Stone, P. W., Harrison, M. I., Feldman, P., Linzer, M, Peng, T., Roblin, D. et al. (2005). Organizational climate of staff working conditions and safety—an integrative model. In *Advances in patient safety: From research to implementation* (Agency for Healthcare Research Quality Publication No. 05-0021). Rockville, MD: Agency for Healthcare Research and Quality.

Stratton, K. M., Blegen, Pepper, G., & Vaughn, T. (2004). Reporting of medication errors by pediatric nurses. *Journal of Pediatric Nursing, 19*(6), 385–392.

Thomas, E. J., Sexton, B. J., Neilands, T. B., Frankel, A., & Helmreich, R. L. (2005). The effect of executive walk rounds on nurse safety climate attitudes: A randomized trial of clinical units. *BMC Health Services Research, 5*(28).

Ulrich, B. T., Buerhaus, P. I., Donelan, K., Norman, L., & Dittus, R. (2005). How RNs view the work environment: Results of a national survey of registered nurses. *Journal of Nursing Administration, 35*(9), 389–396.

Wakefield, B. J., Uden-Holman, T., & Wakefield, D. S. (2005). Development and validation of the Medication Administration Error Reporting Survey. In *Advances in patient safety: From research to implementation* (Agency for Healthcare Research and Quality Publication No. 05-0021). Rockville, MD: Agency for Healthcare Research and Quality.

Weir, C., Hoffman, J., Nebeker, J. R., & Hurdle, J. F. (2005). Nurse's role in tracking adverse drug events: The impact of provider order entry. *Nursing Administration Quarterly, 29*(1), 39–44.

PART V

International Nursing Research

Chapter 12

Nursing Research in Ireland

Geraldine McCarthy, Josephine Hegarty, and
Dawn O'Sullivan

ABSTRACT

This review presents an analysis of research published by Irish nurses during the period 1990–2005. The analysis is the first effort made to identify the main characteristics of Irish nursing research. Overall, 213 published studies were identified for consideration, from which, 152 were included in the review. The studies were published in 60 journals, 4 books, and 8 research reports. Journal articles selected from 6 journals accounted for 52%. Inclusion criteria were quality of research design, sampling (including sample size), data analysis, scientific merit, and authorship. Each article was analyzed based on this schema. The major areas of research identified included clinical practice (56%) (e.g., medical surgical, mental health, intellectual disability, and maternal and child), nursing management and professional issues (19%), and nursing education (25%).

Keyword: nursing research

NURSING RESEARCH IN IRELAND

Irish nursing has been transformed in recent years as a result of the Commission on Nursing (Government of Ireland, 1998), with development of nursing and midwifery schools within universities and other third-level institutions, change to an all-graduate profession, increasing number of graduates taking higher degrees, introduction of clinical career paths, and new structure and responsibilities for nurse managers. The need for a research agenda for nursing and midwifery has become imperative in this rapidly changing environment. *A Research Strategy for all Health Care Professionals* (Department of Health & Children, 2001), and *A National Research Strategy for Nursing and Midwifery* (Department of Health & Children, 2003) have been published. However, research published by nurses in Ireland to date has not been synthesized. This review presents an analysis of published research during the period 1990–2005. It is presented in three major sections: clinical practice, management and professional issues, and education. An introduction and summary is given in each section.

CLINICAL PRACTICE

Eighty-five studies were identified for review under this category; specific areas of research included general nursing (31 studies), mental health (13), intellectual disability (10), maternal and child (31).

General Nursing

Thirty-one studies were identified for analysis, three related to pain, four to the experiencing of coping with cancer, and four on information needs of patients with cardiac conditions. Two studies related to fatigue, seven to infection control, five to older adults, and six to outcomes relating to clinical nurse specialisation in acute care situations.

Pain

O'Connor (1995a, 1995b), in a descriptive quantitative study, investigated assessment of pain in patients with early acute myocardial infarction and compared assessment of both patients and nurses. Findings indicated that nurses underestimated patients' pain in 46% of instances and overestimated in 13% of cases. Nurses documented location and verbal statements about pain but little about pain quality, intensity, or duration. A retrospective analysis of randomly selected patient charts (MacLellan, 1997) examined the documentation of pain in hospital. Results indicated that documentation of pain following surgery was poor and suggested that as-needed prescribing may hinder optimal pain management. Experimental research (MacLellan, 2004) detailed the introduction and evaluation of a nurse-led intervention to improve pain management after surgery. Pain scores ($n = 800$ patients and 9,138 pain scores) were measured in two phases, with results indicating a statistical significant reduction of pain after intervention for major surgical postoperative patients.

Experience of and Coping with Cancer

Two researchers identified situation-specific responses in Irish breast cancer patients. In a cross-sectional correlational study, McCarthy (1999) investigated women's ($n = 86$) responses to the diagnosis and treatment of breast cancer and efforts made to cope and adapt. Participants perceived their situation as either a challenge ($n = 47$) or anticipated threat ($n = 31$); both problem-focused and emotion-focused coping were used, with emotion-focused coping used most often. O'Mahony (2001) explored Irish woman's experience of a recent breast biopsy to gain a deeper understanding of individual experiences. A qualitative phenomenological approach was utilized with a sample of eight women. Themes that emerged related to finding a lump, knowing, not knowing, waiting, and getting back to normal. Wright, Courtney, and Crowther (2002) investigated the effectiveness of autogenic training (AT) a technique of deep breathing and self-hypnosis in 18 patients diagnosed with cancer. Results indicated a significant reduction in anxiety and an increase in fighting spirit compared to before the intervention, with an increased sense of coping and apparent benefits of AT practice. Wright, Courtney, Donnelly, Kenny, and Lavin (2002) retrospectively investigated the perceived benefits of reflexology on quality of life among a sample of 47 clients with cancer. Qualitative data randomly retrieved from recorded evaluations made throughout treatments revealed improvement in functional status and impairment, which subsequently lead to improvement in general health.

Information Needs

Joyce and Mulligan (1994) identified the sources and appropriateness of information received by 50 patients diagnosed as needing coronary artery bypass graft. The majority had not received information about issues such as breathing, ventilators, and wound care on resumption of work. Half had received information about pain, diet, intensive care, and medications, but none reported receiving information about rehabilitation. Medical consultant, other doctors, and nurses were sources of information, but nurses in a lesser capacity than doctors. More recently, two researchers focused on the information needs of patients after a myocardial infarction. Hughes (2000) tested the reliability and validity of two instruments—Cardiac Patients Learning Needs Inventory (CPLNI) and the Information Need Inventory for Patients post-Myocardial Infarction (INIPPI)—in a quantitative cross-sectional study. Thirty-one sequentially admitted patients were randomly allocated to one of two available interview schedules (CPLNI or

INIPPI) and interviewed on two occasions. Findings indicated a higher level of reliability in the modified instrument (INIPPI) than in the CPLNI. Timmins and Kaliszer (2003), using the CPLNI, assessed patients' ($n = 27$) needs immediately and at 6 weeks after a first myocardial infarction, and they made comparisons between these and the perceptions of cardiac nurses ($n = 68$). Findings showed that responses were highly skewed, with two-third in the very important category and less than 1% in the not important/somewhat important categories. In a descriptive study, Quinn, Redmond, and Begley (1996) investigated perceptions of needs, their importance, and fulfilment in relatives ($n = 351$) visiting adult critical care units and critical care nurses ($n = 255$). Ten needs, including receiving information and reassurance, were given equal ratings of importance by both relatives and nurses, and nurses were identified as the most important persons to meet needs.

Fatigue

McCann and Boore (2000) described fatigue and associated factors in 39 renal patients receiving maintenance dialysis in a descriptive correlational study. A high level of fatigue was experienced with corresponding low levels of vitality. Fatigue was associated with presence of symptoms such as sleep problems, poor physical health status, and depression. Glacken, Coates, Kernohan, and Hegarty (2003), using grounded theory, gained an appreciation from 20 patients of what it was like to live with Hepatic C–k associated fatigue. Fatigue was described in terms of living with fatigue (struggling to redefine boundaries in order to regain control), resting and sleeping, pacing and positioning, and mobilizing resources.

Infection Control

Healy (2001) conducted a prospective, observational study in an intensive care unit (ICU) to evaluate a new range of surface-treated catheters in relation to sepsis, thrombosis, and indwelling catheter times. The sample of 86 patients received 119 surface-treated multi-lumen catheters, standard sterile barrier precautions, and follow-on care by nursing staff as per standard ICU protocol. Distal end of catheter was removed aseptically and microbiologically examined. Findings illustrated a range of indwelling time from 1 to 23 days (mean = 8 days), and 8% in situ for longer than ICU protocol; 67% demonstrated colonization, and thrombosis rates were 3.3%. Creamer (2000) investigated duration of cannulation in order to minimise the risk of infection. Data were generated through semi-structured interviews with a sample of 10 nurses from medical and surgical wards. Results demonstrated that effectiveness in practice rests not solely on individual professional practice but were also related to organizational support systems. In a subsequent study, Cramer, McCarthy, Tighe, and Smyth (2002) surveyed peripheral intravenous catheter (PVC) sites (554 PVCs in 397 patients), focusing on the assessment of site for infection. Results demonstrated that just 5% had a site infection. The authors stated that involvement of the infection control nurse in the wards studied may have contributed to the low infection rate. Cramer, Cunney, Humphreys, and Smyth (2002) also reported on a program of continuous surveillance of surgical-site infections, using basis surveillance clinical evidence supported by, but not dependent on, laboratory results. 59,335 surgical sites were surveyed over a 16-year period. Overall infection rate was 4.5%, with 2.4% in clean surgery. Apart from increases in the 3rd, 4th, and 13th years, infection rates remained relatively stable during the 16 years.

Using a quasi-experimental design, Creedon (2005) investigated hand washing in doctors, nurses, and other health care professionals on an ICU. Data were collected using a structured observation schedule ($n = 314$) and a self-report questionnaire ($n = 62$). Findings demonstrate compliance ratings of 51% pre-test and 83% post-test, suggesting that the program led to improved compliance with hand-hygiene guidelines.

Long, Allwright, and Begley (2004), using grounded theory, explored 31 male prisoners' views and experiences of drug injection use in prisons. Purposive sampling consisted of illicit drug injectors ($n = 16$) and noninjectors ($n = 15$) for in–depth interviewing. Participants reported that heroin injecting in prison was common and "out of control." Findings also highlighted that low availability of injecting equipment resulted in sharing needles that received inadequate cleaning between users, increasing the risk of contracting bloodborne viruses. McGrane and Staines (2003) examined nurses' ($n = 120$) understanding of the hepatitis B virus and attitudes and acceptance of the hepatitis B vaccination. Results indicated that participants were aware of the aetiology and infectivity of the virus. Acceptance of the hepatitis B vaccine was high, and reasons for accepting immunization included free cost (81%), caring for clients with hepatitis B (78%), and benefits of the vaccine (75%).

Older Adult

Syron and Shelley (2001) developed an assessment tool for the collection of information about carers' needs and pilot tested it with 66 caregivers of predominantly older people. Major needs identified were financial, housing, social life, and practical support. Almost half of caregivers themselves had chronic health problems and took regular medications. Coffey (2004), in a qualitative study, explored the perceptions of nurses ($n = 40$) and care attendants ($n = 40$) employed in the care of older people regarding the provision of formal training for care using focus groups and open-ended questionnaires. Positive attitudes toward training for care attendants were identified, along with a perceived link between the provision of training and a blurring of boundaries. Findings also disclosed that although nurses were positively disposed to the training of care attendants, this was not accompanied by a desire to become actively involved. Murphy (2002) investigated liaison practices between hospital nurses and public health nurses (PHNs) with regard to home discharges ($n = 256$) of elderly patients, using a quantitative descriptive design. PHNs received discharge liaison information in just 36% of cases, and 67% were contacted within 24 hours. A further 14% of discharged patients were visited after local networks informally brought them to the attention of the PHN. In descriptive research, Moore and Pitman (2000) surveyed all adult inpatients ($n = 297$) in one Irish hospital as part of a strategy to develop a pressure sore prevention policy. Results revealed that 13% of patients had pressure sores on two or more sites, the majority occurring in the 60–99 years age category, with 65% developed post-admission. More recently, Moore and Price (2004) investigated nurses' ($n = 300$) views and practices of pressure ulcer prevention in a cross-sectional survey. The researchers suggested that although nurses held positive attitudes toward prevention of pressure sores, barriers to practice were identified as staffing, time, and patient numbers.

Outcomes Based on Clinical Nurse Specialization

Clinical nurse specialists have recently been formally introduced in Ireland, and just eight studies have been sourced on their contribution. In a prospective descriptive study, O'Neill (1997) wanted to determine whether patients wearing 24-hour Ambulatory Blood Pressure Machine made changes to their daily routine and understood and accepted lifestyle information given by the specialist. Results indicated that 90% knew that they could continue with their usual daily activities. Advice on smoking, alcohol, and exercise was accepted by the majority (78%); however, advice on stress and diet was less well accepted (58%). Minnock (2002) evaluated the feasibility and patient acceptance of a trained rheumatology nurse performing intra-articular injections, with 23 patients using a specialist satisfaction and efficacy measure. Overall satisfaction was rated at 85%, information and explanation of the procedure at 92%, and overall comfort at 75%. In a descriptive correlational study, Minnock, Fitzgerald, and Bresnihan (2003) examined the relationship between quality of life of 58 women with rheumatoid arthritis (RA), their perceived levels of social support, and their primary caregivers' knowledge of the disease. Poor health status was reported for arthritic pain, social activity, and level of tension. The greatest level of dissatisfaction was associated with arthritic pain management (57%), and this received the highest priority for health status improvement. Both patients and caregivers displayed limited knowledge of RA or its treatment. Murphy, Byrne, and Costello (2002) estimated the efficacy of an early supported discharge program on outcomes for 100 patients with exacerbations of chronic obstructive pulmonary disease. Findings revealed that early discharge was a safe and effective alternative to hospital stay. Diabetes nurse specialists' knowledge of the purpose and utility of documentation and their attitude to documentation was investigated by Clarke (2002). A descriptive quantitative design revealed that the majority had a negative attitude toward documentation unrelated to the documentation format used, or knowledge of the purpose and utility of documentation. In an observational study, Ryder, Travers, Timmons, Ledwidge, and McDonald (2003) examined the feasibility of a specialist heart failure nurse–supervised rapid titration of angiotensin-converting enzyme inhibitor in 52 sequential class 1V heart failure patients admitted to the cardiology service. Results demonstrated that the service was feasible and safe and possibly decreased length of hospital stay and out patient department visits.

Summary

Thirty-one studies relating to diverse topics were reviewed in this section. Infection control received the most attention, and studies relating to fatigue received the least. Designs utilized were qualitative (5), quantitative (24), and mixed approaches (2).

Mental Health

Thirteen research publications were identified for review: one examining career choice, three examining stress and coping, four examining role, and five examining clinical studies (e.g., experiences of acute mental health care, modification of behavior, safety and quality of community services).

Wells and McElwee (2000) examined reasons for career choice among students completing second level school education, psychiatric nursing students, and social care students using a focus group approach. Results indicated that students rely on stereotypical views as part of the decision-making process in shaping occupational decisions. School leavers conceptualized psychiatric nursing as being a job involving menial and physical tasks. Social care students saw psychiatric nursing as lacking autonomy and institutional in nature. Psychiatric nurses felt themselves exploited and second-class compared to general nurses. Ryan and Quayle (1999) investigated stress and coping in psychiatric nursing using a stratified random sample of 179 psychiatric nurses employed in one health board area. Participants reported low levels of stress related to organizational issues rather than matters intrinsic to work. These results were replicated in a later study (Murphy, 2004) of nonpsychiatric staff members (nephrology nurses) who reported stress arising from job content, resource issues, professional working relationships, and extrinsic factors. Tully (2004) measured levels of distress, sources of stress, and ways of coping of a convenience sample ($n = 35$) of psychiatric nursing students.

The investigator found high levels of distress, with students using coping methods such as comfort eating, wishing things were different, smoking, or taking medication. Limited coping skills and preparing to become a nurse were found to be significantly stressful and a possible risk to the well being of students.

Gijbels (1995), in a descriptive qualitative study, examined the perceived therapeutic skills of mental health nurses in an acute admission unit. Results indicated that nurses performed a variety of roles, including elements of caretaker, role model, container, custodian, mediator, informer, coordinator, manager, and administrator, with few suggesting that of an independent therapeutic agent. The unique role was seen as "being there" at the "coalface" available over a 24-hour period. Based on the results, the researcher suggested that nurses valued and possessed a range of therapeutic skills and qualities but were unable to draw on these, leaving them to draw on administrative, coordinating, and managerial skills. In an effort to clarify the nature and scope of psychiatric nursing function, Cowman, Farrelly, and Gilheany (2001) described the role and function of psychiatric nurses in clinical practice. A descriptive qualitative research design was utilized, including 155 nurses from 13 settings in one geographic area. Nine categories of nursing role were identified: assessment of needs and evaluating care, planning care, nurse-patient caring interactions, pharmacological interventions, education, documenting information, coordinating services, communicating with other professionals, and administration. Through interviews with eight registered nurses (RNs), Deady (2005), explored the nature of the subjective experience of mental health nursing. Results indicated that many of the personal and professional values, attitudes, and beliefs expressed reflected a humanistic philosophy of caring. The notion of caring was a strong feature, and this caring role appeared to take place through the development of an interpersonal relationship that was not formalized. Murphy, Cooney, Casey, Connor, O'Connor, and Dineen (2000) wanted to determine whether the Roper, Logan, and Tierney Model of Nursing (2000) was appropriate for planning nursing care for mentally ill clients. Data collected from 237 care plans and through interviews with 20 nurses evaluated the extent to which the model was used to assess, plan, and implement care in nursing documentation. Little evidence that the model guided care planning was found, and nurses considered the model constraining and physically orientated.

In a phenomenological study, Farrelly (1999) explored patients' experiences of acute mental health care. A purposeful sample of eight ex-patients after a first voluntary admission to a public psychiatric ward but discharged for no more than 1 month participated. Six themes emerged: encounters with other patients, pharmacological and other therapies, loss of control and freedom; staff attitudes, someone to talk to, and personal amenities. Clancy, Taylor, and O'Sullivan (2002) sought to validate a scale for assessing the risk of violence at the time of psychiatric hospitalization. The checklist was completed by a nurse for each of 116 patients admitted over a 2-month period to a psychiatric admission unit. Results indicated that a history of violence prior to admission and a diagnosis of schizophrenia or mania were significantly associated with aggressive behavior. Patton (2003), in a qualitative descriptive study, examined the technique of Reality Orientation (RO) and how it influenced violence and aggression within an acute psychiatric service. Data were collected, via semi-structured interviews, from 12 staff in an inner city acute psychiatric unit. Results indicated that RO was defined as the here and now—patients who need orientation, orientation assessment, truth telling, when not to implement, associated therapies, and techniques and effectiveness.

Utilizing a descriptive survey design, Cowman and Walsh (2004) described safety and security measures in psychiatry acute admission wards in 37 psychiatric hospitals. A wide variation in practices was found with no overall policy or agreement on best practice in terms of safety or security. Twenty percent of wards had access to neither an ICU nor a seclusion room; 27% of wards always had the door locked; patient-searching practices and testing for illegal drugs and alcohol on admission and when returning from weekend leave varied between 4% and 27%. Cusack (1994) investigated the quality of community services for 29 individuals with a mental illness transferred from institutionalized residences to high-support hostels. Ninety-six percent of respondents preferred community living and reported satisfaction with deinstitutionalized care, yet difficulty in community integrating.

Summary

Thirteen studies focusing on mental health issues were reviewed. In the majority, data were collected from either staff or student nurses and related to their experiences. Just two studies used data from the individual receiving care. Seven used qualitative designs, and six quantitative designs.

Intellectual Disability Nursing

Intellectual disability nursing is a specific branch of nursing in Ireland. Students receive a bachelor of science degree and registration as an intellectual disability nurse. Research endeavors in this area are growing, with an emphasis on patients' or careers' perspectives. Ten studies were identified for inclusion in this section, most of them from one research center directed by Cosgrave.

In one of the first studies by this group, Cosgrave, McCarron, Anderson, Tyrrell, Gill, and Lawlor (1998) tested the validity and reliability of the Test for Severe Impairment (TSI) among 60 individuals with Down syndrome. The researchers advocated the usefulness of the TSI for monitoring the progression of dementia. Cosgrave, Tyrrell, McCarron, Gill, and Lawlor (1999a) investigated whether there was a relationship between age of menopause and onset of dementia in 143 women with Down syndrome. Dementia and moderate intellectual disability was present in 14 women, and age of menopause significantly correlated with the age at onset of dementia for 12 women. Using a cross-sectional design, the researchers explored aggression and adaptive and maladaptive behaviors in 29 older persons with Down syndrome and dementia, and 99 people without dementia (Cosgrave, Tyrrell, McCarron, Gill, & Lawlor, 1999b). Dementia was higher among older individuals; however, it was not found to be a predictor of aggressive or maladaptive behavior. Lower levels of adaptive behavior occurred in individuals with both dementia and lower levels of cognitive functioning. In a 5-year follow-up study, Cosgrave, Tyrrell, McCarron, Gill, and Lawlor (2000) investigated the onset of dementia in relation to age, duration, and clinical features among 80 females with Down syndrome. On initiation of the study, 7 subjects had dementia, which developed in a further 28 subjects by completion. Increasing age was associated with onset of dementia. Memory loss followed by spatial disorientation and increased dependence were the most common presenting symptoms. McCarron, Gill, Lawlor, and Beagly (2002) tested the usefulness of the Caregiver Activity Survey-Intellectual Disability scale in measuring the amount of time caregivers spent with 30 persons with dementia ($n = 16$) and without dementia ($n = 14$) in conjunction with Down syndrome and Alzheimer disease. Findings support the usefulness of the measurement tools in assessing the amount of time spent caring for these individuals.

Other researchers investigated the interactions of people with profound learning disabilities (Griffiths & Cowman, 1999) and, using a triangulation approach, collected data from two randomly selected individuals, using nonparticipant observation, and completed semi-structured interviews with key caregivers of these individuals. Observational data demonstrated that individuals with profound learning disabilities interacted differently in various settings and to the amount of stimulation received, which was supported by findings from interviews. O'Halloran (1996) explored the decision-making experiences of five adults with learning disabilities living in a community residence. Participants reported appreciating opportunities to make decisions; however, the decisions made were considered minor. Also, clients indicated contentment with both activity and passivity in the decision-making process. Sheerin (2004) investigated the key nursing interventions provided by intellectual disability nurses in residential care. Consensus of 38 interventions was reached, which were correlated with North American Nursing Diagnosis Association nursing diagnoses including anger control assistance, emotional support, and safety enhancement. Using a phenomenological case study approach, Hartrey and Wells (2003) investigated the meaning of respite care among a convenience sample of two mothers of children with learning disabilities. Diary documentation, a taped narrative, and written reflections were used to gather data. Three categories emerged that addressed emotional, social, and physical meanings. Although providing psychological and physical relief in addition to opportunities for social engagement, placing their children in respite care led to feelings of guilt among mothers. Courell (1997), using semi-structured interviews, investigated four caregivers' and four nurses' experiences regarding the hospitalization of adults with severe learning difficulties. Five themes emerged from each respondent group: communication, training, time/resources, planning, and effect of hospitalization. Findings suggest that nurses experienced difficulties communicating with adults with severe learning difficulties, which resulted in concern among caregivers. Other concerns included lack of time to effectively care for this group of patients and no prior information concerning admission.

Summary

Ten studies were reviewed in this section: six investigated phenomena from patients' perspectives, three studied caregivers, and just one studied nurses. Four studies used quantitative designs; three, qualitative, and three, mixed. Five studies investigated dementia in persons with Down syndrome. Of that five, one focused on each of the following areas: interactions of people with a profound learning disability; decision-making experiences of adults with learning disabilities; key nursing interventions provided by intellectual disability nurses; the meaning of respite care to mothers of children with learning disabilities; and the experiences of caregivers and nurses regarding the hospitalization of adults with severe learning difficulties.

Maternal and Child

Thirty-one maternal and child studies are reviewed in this section relating to health behaviors of women, role of the midwife, third stage of labor, neonatal resuscitation, sudden infant death syndrome (SIDS), breastfeeding, and first-time mothers.

Lynch (1993), using questionnaires administered to 40 women and 40 midwives at antenatal clinics, explored awareness of the effects of alcohol on fetal development and perceptions of educational provision on the topic. The investigator found that 95% of pregnant women drank alcohol prior to pregnancy, and 65% drank after becoming pregnant. Just 5% understood the importance of abstaining from alcohol, and 25% perceived that midwives provided pertinent information. Preconceptual clinics were not used to any extent.

Hyde (1996, 1999a) investigated variations in contraceptive behavior among unmarried Irish women. The convenience sample comprising 51 women attending a prenatal hospital clinic was interviewed on two occasions. Behaviors ranged between fertility denial, destiny dependence, progressive occasional or intermittent risk-taking, calculated risk-taking, and contraceptive failure or misuse.

O'Connell and Cronin (2002), using a questionnaire completed by 15 domiciliary midwives, investigated midwifery practice in Ireland relating to women seeking home births and the outcome of home births from 1993 to 1997. Results show that 585 women planned to give birth in their homes with assistance from the midwife, and 500 women achieved this objective. Spontaneous delivery rate for women who commenced labor at home was 97%, and these women gave birth without medication or other interventions. Five hundred forty-four women breastfed their babies, and 538 continued to breastfeed at 6 weeks.

Hyde and Roche-Reid (2004), in interviews with 12 midwives, found that the midwives' role in facilitating women's choice through communicative action was impeded by the colonization of labor and childbirth by a "technocratic system of obstetrics." Lawler and Sinclair (2003) provided insight into the life of women who have lived through postnatal depression. A phenomenological approach with a purposeful sample of seven women revealed that all women experienced a loss of former self. They vividly described sorrow and brokenness and struggled to come to terms with their new image. In a phenomenological study of the experiences of student midwives, Begley (2003) interviewed on three occasions 31 volunteer midwifery students and analyzed diary recordings of 19 midwifery students regarding caring for women suffering a stillbirth, miscarriage, or neonatal death. Three themes emerged from the data: (1) "you don't know what to say," relating to the students' experiences of caring for bereaved couples; (2) "they wrapped him in a blanket," referring to care received; and (3) "crying like a fool," to describe their own feelings.

Third Stage of Labor

Begley (1990b) conducted a randomized controlled trial (RCT) of 1,429 women to compare active management of the third stage of labor (using intravenous Ergometrine 0.5 mg) with a method of physiological management in women at low risk of hemorrhage. The active management group had a higher incidence of manual removal of placenta; problems such as nausea, vomiting, and severe after birth pains; hypertension; and secondary postpartum hemorrhage. The incidence of postpartum and postnatal hemoglobins less than 10 gm/dl was higher in the physiological group. The routine use of Ergometrine during the third stage of labor in women with low risk of hemorrhage did not appear necessary and appeared to have adverse effects.

Subsequently, Begley (1993) investigated women's views of the third stage of labor. Two hundred women who delivered consecutively over a 2-month period (114 from the physiological group; no routine oxytoxin was given) and 86 from the active group (IV ergometrine 0.5 mg given immediately after delivery) participated. No differences were found in how long it took to deliver the placenta, degree of tiredness, amount of lochia, or after-birth pains. The degree of discomfort felt during the delivery showed differences in the "very uncomfortable" value for 9% in the active group and 3% in physiological group. Physiological management of the third stage, as practiced, did not appear to cause women any problems and did cause slightly less discomfort than active management.

Neonatal Resuscitation

Ryan, Clark, Malone, and Ahmed (1999) evaluated the introduction of the neonatal resuscitation program (NRP) into the delivery room of a maternity hospital. A prospective controlled observational study was conducted of 51 deliveries before and 51 deliveries following the training of delivery room staff in NRP. The sample comprised 33 nurse-midwives and 11 doctors. Improvements took place in delivery room preparation, the evaluation and management of the newborn infant, and thermal protection at birth. There was no significant difference in the use of endotracheal intubations, chest compression, chest complications, or medications. Fifteen of the 51 infants became hypothermic prior to the introduction of NRP, but none of the infants developed hypothermia in the post-NPR part of the study.

Sudden Infant Death Syndrome

Six studies have been conducted on SIDS, and the results from recent studies indicate changes over time in childcare practice. McGarvey, McDonnell, Chong, O'Regan, and Matthews (2003), in a 5-year population-based case control study, investigated risk factors associated with sleeping environments of Irish infants. A total of 203 SIDS cases and 622 control infants born 1994–1998 were studied. In a multivariate analysis, co-sleeping significantly increased the risk of SIDS, both as a usual practice and during the last sleep period. The associated risk was dependent on maternal smoking and was not significant for infants who were over 20 weeks of age or placed back in their own cot/bed to sleep. Matthews, McDonnell, McGarvey, Loftus, and O'Regan (2004), using the same data, investigated the influence of analytical design on the variability in a study. A maternal urinary tract infection during pregnancy remained a powerful and consistent risk factor. Risk also included social deprivation, maternal cigarette smoking and drinking during pregnancy, a slightly reduced birth weight, parental report of the baby being ill during the interval between birth and death, and in the last sleep period being placed prone to sleep or co-sleeping.

McDonnell, Mathews, McGarvey, Mehanni, and O'Regan (2002) employed a population-based case control study and demonstrated that cigarette smoke exposure increases the risk of SIDS in Irish infants almost fourfold and in a dose-dependent fashion. Mehanni, Kiberd, McDonnell, and O'Regan (1999) compared data from parents interviewed in 1994 ($n = 153$) and 1996 ($n = 132$) regarding sources of information for the prevention of SIDS and the extent of parental change in infant care practices as recommended. Results indicated that the media and public health nurses continued as main sources of information. A significant number of young (64%) and new (58%) parents were uninterested or unable to access relevant literature, indicating a gap in service provision. There was no significant difference in the percentage of parents who smoked or in the uptake of breast-feeding and the manner in which parents clothed children.

However, this contradicts findings from researchers exploring epidemiological factors associated with SIDS in Ireland (Matthews, Kiberd, Maha, Cullen, McDonnell, O'Regan, 2000). In this study, the researchers found a dramatic decrease in SIDS from 2.2/1,000 live births in the 1980s to 0.8/1,000 live births in the years 1993 to 1997.

A study by Sheehan, McDonnell, Doyle, Matthews, and Devaney (2003) evaluated the quality and value of infant postmortem reporting. Two hundred forty-five reports from 1994 to 1996 and 1998 to 2000 in Ireland were evaluated using the SIDS register. Quality of necropsies was below the minimum accepted standards, and those performed in regional centers were significantly higher than those performed elsewhere.

Breastfeeding

Clarke (1996) investigated whether there was a difference in breastfeeding rates within a 6-month period following a specific educational course. Retrospective quantitative review of the monthly initiation and discharge breastfeeding rates was taken from ward diaries. Results illustrated a positive difference in the breast-feeding rate before and after a breast-feeding program, with breast initiation rates up 4% and discharge breastfeeding rates up 8% (overall rates 48% to 56%).

Begley (1990a) investigated whether Ergometrine had an effect on the duration of breastfeeding in a randomised RCT. Three hundred thirty-six women randomly assigned to one of two groups (active management or physiological management) completed two questionnaires administered on the third postnatal day and at a 6-week visit. The incidence of women ceasing to breastfeed before the baby was 4 weeks of age was higher (38%) in the Ergometrine group then in the non-Ergometrine group (27%). Reasons given for stopping breastfeeding for 77% of Ergotamine group compared with 47% of the non-Ergometrine group was "hungry baby/insufficient milk," a difference that was highly significant. Overall, Ergometrine was associated with a negative effect on the establishment of breast-feeding.

First-Time Mothers

In a qualitative study, Cronin and McCarthy (2003) interviewed 13 young first-time mothers to identify needs, perception, and experiences in the postnatal period. Findings revealed that attendance at antenatal classes was variable and perceptions of being unprepared for birth and motherhood prevailed. Participants appeared shocked at the amount of pain experienced during birth and experienced little rest during hospitalization. Physical and emotional support and preparation for childcare was received from midwives; and breastfeeding, although promoted by midwives, was not acceptable due to socio-environmental factors. The maternal mother played a key role in providing direct childcare, advice, and emotional help to the young mother. Maternal depression, loneliness, living at home with limited space, and difficulty in "letting go" of baby to return to school were reported. Leahy Warren (2005), using a descriptive correlation design, explored the relationship between social support and confidence in infant care practices in 135 first-time mothers. Both appraisal and informational support showed a significant relationship with infant care practices. The primary sources of appraisal support were husbands/partners and maternal mothers.

Based on data collected through interviews with 51 unmarried pregnant women, Hyde (1997a) reported several factors surrounding experiences during pregnancy and in the first few weeks of motherhood. The differing responses of the respondents' fathers and mothers to their nonmarital pregnancy suggested opposing priorities with regard to the daughters' role within society. Mothers wanted their daughters to experience life beyond the traditional mothering role, and fathers were anxious that daughters would subscribe to the traditional woman's role. Participants perceived the public's perception of a pregnant woman's status as dependant on her age and male partnership status (Hyde, 2000a) and were surprised at the high level of positive public responses to their pregnancy, which is contrary to the widespread negative media image (Hyde, 2000b). However, the participant's nonmarital status was central when tension was apparent in social interactions. The manner in which knowledge of the pregnancy was managed within social interactions resembled the notion of "mutual pretense awareness" (i.e., both parties being aware of the pregnancy but failing to acknowledge it in their interactions) (Hyde, 1998 p. 636). Encounters between medical personnel and the unmarried pregnant women (Hyde, 1997b) illustrate how discussions focused on medical practitioners introducing the concept of adoption, respondents being pressured to see a social worker, and social arrangements for childcare and their capacity to parent questioned. For the mothers who returned to live in the family home after birth, the relationship between the new mother and her father had been reshaped to some extent, with the woman gaining more bargaining leverage (Hyde, 1999b). Hyde (2003) also explored gender relations between unpartnered mothers and the fathers of their children. Interestingly, women who were not supported by their partners believed that they had gained something, which they considered the child's father had lost.

Child

Collier (1993) investigated home accidents among children ages 0–9 years. Random sampling of children presenting in an Accident and Emergency department yielded 100 parents for inclusion, and 81 of these completed the questionnaire. Based on the findings, Collier suggested that males had a higher accident rate; most accidents occurred in children aged between 1 and 2 years of age, the child was either the first or second child in the family, falls were most prevalent, and the majority of accidents (72%) were classified as mild. Retrospectively, 49% of respondents recalled that they had received home safety advice but rarely attributed this to health professionals.

Hanafin (1998) examined school/nursing/medical examination records of 6,206 children to assess socio-demographic factors associated with reported nocturnal enuresis. Parents of children aged 4–14 years reported enuresis prevalence of 11%. Age, large family size, and low ordinal position in the family were statistically significantly associated with reported prevalence.

Hyde, Treacy, Whitaker, Abaunza, and Knox (2000) explored children's ($n = 78$) understanding and experiences of illegal drug use, smoking, and alcohol consumption as part of a larger, comparative, longitudinal study in the Republic of Ireland, Northern Ireland, and Spain through in-depth interviewing. Most participants were aware of at least two drug names, the use of illegal drugs in their environment, and negative side effects. Three male participants had smoked cannabis. As part of the same study, Hyde, Treacy, Boland, Whitaker, Abaunza, and Knox (2001) discussed the findings concerning alcohol consumption, which revealed a progression from covert unsanctioned consumption to overt unsanctioned consumption to overt sanctioned consumption to peer-unsanctioned consumption.

Savage and Callery (2005) explored 32 children and their parents' perspectives on dietary management of cystic fibrosis. Using a mixed methods ethnographic design, they found differences between parents' and children's perspectives in managing diet, a factor that health care professionals need to be aware of.

Summary

Thirty-one studies were reviewed in this section. Six related to generic topics such as effect of alcohol on fetal development, home birth, role of midwife, and contraceptive practices; two to the third stage of labor; one to neonatal resuscitation; two to breastfeeding, six to SIDS; nine to first-time mothers; and five to children. Topics again were diverse with investigators drawn from a variety of professional backgrounds.

MANAGEMENT AND PROFESSIONAL ISSUES

Management and professional issue studies were analysed in relation to perceptions of managerial functions, identification of managerial competencies, middle managers' involvement in developing strategy, nurses' expectations of the content and delivery of a nursing management degree, patient satisfaction with nursing care, and turnover in nursing and midwifery. Professional issues investigated included empowerment, image of Irish nursing, and the nurse's role.

Carney (1993) identified 39 important indicators of managerial skills and examined and compared the perceptions of two groups of Irish nurses, 3rd-year student nurses ($n = 50$) and RNs ($n = 50$), regarding the relative importance they assigned to these skills. Overall, both RNs and students scored creative decision-making, leadership skills, and organization of resources as not "critically necessary." However, management skills associated with actual nursing care (e.g., planning individual patient care, evaluation of care and recognizing changes in patients conditions) scored high. Overall, the researcher concluded that there appears to be little understanding of the managerial function among student and qualified nurses.

At the request of the national government, Rush, McCarthy and Cronin (2001) conducted a multisite study using multiple research methods to identify the competencies expected of top, middle, and frontline managers in nursing and expressed these in terms of behavioral (positive or negative) indicators. The researchers identified specific competencies at three levels: first-line manager, mid-level manager, and director of services.

Carney (2004a, 2004b), using semi-structured telephone interviews, investigated the level of involvement that middle manager heads of departments had in strategy development in acute hospitals and identified whether professional clinicians ($n = 13$) were more involved than nonclinician managers ($n = 12$). Carney found that nonclinician managers perceived themselves as more involved in strategy development than professional clinicians ($p < 0.05$). Professional clinicians perceived that their expertise was not recognized or appreciated by nonclinicians or by senior management ($p < 0.05$).

Joyce (2005), in an action research study using focus group interviews, questionnaires, document analyses, and a reflective diary, explored nurses' ($n = 117$) expectations of the content and delivery of a nursing management degree program and the program's ability to enable the students to meet leadership and management needs. Results indicated that nurses commencing the management degree program were unsure of their educational needs and might not know what they need to know in light of the many changes taking place in management.

McCarthy (1992) measured patient satisfaction with nursing care using an established scale among 133 patients in four wards. Results indicated high satisfaction, with little difference between wards. However, dissatisfaction was expressed in relation to continuation of care, conflicting advice between doctor and nurse, patient education from the nurse regarding treatments, and medication. Turnover of nurses and midwives became a national issue in Ireland in the late 1990s. McCarthy, Tyrrell, and Lehane (2003) estimated turnover rates among RNs and identified underlying reasons. Participants were drawn from 128 health care services and, of 3,243 mailed questionnaires, 1,921 were returned over a 1-year period, for a 59.2% response rate. Telephone interviews were also conducted with 140 participants from the original sample. The mean turnover rate was 12%, with considerable variation across sites. Reasons for leaving included the following: to pursue other employment in nursing (35%), to travel abroad (21%), and a desire to undertake further study (12%). It appeared that a considerable number of nurses could have been retained if retention strategies focusing on promotion of greater autonomy, professional development, managerial support, or improved professional practice environment had been introduced.

Professional Issues

Scott, Matthews, and Corbally (2003) explored the meaning of empowerment from the perspective of nurses and midwives and identified the factors that enhanced or inhibited empowerment. Using focus groups and a national survey, the researchers found a moderately empowered work force. Factors perceived to enhance empowerment included education, skills, and self-confidence. Factors considered to inhibit empowerment were poor management styles, lack of education, and lack of both recognition and support from management.

Timmins and McCabe (2005) surveyed the assertive behaviors of nurses and midwives ($n = 391$) and explored barriers and facilitators to the use of assertive skills in the workplace. Assertive behaviors were used more frequently with colleagues than with management or medical personnel. Responsibility to patients emerged as a supporting factor, and managers and work atmosphere viewed as obstacles. Clarke and O'Neill (2001), in an analysis of how the *Irish Times* portrayed Irish nursing during the 1999 nurses strike, examined articles, comments, and letters to the editor of one newspaper during the industrial action. The researchers found that the technical skills of caring appeared to be valued at the expense of comfort and compassionate care.

In a documentary analysis of primary source materials from 1920 to 1980, Fealy (2004) found that the Irish public discourse for most of the 20th century was laudatory with respect to nursing, and the good nurse was depicted as nurse-as-woman, good Catholic nurse, good practical nurse, and good Irish nurse. The image changed over time with respect to the role of the nurse.

Rose (1997), through survey, determined the number of staff (nursing staff $n = 27$; attendants $n = 9$) members who suffered physical or verbal abuse, and the frequency of abuse sustained, while on duty in one Irish accident and emergency department. The investigator found that 60% of the respondents had experienced physical violence, and 91% feared that they might be physically abused at work. Many incidents went unreported and sick leave following abusive encounters was reported in 27% of cases.

Flynn and Sinclair (2005), using a case study, explored the relationship between nursing protocols and nursing practice. Interview data from 17 nurses indicated that nurses adapt clinical protocols as they see fit, demonstrating the importance placed on personal autonomy and judgment.

Role

Larkin (1998) explored the experiences of palliative care nurses through in-depth bilingual interviews. Using Irish poetry with 16 RNs, five expressions of unique commonality, which encapsulated the essence of being an Irish palliative care nurse, were derived: Dluchaidreamh (closeness), Anam chara (soul-friend), Gramhar (loving), Aire (Caring), and Spioraid (spirit).

In another qualitative study, O'Meara Kearney (1999) used focus group interviews with 16 nurses to develop a conceptual description of how they perceived the role of the nurse. Three themes emerged from the data. These were developing interactive-supportive relationships, knowledgeable caregivers, and pulling everything together.

In a grounded theory study, O'Flynn, Caffrey, and Higgins (2003) used unstructured interviews to explore therapists' ($n = 12$) experience of working with a policy that required them to report risk to children based on information received from adult clients who have been sexually abused as children. Therapists' considered working with the policy to be a highly complex, dynamic, and emotional process. Kavanagh and McBride (2003) evaluated the service provided by the accident and emergency (A&E) liaison nurse in one hospital using a survey that was completed by 45 A&E staff and 60 general practitioners (GPs). The researchers found that GPs and A&E staff frequently utilized the liaison service, which they perceived to improve internal and external communications (95%), and the continuity (91%) and quality (86%) of patient care.

McCabe (2004) explored nurse-patient communication using a sample of eight inpatients in a hermeneutic phenomenological study. McCabe found that nurses communicate well with patients when using a patient-centered approach. Hanafin and Cowley (2003) surveyed the public health nursing service in Ireland and respondents' ($n = 615$) perceptions of the quality of service provided. The investigators found that public health nurses (PHNs) working with families with infants communicated with a number of other professionals, but the PHNs could not always directly refer clients. Substantial variations occurred in the amount of feedback PHNs received from other professionals.

Using a triangulation approach, Begley, Brady, Byrne, MacGregor, Griffiths, and Horan (2004) investigated the role and workload of PHNs and tested a workload/caseload tool specific to community nursing. The research team found that the role of the PHN was diverse and intense. Concerns related to role ambiguity consequential of ongoing development of community services, hierarchical management structures, and work overload emerged. Brady Nevin (2005) investigated Irish endoscopy nurses' ($n = 70$) perceptions of advancing their practice to include endoscopic procedures and to highlight perceived barriers to the implementation of advanced practice. Irish endoscopy nurses positively perceived the advancement of their practice and identified lack of adequate preparation and support, risk of litigation, and fragmented roles as barriers to the role of advanced nurse practitioner in endoscopy. Dowling (2000) explored the perceptions of the clinical nurse specialist role using interviews and a short rating scale on a stratified random sample of 15 general nurses and five ward sisters. Consultant and research roles were ranked low, yet specialists were deemed the best qualified to educate patients, and nurses were contacted to visit patients when RNs did not have the time.

The National Council for the Professional Development of Nursing and Midwifery (NCNM) is responsible for career path progression in nursing and midwifery in Ireland. In (2004) the Council evaluated the effectiveness of the role of the clinical nurse/midwife specialist. It found that the role exists on a developmental continuum. Although clinical aspects were found to be well developed and respected, educational and audit aspects of the role required further development. Concerns related to role preparation, inadequate resources, and role ambiguity were articulated. Richmond (2004), using a qualitative methodology, investigated general nurses' view of the role of the clinical nurse specialist in a regional hospital and compared results with the core concepts identified by the NCNM. Overall, four core concepts nominated by the NCNM (clinical focus, patient advocate, education/training, consultancy) were identified. The core concept of audit was not included.

Wilkin and Slevin (2004), using a descriptive, qualitative approach, explored the meaning of caring to ICU nurses ($n = 12$). Caring was synonymous with nursing and was identified as a process of competent physical and technical action imbued with affective skills. Based on preliminary content analysis of primary-source historical documentation, Meehan (2003) proposed a careful nursing model, with key concepts identified as disinterested love, contagious calmness, creation of a restorative environment, skill in fostering safety and comfort, nursing interventions, participatory-authorities management, trustworthy collaboration, and nurses caring for themselves. Surlis and Hyde (2001) investigated HIV patients' experience of stigma during hospitalisation and nursing care. A volunteer sample of 10 former inpatients of hospitals participated in interviews. Using Goffman's conceptualization of stigma, results suggested that some patients experienced stigma from nurses, and such stigma was stratified according to the means by which the disease had been contacted, with drug users expressing the greatest experience of stigma.

A number of studies focused on health promotion. For example, Hope, Kelleher, and O'Connor (1998) conducted a cross-sectional survey of lifestyle practices and the health-promoting environment of qualified and student nurses ($n = 729$). The investigator found that student nurses consumed more alcohol, had a higher incidence of smoking, and tried illicit drugs more often than staff nurses, while a greater number of qualified nurses experienced higher workplace stress levels. Treacy and Collins (1999) investigated randomly selected hospital nurses' ($n = 47$) understandings of health promotion and perceptions of health-promoting practice using a grounded theory design. They found that the concept of health promotion lacked clarity and shared understanding. Although health promotion was perceived to be secondary to other aspects of care, several health-promoting activities were considered a routine part of their role.

Summary

In this review, six studies related to management and 22 to professional issues were reviewed. Topics were disparate, and it appears that management issues have received little attention. Sixteen studies focused on different aspects of the nurses' role, as perceived mostly by nurses, with just two studies including patients in their sample.

RESEARCH ON NURSE EDUCATION

Thirty-seven studies were reviewed in this section, with seven relating to post-graduate education and 30 to undergraduate nurse education. Six studies utilized a mixed-method approach; 17, a quantitative approach; and 14, a qualitative approach. Twenty-one studies used surveys, and two used a case-study design. Sampling could have been described in greater detail in most of the studies, with only six studies utilizing probability sampling.

Postgraduate Nurse Education

The NCNM (2004) reported on the continuing professional development of nurses and midwives. The focus groups ($n = 34$) and subsequent questionnaires ($n = 2,005$) concentrated on the concept of competence, its achievement and maintenance, and the career choices available to nurses and midwives. Ratings of competence by respondents showed 40% assessed themselves as proficient; 14%, as expert; and 1%, as novice professionals. Recommendations that emerged focused on the achievement of five objectives, which included the development of a wide range of education activities for nurses and midwives. In another survey ($n = 136$), McCarthy and Evans (2003) reaffirmed the need for continuing education for nurses and midwives, with the requirement for more time allocated by the employer for course attendance and study. Delamere (2002), in a descriptive survey with a purposeful sample of 68 nurses, demonstrated that a postregistration course could have positive effects on nursing practice. In a small action research study (Elliott & Higgins, 2005), the development and evaluation of a self- and peer-assessment strategy designed to promote postgraduate student ($n = 20$) participation in group projects was investigated. Students ($n = 14$) found the strategy was effective in ensuring fairness and equity in the grading of projects. Clarke and Graham (1996) examined, by interview, the use of reflection and reflective diaries by RNs ($n = 7$) as part of a short course. Participants derived personal and professional benefit from the process. One Irish descriptive survey focused on postregistration nursing students ($n = 120$) experience and attitudes toward computers (Curtis, Hicks, & Redmond, 2002). Overall, the students felt that more encouragement and training were required to assist in computer use. The experience of distance education programs by nurses ($n = 15$) was the subject of a qualitative study conducted by Hyde and Murray (2005). The researchers found that the experience was positive for students.

Undergraduate Nurse Education

Cowman (1995, 1996, 1998) investigated the differences in learning strategies used and course experience of the total student nurse population in 1991 in Northern Ireland and the Republic of Ireland ($n = 1,122$). Significant differences were observed between students' teaching and learning preferences in the different branches of nursing (general, psychiatric, and intellectual disabilities). Generally, students preferred teacher-structured strategies (Cowman, 1995). Clarke, Gobbi, and Simmons (1999) conducted an evaluation case study of the first pilot registration/diploma nursing program introduced in Ireland. Eight major methods were employed in the case study for collection of data. The researchers demonstrated differences of opinion concerning the nature, purpose, and scheduling of tuition in the biological and social sciences. Difficulties existed with the An Bord Altranais (Irish Nursing Board) method of assessment of clinical nursing skills; and students reported that practice was the main catalyst for their learning, and clinical placement coordinators made a large contribution to student learning.

McCarthy and Cronin (2000), utilizing a quantitative cross-sectional design, administered a researcher-constructed questionnaire to 727 diploma student nurses (response rate 75%). The study investigated the characteristics of the total 1998 cohort of student nurses and compared the results to a similar 1988 study. The majority of students' families supported nursing as a career choice, reinforcing the notion that the choice of nursing as a career was held in high regard. The most notable changes over the 10 years were the increase in male applicants for nursing and the older profile of student nurses.

Drennan (1999), utilizing a descriptive survey design, evaluated the theoretical component of the first year of the diploma in nursing program in two schools of nursing and their partnered institutes of higher education. Drennan suggested that the program was overassessed and students reported difficulties, particularly in relation to the biological science component of the course. McKee (2002), utilizing a quantitative descriptive correlational design, addressed the question of difficulty with the bioscience component. Study skills, attendance, and lack of previous theoretical biological sciences were found to have contributed significantly to the examination results in biological science.

Tyrell (1997) studied first- and third-year certificate student nurses' ($n = 76$) knowledge and attitudes toward assessment of acute pain using a researcher-developed questionnaire. The majority of the students felt they lacked knowledge and confidence in this area. Tuohy (2002) used an ethnographic approach with eight students to understand how students communicate with older people. Recommendations made for facilitating improvement in student nurse-older patient communication included a more person-centred approach to patient care, increased education on interpersonal skills, a need for preceptors to facilitate student learning in the area of communication, and increased facilitation of reflective practice.

Using a descriptive, exploratory survey design, Nicholl and Higgins (2004) reported on how a group of nurse teachers perceived and interpreted reflective practice in preregistration nursing curricula in all the schools of nursing involved in the diploma in nursing ($n = 40$), with a response rate of 50%. Results indicated a variation in hours assigned to reflection within the curriculum and the positioning of reflection within the curricula. O'Connor, Hyde, and Treacy (2003), based on interview data collected from 11 nurse teachers, noted that nurse teachers felt that reflection was a way of learning from experiences; however, it was noted that reflective practice was compartmentalized within preregistration nursing curricula.

Evans and Kelly (2004) utilized a descriptive survey design to examine the stress experience and coping abilities of a convenience sample of 52 diploma student nurses. Key stressors were identified as examinations, level and intensity of academic workload, the theory-practice gap, and poor relationships with clinical staff. Timmins and Kaliszer (2002b), using a survey design, explored the attitudes of those involved in nurse education ($n = 57$) to absenteeism among diploma student nurses. The researchers found that the majority of nurse educators agree that student nurse attendance at both the clinical and theoretical aspects of the program is a problem, and nurse educators recommend the monitoring of attendance during lectures. Retrospective analysis of student attendance records ($n = 70$) showed a time-lost index of 4% (Timmins & Kaliszer, 2002a). A survey of the students ($n = 110$) revealed that academic commitments, financial constraints, relationship with clinical and education staff, finances, and the death of a patient

(Timmins & Kaliszer, 2002c, 2002d) influenced absenteeism. The authors recommended accurate monitoring and the use of appropriate preventive strategies to reduce absenteeism (Timmins & Kaliszer, 2002d).

A descriptive, quantitative, comparative survey design was conducted to measure perceived levels of assertiveness and students' reported self esteem (Begley & White, 2003; Begley & Glackin, 2004). In general, students' ($n = 72$) reported level of assertiveness and self esteem rose as they approached completion of the 3-year program. Students' self-esteem could be increased by the use of frequent positive feedback and by improving job satisfaction.

Using a grounded theory approach, Brown (1993) investigated student and teacher perceptions of power distribution in their relationship. Results indicated that power operated in three planes with differing emphasis. In a descriptive survey design, students who participated in a university-welcoming program tailored to the needs of mature students demonstrated significantly stronger theoretical progression than those who had not (Fleming & McKee, 2005).

Landers (2001), in a qualitative, descriptive study, ascertained 10 first-year certificate students' views on the link between theory and clinical practice. The research highlighted the need for nurse tutors to support student nurses on clinical placements and, where possible, reconciliation between the divergences of what is taught and practiced. Fealy (1999), utilizing an interpretative phenomenological approach, interviewed six registered general nurses in an exploration of the discourse on the theory-practice relationship. All conceptualized the theory practice relationship using the "applied science" approach, and five of the six articulated the "practical" approach. The appropriateness of the clinical learning environment has been the focus of many Irish studies. Savage (1998, 1999) reported on first-, second-, and third-year student nurses' views on the influence of staff nurses in creating a ward-learning environment. Findings demonstrated that less than half of the respondents reported favorable ward-learning environments. Landers (1996) appraised 25 student nurses' experiences in theatre placement. Students' stress associated with their theatre placement was due to the alien environment, the isolation of the theatre department, and their lack of knowledge about theatre.

Efforts to facilitate learning in clinical practice are diverse, but one of the main factors that assists students with learning is their supernumerary (i.e., surplus to the rostered compliment) status as diploma students. Joyce (1999) utilized an action research approach, employing phenomenological methods to develop a framework for implementing supernumerary learning in a diploma in nursing program in an Irish hospital. The framework developed incorporates the notion of differing levels of skill (Steinaker & Bell, 1979, experiential taxonomy), knowledge, and attitude acquisition over time with the corresponding role of the supervisor. Joyce's (1999) recommendations included the need for longitudinal studies with larger sample sizes, possibly utilizing the framework developed to move the action research process into the final phase of implementation, observation and reflection on the experience of using such a framework to support supernumerary learning. O'Callaghan and Slevin (2003) investigated the experiences of 10 RNs facilitating supernumerary nursing students. RNs appeared to have differing interpretations of the term supernumerary status, varying from students being perceived as an extra help to being in a pure observational role. Hyde and Brady (2002) and Brady and Hyde (2002) explored 16 staff RNs' attitudes and perceptions of their role in facilitating learning for student nurses in clinical areas. The researchers found that RNs felt that supernumerary students were overly focused on theory, and the student's role was misconstrued as being solely observational and not as a team member.

The Clinical Placement Coordinator (CPC) role in the support of student nurses nationally was studied using random cluster sampling and mixed methods approach (Dreenan, 2002). Core elements of the CPC role were identified as student support and practice development. First- and third-year student nurses' perceptions of the clinical learning environment were researched by Condell, Eliott, and Nolan (2001). The survey showed that students favored active participation within the clinical setting as the best method of learning. Morgan and Collins (2002), using a phenomenological approach, found that during a first clinical placement, students learned a variety of clinical skills from ward sisters, staff nurses, clinical placement coordinators and other students. The staff nurse was identified as the key person involved in teaching students clinical skills in practice. The attitudes of RNs to students on clinical practice placements have been found to affect students' learning (Morgan 2002, 2004). Kelly (2002) examined the experience of qualified nurses in assessing student's clinical skills using a constructivist approach. The researchers demonstrated that nurses believed that clinical staff have an important role to play in clinical assessment of students, but they need appropriate support from managerial and educational staff to fulfil this role.

The views of 10 nurse managers toward diploma student nurses during their first clinical placement were ascertained using a grounded theory approach (Begley & Brady, 2002). In general, managers felt that there was adequate preparation of staff nurses and students for the first clinical placement, and students demonstrated interest and ample ability. Higgins and McCarthy (2005) explored six psychiatric student nurses' experiences of mentorship during their first practice placement. Students generally viewed mentorship in a positive light.

Begley conducted a comprehensive longitudinal study of midwifery training using triangulation methods (1999b). Information was gathered from 125 student midwives using a variety of approaches. Students inevitably had good days and bad days. Good days were associated with giving nursing care to women and ensuring job satisfaction, and bad days were linked with staff relationships (Begley, 1998). Begley (2001b, 2001c) stated that the perceived gap between qualified nursing staff and students was due to a number of factors: previous learning not being acknowledged, an unwelcoming atmosphere, the perceived rudeness of some staff, and difficult interpersonal relationships. However, the students still appreciated the midwife for expertise shown (Begley, 2001a). Begley (2002) described the hierarchical nature of midwifery nursing practice, which may be due to the dominance of females within the profession and the tendency of hospitals to employ their own graduates. Student midwives articulated the view that their educational needs were often denied, as they were given little clinical training or guidance—their status being akin to that of a junior employee (Begley, 1999a, 1999c). Begley (1999d) recommended that student midwives receive more support in the clinical environment and that the duration of theoretical input for student midwives be increased, which has been achieved by increasing the number of theoretical weeks (Government of Ireland, 1998).

Summary

Thirty-seven studies (54 publications) in the area of nurse education were reviewed, seven in the area of postgraduate education and 30 in undergraduate nurse education. Eight of the undergraduate studies examined theoretical matters, two investigated the theory practice gap, thirteen focused on the facilitation of learning in the clinical environment, and seven related to student profile/characteristics and student issues. What is notable about research in the area of nurse education is the disparity of the research topics and the lack of cohesiveness in research in this area. The paucity of research in the area of postgraduate nurse education is striking, and this needs to be addressed as a matter of urgency. There is also a notable lack of research, which looks at the short- and long-term outcomes/benefits of both undergraduate and postgraduate education.

CONCLUSION

The review presented in this chapter is representative of the endeavors made by nurses and midwives in Ireland to establish a research base. Over the past 15 years, nurses have conducted research alone ($n = 124$) or in collaboration with other health care professionals ($n = 26$). The 150 studies reviewed were drawn from 60 journals, 4 books, and 8 research reports. Research has focused primarily on clinical issues (56%). Other major foci have been education (25%) and management (19%). Studies used quantitative (50%), qualitative (39%), or mixed approaches (11%). The method of sampling used was predominantly convenience. Both descriptive (38%) and inferential statistics (62%) were used, and most research lacked an underpinning theoretical framework.

It is apparent that considerable research has been conducted, particularly in the past five years. It is evident also from the review that research endeavors have been disparate and that efforts need to be concentrated on specific topics. To focus minds, two major studies on research priorities have been commissioned and recently completed. Research priorities have been developed for the Southern Region of Ireland (McCarthy, Savage, & Lehane, 2005). Based on focus groups and a questionnaire completed by 474 nurses, results identified research priorities to be the effect of staff shortages on retention of RNs/registered midwives, quality of life of chronically ill patients, stress and bullying in the workplace, assessment and management of pain, skill mix and staff burnout, cardiopulmonary resuscitation decision making, coordination of care between hospital and primary care settings, medication errors, and promoting healthy lifestyles. Respondents also indicated that these priorities warranted immediate attention. A national study has also reported similar results (Meehan, Butler, Drennan, Johnson, Kemple, & Treacy, 2006). A three-round decision Delphi survey ($n = 780$ nurses and 142 midwives) was followed by group workshops that identified key short-term priorities as care delivery outcomes, recruitment and retention of nurses, communication in clinical practice and nursing input into health policy and decision making, preparation of midwives for practice, promotion of women-centered and evidence-based midwifery care, and promotion of the distinctiveness of midwifery.

A number of Irish journals publishing research papers have been launched over the years, but unfortunately, many have ceased to exist. These include *Nursing Review* (1981–2000); *The All Ireland Journal of Nursing and Midwifery* (2000–2003), and *The Irish Nursing Forum and Health Services* (1986–2001). The following are still published: *World of Irish Nursing* (1972–), *Irish Nurse* (1998–), *The Irish Practice Nurse* (1999–), and *Irish Journal of Anaesthetic and Recovery Nursing* (2003–).

After conducting this review, we conclude that although significant progress has been made over time, research endeavors have been disparate. The challenge now is to concentrate research in specific areas, capitalize and build on research conducted to date, and ensure that practice is evidence based. These challenges should be met through recent change to an all-graduate profession, increasing career opportunities that incorporate research and the establishment of strengthened managerial roles for nurse and midwives.

REFERENCES

Begley, C. M. (1990a). The effect of ergometrine on breast feeding. *Midwifery*, 6(2), 60–72.

Begley, C. M. (1990b). A comparison of "active" and "physiological" management of the third stage of labour. *Midwifery*, 6(1), 3–17.

Begley, C. M. (1993). Women's views of the third stage of labour. *Nursing Review*, 12(1) 14–17.

Begley, C. M. (1998). Student midwives' experiences in the first three months of their training "good days and bad days." *Nursing Review*, 16(3/4), 77–81.

Begley, C. M. (1999a). Student midwives' views of their working role during midwifery training "thrown in at the deep end." *Nursing Review, 17*(3), 76–81.

Begley, C. M. (1999b). A study of student midwives' experiences during their two-year education programmed. *Midwifery, 15,* 194–202.

Begley, C. M. (1999c). Student midwives' views of "learning to be a midwife" in Ireland. *Midwifery, 15,* 264–273.

Begley, C. M. (1999d). Student midwives' experiences during their training programme. In M. Treacy, & A. Hyde (Eds.), *Nursing Research Design and Practice.* Dublin: University College Dublin Press.

Begley, C. M. (2001a). Student midwives views of student/staff relationships in the first 3 months of clinical practice: "They all have their moments." *All Ireland Journal of Nursing and Midwifery, 1*(4), 128–134.

Begley, C. M. (2001b). "Giving Midwifery care": Student midwives' views of their working role. *Midwifery, 17,* 24–34.

Begley, C. M. (2001c). "Knowing your place": Student midwives' views of relationships in midwifery in Ireland. *Midwifery, 17,* 222–233.

Begley, C. M. (2002). "Great fleas have little fleas": Irish student midwives' views of the hierarchy in midwifery. *Journal of Advanced Nursing, 38*(3), 310–317.

Begley, C. M. (2003). "I cried" I had to: Student midwives' experiences of still birth, miscarriage and neonatal death. *Evidence Based Midwifery, 1*(1), 20–26.

Begley, C. M., & Brady, A. (2002). Irish Diploma in Nursing student's first clinical allocation: The views of nurse managers. *Journal of Nurse Management, 10,* 339–347.

Begley, C. M., Brady, A. M., Byrne, G., MacGregor, C., Griffiths, C., & Horan, P. (2004). *A study of the role and workload of the Public Health Nurse in the Galway community area.* University of Dublin, Trinity College: School of Nursing and Midwifery.

Begley, C. M., & Glacken, M. (2004). Irish nursing students' changing levels of assertiveness during their preregistration programmed. *Nurse Education Today, 24,* 501–510.

Begley, C. M., & White, P. (2003). Irish nursing students' changing self–esteem and fear of negative evaluation during their pre-registration programmed. *Journal of Advanced Nursing, 42*(4), 390–401.

Brady, D., & Hyde, A. (2002). Certificate-trained staff nurses' perceptions of the changes in nursing education in Ireland from certificate to diploma level. *Journal of Continuing Education in Nursing, 33*(5), 231–237.

Brady Nevin, C. (2005). Mini Doctors or advanced nurse practitioners? Irish endoscopy nurses' perceptions regarding the development of advanced practice in endoscopy. *Gastroenterology Nursing, 28*(4), 1–7.

Brown, G. (1993). Accounting for power: Nurse teachers' and students' perceptions of power in their relationship. *Nurse Education Today, 13,* 111–120.

Carney, M. (1993). Management skills the nurses' perception. *Nursing Review, 11*(3/4), 4–8.

Carney, M. (2004a). Middle manager involvement in strategy development in non-profit organizations: The director of nursing perspective—how organizational structure impacts on the role. *Journal of Nursing Management, 12*(1), 13–21.

Carney, M. (2004b). Perceptions of professional clinicians and non-clinicians on their involvement in strategic planning in health care management; Implications for interdisciplinary involvement. *Nursing and Health Sciences, 6,* 321–328.

Clancy, M., Taylor, M., & O'Sullivan, K. (2002). Prospective short-term study on the prediction of aggressive behaviour: Validation of a screening checklist. *The All Ireland Journal of Nursing and Midwifery, 2*(3), 36–40.

Clarke, A. (2002). The influence of documentation format on diabetes nurse specialists' knowledge of the purpose and utility of documentation and their attitude to documentation. *The All Ireland Journal of Nursing and Midwifery, 2*(6), 41–47.

Clarke, D., & Graham, M. (1996). Reflective practice the use of reflective diaries by experienced registered nurses. *Nursing Review, 15*(1), 26–29.

Clarke, J., Gobbi, M., & Simons, H. (1999). Evaluation case study of the registration/diploma nursing programmed. In M. Treacy, & A. Hyde (Eds.), *Nursing Research Design and Practice*. Dublin: University College Dublin Press.

Clarke, J., & O'Neill, C. S. (2001). An analysis of how The Irish Times portrayed Irish nursing during the 1999 strike. *Nursing Ethics, 8*(4), 350–359.

Clarke, N. (1996). Breastfeeding: a co-ordinated approach. *Nursing Review, 15*(1), 22–25.

Coffey, A. (2004). Perceptions of training for care attendants employed in the care of older people. *Journal of Nursing Management, 12*, 322–328.

Collier, N. (1993). A study of home accidents involving young children 0–9 years in the settled community in community care area eight, Eastern Health Board. *Nursing Review, 12*(1), 25–30.

Condell, S., Elliott, N., & Nolan, L. (2001). Perceptions of the clinical learning environment: A supernumerary student survey. *All Ireland Journal of Nursing and Midwifey, 1*(4), 148–151.

Cosgrave, M. P., McCarron, M., Anderson, M., Tyrrell, J., Gill, M., & Lawlor, B. A. (1998). Cognitive decline in Down syndrome: A validity/reliability study of the Test for Severe Impairment. *American Journal on Mental Retardation, 103*(2), 193–197.

Cosgrave, M. P., Tyrrell, J., McCarron, M., Gill, M., & Lawlor, B. A. (1999a). Age at onset of dementia and age of menopause in women with Down's syndrome. *Journal of Intellectual Disability Research, 43*(6), 461–465.

Cosgrave, M. P., Tyrrell, J., McCarron, M., Gill, M., & Lawlor, B. A. (1999b). Determinants of aggression, and adaptive and maladaptive behavior in older people with Down's syndrome with and without dementia. *Journal of Intellectual Disability Research, 43*(5), 393–399.

Cosgrave, M. P., Tyrrell, J., McCarron, M., Gill, M., & Lawlor, B. A. (2000). A five year follow up study of dementia in persons with Down's syndrome: Early symptoms and patterns of deterioration. *Irish Journal of Psychological Medicine, 17*(1), 5–11.

Courell, D. (1997). The hospitalization of people with severe learning difficulties . . . the experience of carers and nursing staff. *Nursing Review, 16*(1), 21–23.

Cowman, S. (1995). The teaching/learning preferences of student nurses in the Republic of Ireland: Background issues and a study. *International Journal of Nursing Studies, 32*(2), 126–136.

Cowman, S. (1996). Student evaluation: A performance indicator of quality in nurse education. *Journal of Advanced Nursing, 24*, 625–632.

Cowman, S. (1998). The approaches to learning of student nurses in the Republic of Ireland and Northern Ireland. *Journal of Advanced Nursing, 28*(4), 899–910.

Cowman, S., Farrelly, M., & Gilheany, P. (2001). An examination of the role and function of psychiatric nurses in clinical practice in Ireland. *Journal of Advanced Nursing, 34*(6), 745–753.

Cowman, S., & Walsh, J. (2004). Focus safety and security procedures in psychiatric acute admission wards. *Nursing Times Research, 9*(3), 185–193.

Cramer, E., Cunney, R. J., Humphreys, H., & Smyth, E. G. (2002). Sixteen years surveillance of surgical sites in an Irish hospital. *Infection Control and Hospital Epidemiology, 23*(1), 36–40.

Cramer, E., McCarthy, G., Tighe, I., & Smyth, E. (2002). A survey of nurses' assessment of peripheral intravenous catheters. *British Journal of Nursing, 11*(15), 999–1006.

Creamer, E. (2000). Examining the care of patients with peripheral venous cannulas. *British Journal of Nursing, 9*(20), 2128–2144.

Creedon, S. (2005). Health care worker's hand decontamination practices: Compliance with recommended guidelines. *Journal of Advanced Nursing, 51*(3), 208–216.

Cronin, C., & McCarthy, G. (2003). First time mothers—identifying their needs, perceptions and experiences. *Journal of Clinical Nursing, 12,* 260–267.

Curtis, E., Hicks, P., & Redmond, R. (2002). Peer reviewed research page, nursing students experiences and attitudes to computers: A survey of a cohort of students on a bachelor in nursing studies course. *Information Technology in Nursing, 14*(2), 7–17.

Cusack, E. (1994). "Is community best? Why not ask the patient?" *Nursing Review, 13*(1), 22–27.

Deady, R. (2005). A phenomenological study of attitudes, values and beliefs of Irish trained psychiatric nurses. *Psychiatric Nursing, 3*(1), 9–12.

Delamere, S. (2002). HIV/AIDS post-registration education: An evaluation of the impact on nursing practice. A descriptive study. *The All Ireland Journal of Nursing and Midwifery, 2*(7), 46–50.

Department of Health and Children (2001). *Making knowledge work for health: A strategy for health research.* Dublin: Government Publications.

Department of Health and Children (2003). *A research strategy for nursing and midwifery in Ireland.* Dublin: Government Publications.

Dowling, M. (2000). Nurses' perceptions of the clinical nurse specialist (CNS) role. *Nursing Review, 17*(4), 96–99.

Drennan, J. (1999). Diploma in nursing studies: An evaluation of the first year curriculum. *Nursing Review, 17*(3), 64–70.

Drennan, J. (2002). An evaluation of the role of the Clinical Placement Coordinator in student nurse support in the clinical area. *Journal of Advanced Nursing, 40*(4), 475–483.

Elliott, N., & Higgins, A. (2005). Self and peer assessment—does it make a difference to student group work? *Nurse Education in Practice, 5,* 40–48.

Evans, W., & Kelly, B. (2004). Pre-registration diploma student nurse stress and coping measures. *Nurse Education Today, 24*(6), 473–482.

Farrelly, M. (1999). Patients' experiences of in-patient mental health care. In M. Treacy, & A. Hyde (Eds.), *Nursing Research Design and Practice.* Dublin: University College Dublin Press.

Fealy, G. (1999). The theory-practice relationship in nursing: The practitioners' perspective. *Journal of Advanced Nursing, 30*(1), 74–82.

Fealy, G. (2004). "The good nurse": Visions and values in images of the nurse. *Journal of Advanced Nursing, 46*(6), 649–656.

Fleming, S., & McKee, G. (2005). The mature student question. *Nurse Education Today, 25*, 230–237.

Flynn, A., & Sinclair, M. (2005). Exploring the relationship between nursing protocols and nursing practice in an Irish intensive care unit. *International Journal of Nursing Practice, 11*, 142–149.

Gijbels, H. (1995). Mental health nursing skills in an acute admission environment: Perceptions of mental health nurses and other mental health professionals. *Journal of Advanced Nursing, 21*, 460–465.

Glacken, M., Coates, V., Kernohan, G., & Hegarty, J. (2003). The experience of fatigue for people living with hepatitis C. *Journal of Clinical Nursing, 12*, 244–252.

Griffiths, C., & Cowman, S. (1999). Towards understanding the interactions of people with a profound learning disability: A pilot study. *Nursing Review, 17*(1/2), 35–39.

Government of Ireland (1998). *Report on the Commission on Nursing. A Blueprint for the Future*. Dublin: The Stationary Office.

Hanafin, S. (1998). Sociodemographic factors associated with nocturnal enuresis. *British Journal of Nursing, 7*(7), 403–408.

Hanafin, S., & Cowley, S. (2003). Multidisciplinary communication in the Irish Public Health Nursing Service: A study. *British Journal of Community Nursing, 8*(12), 544–549.

Hartrey, L., & Wells, J. S. G. (2003). The meaning of respite care to mothers of children with learning disabilities: Two Irish case studies. *Journal of Psychiatric and Mental Health Nursing, 10*, 335–342.

Healy, M. (2001). Can surface treated central venous catheters provide benefits for both patients and hospital staff. *All Ireland Journal of Nursing and Midwifery, 1*(4), 153–156.

Higgins, A., & McCarthy, M. (2005). Psychiatric nursing student's experiences of having a mentor during their first practice placement: An Irish perspective. *Nurse Education in Practice, 5*(4), 218–224.

Hope, A., Kelleher, C. C., & O'Connor, M. (1998). Lifestyle practices and the health promoting environment of hospital nurses. *Journal of Advanced Nursing, 28*(2), 438–447.

Hughes, M. (2000). An instrument to assist nurses identify patients' self perceived informational needs post myocardial infarction. *All Ireland Journal of Nursing and Midwifery, 1*(1), 13–17.

Hyde, A. (1996). Unmarried pregnant women's accounts of their contraceptive practice. A qualitative analysis. *Irish Journal of Sociology, 6*, 179–211.

Hyde, A. (1997a). Gender differences in the response of parents to their daughter's nonmarital pregnancy. In A. Byrne, & M. Leonard (Eds.), *Women and Irish society: A sociological reader*. Belfast: Beyond the Pale Publications.

Hyde, A. (1997b). The medicalisation of childbearing norms: Encounters between unmarried pregnant women and medical personal in an Irish context. In A. Cleary, & M. P. Treacy (Eds.), *The sociology of health and illness in Ireland*. Dublin: University College Dublin Press.

Hyde, A. (1998). From mutual pretence awareness to open awareness. Single pregnant women's public encounters in an Irish contest. *Qualitative Health Research, 8*(5), 634–643.

Hyde, A. (1999a). Variations in contraceptive behaviour among unmarried Irish women. In, L. F. Heber, & T. George (Eds.), *International perspectives on women, health and culture: A world-wide anthology*. Wiltshire: Mark Allen Publishing Group.

Hyde, A. (1999b). Matrilocality and female power: Single mothers in extended households. *Womens' Studies International Forum*, 22(6), 597–605.

Hyde, A. (2000a). Age and partnership as public symbols: Stigma and non-marital motherhood in an Irish Context. *European Journal of Women's Studies*, 7, 71–89.

Hyde, A. (2000b). Single pregnant women's encounters in public: Changing norms or performing roles? *Irish Journal of Applied Social Studies*, 2(2), 84–105.

Hyde, A. (2003). Resistance to male dominance in the social organisation of reproduction: The case of unmarried women. *Irish Journal of Feminist Studies*, 5(1–2), 5–19.

Hyde, A., & Brady, D. (2002). Staff nurses' perceptions of supernumerary status compared with rostered service for Diploma in Nursing Students. *Journal of Advanced Nursing*, 38(6), 624–632.

Hyde, A., & Murray, M. (2005). Nurses' experiences of distance education programmes. *Journal of Advanced Nursing*, 49(1), 87–95.

Hyde, A., & Roche-Reid, B. (2004). Midwifery practice and the crisis of modernity: Implications for the role of the midwife. *Social Science and Medicine*, 58(12), 2613–2623.

Hyde, A., Treacy, M., Whitaker, T., Abaunza, P. S., & Knox, B. (2000). Young peoples' perceptions of and experiences with drugs. Findings from an Irish study. *Health Education Journal*, 59(2), 18–28.

Hyde, A., Treacy, M., Boland, J., Whitaker, T., Abaunza, P. S., & Knox, B. (2001). Alochol consumption among 11–16 year olds: "Getting around" structural barriers? *National and Health Sciences*, 3, 237–245.

Joyce, P. (1999). Implementing supernumerary learning in a pre-registration diploma in nursing programmed: An action research study. *Journal of Clinical Nursing*, 8, 567–576.

Joyce, P. (2005). Developing a nursing management degree programmed to meet the needs of Irish nurse managers. *Journal of Nursing Management*, 13(1), 74–82.

Joyce, P., & Mulligan, A. (1994). Inpatient preparations of patients for coronary artery bypass graft surgery prior to transfer to another hospital where surgery is performed. *Nursing Review*, 12(2), 27–29.

Kavanagh, L., & McBride, L. K. (2003). Making the link—an impact evaluation of one Dublin hospital's accident and emergency department's liaison nurse service. *Accident and Emergency Nursing*, 11(1), 39–48.

Kelly, M. (2002). The experience of qualified nurses in assessing student nurses' clinical skills. *The All Ireland Journal of Nursing and Midwifery*, 2(3), 47–53.

Landers, M. (1996). Student nurse's appraisal of their theatre experience. *Nursing Review*, 14(3/4), 13–15.

Landers, M. (2001). Students' views of the theory gap in nursing. *All Ireland Journal of Nursing and Midwifery*, 1(4), 142–147.

Larkin, P. J. (1998). Cultural awareness. The lived experience of Irish palliative care nurses. *International Journal of Palliative Nursing*, 4(3), 120–126.

Lawler, D., & Sinclair, M. (2003). Grieving for my former self: A phenomenological hermeneutical study of women's lived experience of postnatal depression. *Evidence Based Midwifery*, 1(2), 36–41.

Leahy Warren, P. (2005). First-time mothers: Social support and confidence in infant care. *Journal of Advanced Nursing, 50*(5), 479–488.

Logan, W. W., Tierney, A. J., & Roper, N. (2000). *Roper-Logan-Tierney Model of Nursing.* London: Churchill Livingstone.

Long, J., Allwright, S., & Begley, C. (2004). Prisoner's views of injecting drug use and harm reduction in Irish prisons. *International Journal of Drug Policy, 15*, 139–149.

Lynch, G. (1993). The education needs of women in Ireland in relation to the effects of alcohol on fetal development. *Nursing Review, 11*(3/4), 19–21.

Matthews, T., Kiberd, B., Maha, M., Cullen, A., McDonnell, M., & O'Regan, M. (2000). The current epidemiology of SIDS in Ireland. *Irish Medical Journal, 93*(9), 264–268.

Matthews, T., McDonnell, M., McGarvey, C., Loftus, G., & O'Regan, M. (2004). A multivariate "time based" analysis of SIDS risk factors. *Archives of Diseases in Childhood, 89*(3), 267–271.

MacLellan, K. (1997). A chart audit reviewing the prescription and administration trends of analgesia and the documentation of pain, after surgery. *Journal of Advanced Nursing, 26*, 345–350.

MacLellan, K. (2004). Postoperative pain: Strategy for improving patient experiences. *Journal of Advanced Nursing, 46*(2), 179–185.

McCabe, C. (2004). Nurse-patient communication: An exploration of patients' experiences. *Journal of Clinical Nursing, 13*, 41–49.

McCann, K., & Boore, J. R. P. (2000). Fatigue in persons with renal failure who require maintenance haemodialysis. *Journal of Advanced Nursing, 32*(5), 1132–1142.

McCarron, M., Gill, M., Lawlor, B., & Beagly, C. (2002). A pilot study of the reliability and validity of the Caregiver Activity Survey-Intellectual Disability (CAS-ID). *Journal of Intellectual Disability Research, 46*(8), 605–612.

McCarthy, A., & Evans, D. (2003). *A study on the impact of continuing education for nurses and midwives who completed post registration courses.* Cork: Nursing and Midwifery Planning and Development Unit.

McCarthy, G. (1992). Patient satisfaction with nursing care at Beaumont Hospital. *Nursing Review, 11*(1/2), 4–7.

McCarthy, G. (1999). A study of Irish women diagnosed with breast cancer. In M. Treacy, & A. Hyde (Eds), *Nursing Research Design and Practice.* Dublin: University College Dublin Press.

McCarthy, G., & Cronin, C. (2000). Typical students. *World of Irish Nursing, 8*(2), 11–13.

McCarthy, G., Savage, E., & Lehane, E. (2005). *Nursing and midwifery research priorities in the Southern Health Board area.* Cork: Nursing and Midwifery Planning and Development Unit.

McCarthy, G., Tyrrell, M., & Lehane, E. (2003). Turnover in nursing and midwifery: The Irish experience. *Nursing Times Research, 8*(4), 249–263.

McDonnell, M., Mathews, T., McGarvey, C. Mehanni, M., & O'Regan, M. (2002). Smoking: The major risk factors for SIDS in Irish infants. *Irish Medical Journal, 95*(4), 111–113.

McGarvey, C., McDonnell, M., Chong, A., O'Regan, M., & Matthews, T. (2003). Factors relating to the infants last sleep environment in sudden infant death syndrome in the Republic of Ireland. *Archives of Diseases in Childhood, 88*(12), 1058–1064.

McGrane, J., & Staines, A. (2003). Nursing staff knowledge of the hepatitis B virus including attitudes and acceptance of hepatitis B vaccination: Development of an effective program. *American Association of Occupational Health Nursing Journal, 51*(8), 347–352.

McKee, G. (2002). Why is biological science difficult for first–year nursing students? *Nurse Education Today, 22,* 251–257.

Meehan, T. C. (2003). Careful nursing: a model for contemporary nursing practice. *Journal of Advanced Nursing, 44*(1), 99–107.

Meehan, T. C., Butler, M., Drennan, J., Johnson, M., Kemple, M., & Treacy, P. (2006). *Nursing and midwifery research priorities for Ireland.* Dublin: National Council for the Professional Development of Nursing and Midwifery.

Mehanni, M., Kiberd, B., McDonnell, M., & O'Regan, M. (1999). Reduce the risk of cot death guidelines. The effect of a revised intervention programmed. *Irish Medical Journal, 92*(2), 266–269.

Minnock, P. (2002). Intra–articular injections in specialist rheumatology nursing practice. *The All Ireland Journal of Nursing and Midwifery, 2*(4), 32–35.

Minnock, P., Fitzgerald, O., & Bresnihan, B. (2003). Quality of life, social support and knowledge of disease in women with rheumatoid arthritis. *Arthritis and Rheumatism, 49*(2), 221–227.

Moore, Z., & Pitman, S. (2000). Towards establishing a pressure sore prevention and management policy in an acute hospital setting. *All Ireland Journal of Nursing and Midwifery, 1*(1), 7–11.

Moore, Z., & Price, P. (2004). Nurses' attitudes, behaviours and perceived barriers towards pressure ulcer prevention. *Journal of Clinical Nursing, 13,* 942–951.

Morgan, R. (2002). Giving students the confidence to take part. *Nursing Times, 98*(35), 36–37.

Morgan, R. (2004). Nursing students' perceptions of staff nurses attitudes towards them during their first practice placement. *Irish Nurse, 7*(12), 18–19.

Morgan, R., & Collins, R. (2002). What clinical skills do student nurses learn and from whom do they learn during their first clinical placement? *The All Ireland Journal of Nursing and Midwifery, 2*(7), 30–34.

Murphy, C. (2002). Liaison between hospital nurses and public health nurses on the discharge of elderly patients from hospital to home. *The All Ireland Journal of Nursing and Midwifery, 2*(1), 33–37.

Murphy, F. (2004). Stress among nephrology nurses. Northern Ireland. *Nephrology Nursing Journal, 31*(4), 423–431.

Murphy, K., Cooney, A., Casey., Connor, M., O'Connor, J., & Dineen, B. (2000). The Roper, Logan and Tierney (1996) Model: Perceptions and operationalization of the model in psychiatric nursing within a Health Board in Ireland. *Journal of Advanced Nursing, 31*(6), 1333–1341.

Murphy, N., Byrne, C., & Costello, R. W. (2002). An early supported discharge programmed for patients with exacerbations of chronic obstructive pulmonary disease (COPD) in Ireland. *The All Ireland Journal of Nursing and Midwifery, 2*(6), 30–34.

National Council for the Professional Development of Nursing and Midwifery. (2004). *An evaluation of the effectiveness of the role of the clinical nurse/midwife specialist.* Dublin: National Council for the Professional Development of Nursing and Midwifery.

National Council for the Professional Development of Nursing and Midwifery. (2004). *Report on the continuing professional development of staff nurses and staff midwives.* Dublin: National Council for the Professional Development of Nursing and Midwifery.

Nicholl, H., & Higgins, A. (2004). Reflection in preregistration nursing curricula. *Journal of Advanced Nursing, 46*(6), 578–585.

O'Callaghan, N., & Slevin, E. (2003). An investigation of the lived experiences of registered nurses facilitating supernumerary nursing students. *Nurse Education Today, 23,* 123–130.

O'Connell, R., & Cronin, M. (2002). Home birth in Ireland 1993–1997. A review of community midwifery practice. *The All Ireland Journal of Nursing and Midwifery, 2*(2), 41–46.

O'Connor, A., Hyde, A., & Treacy, M. (2003). Nurse teachers constructions of reflection and reflective practice. *Reflective Practice, 4*(2), 107–119.

O'Connor, L. (1995a). Pain assessment by patients and nurses, and nurses' notes on it in early acute myocardial infarction (Part 1). *Intensive and Critical Care Nursing, 11,* 183–191.

O'Connor, L. (1995b). Pain assessment by patients and nurses, and nurses' notes on it, in early acute myocardial infarction (Part 2). *Intensive and Critical Care Nursing, 11,* 283–292.

O'Flynn, M., Caffrey, S., & Higgins, A. (2003). Therapist's experiences of the obligation to report when working with adult survivors of child sexual abuse. *The Irish Journal of Psychology, 24*(1), 58–69.

O'Halloran, S. (1996). The decision making experiences of adults living in a community based residence. *Nursing Review, 14*(3/4), 25–27.

O'Mahony, M. (2001). Women's lived experiences of breast biopsy: A phenomenological study. *Journal of Clinical Nursing, 10,* 512–520.

O'Meara-Kearney, A. (1999). The role of the professional general nurse. In M. Treacy, & A. Hyde (REds.), *Nursing Research Design and Practice.* Dublin; University College Dublin Press.

O'Neill, V. (1997). 24 hour ambulatory blood pressure monitoring. Is it patient friendly? Does the client understand the significance of lifestyle advise. *Nursing Review, 15*(3/4), 93–95.

Patton, D. (2003). How reality orientation may impact upon violence and aggression within acute psychiatric care. *International Journal of Psychiatric Nursing Research, 8*(3), 972–984.

Quinn, S., Redmond, K., & Begley, C. M. (1996). The needs of relatives visiting critical care units. *Nursing Review, 15*(1), 9–14.

Richmond, J. (2004). General nurse perceptions of the role of the clinical nurse specialist in Ireland. *Cancer Nursing Practice, 3*(6), 33–39.

Rose, M. (1997). A survey of violence toward nursing staff in one large Irish accident and emergency department. *Journal of Emergency Nursing, 23*(3), 214–219.

Rush, D., McCarthy, G., & Cronin, C. (2000). *Report on Nursing Management Competencies.* Dublin: Office for Health Management.

Ryan, C. A., Clark, L. M., Malone, A., & Ahmed, S. (1999). The effect of a structured neonatal resuscitation program on delivery room practices. *Neonatal Network: The Journal of Neonatal Nursing, 18*(1), 25–30.

Ryan, D., & Quayle, E. (1999). Stress in psychiatric nursing fact or fiction. *Nursing Standard, 14*(8), 32–35.

Ryder, M., Travers, B., Timmons, L., Ledwidge, M., & McDonald, K. (2003). Specialist nurse supervised in–hospital titration to target dose ACE inhibitor—is it safe and feasible in a community heart failure population? *European Journal of Cardiovascular Nursing, 2*(3), 183–188.

Savage, E., & Callery, P. (2005). Weight and energy: Parent's and children's perspectives on managing cystic fibrosis diet. *Archives of Diseases in Childhood, 90,* 249–252.

Savage, E. B. (1998). The ward learning environment for student nurses: A study to determine the influence of staff nurses. Part 1. *Nursing Review, 16*(3/4), 82–86.

Savage, E. B. (1999). The ward learning environment for student nurses: A study to determine the influence of staff nurses: Part 2. *Nursing Review, 17*(3), 57–63.

Scott, A., Matthews, A., & Corbally, M. (2003). *Nurses' and midwives' understanding and experiences of empowerment in Ireland.* Dublin: Department of Health and Children.

Sheehan, K. M., McDonnell, M., Doyle, E. M., Matthews, T., & Devaney, D. (2003). The quality and value of sudden infant death necropsy reporting in Ireland. *Journal of Clinical Pathology, 56,* 753–757.

Sheerin, F. (2004). Identifying the foci of interest to nurses in Irish intellectual disability services. *Journal of Learning Disabilities, 8*(2), 159–174.

Steinaker N. W., & Bell, M. R. (1979). *The experiential taxonomy: A new approach to teaching and learning.* New York: Academic Press.

Surlis, S., & Hyde, A. (2001). HIV-Positive Patients' Experiences of Stigma During Hospitalization. *Journal Of The Association of Nurses in AIDS Care, 12*(6), 68–77.

Syron, M., & Shelley, E. (2001). The needs of informal carers: A proposed assessment tool for use by public health nurses. *Journal of Nursing Management, 9*(1), 31–38.

Timmins, F., & Kaliszer, M. (2002a). Absenteeism among nursing students–fact or fiction. *Journal of Nursing Management, 10,* 251–264.

Timmins, F., & Kaliszer, M. (2002b). Attitudes to absenteeism among diploma nursing students in Ireland–an exploratory descriptive study. *Nurse Education Today, 22,* 578–588.

Timmins, F., & Kaliszer, M. (2002c). Aspects of nurse education programmes that frequently cause stress to nursing students–fact-finding sample survey. *Nurse Education Today, 22,* 203–211.

Timmins, F., & Kaliszer, M. (2002d). Is stress and job satisfaction associated with absenteeism in the student nurse population? *The All Ireland Journal of Nursing and Midwifery, 2*(5),78–86.

Timmins, F., & Kaliszer, M. (2003). Information needs of myocardial infarction patients. *European Journal of Cardiovascular Nursing, 2,* 57–65.

Timmins, F., & McCabe, C. (2005). Nurses' and midwives' assertive behaviour in the workplace. *Journal of Advanced Nursing, 51*(1), 38–45.

Touhy, D. (2002). Student nurse–older person communication. *Nurse Education Today, 23,* 19–26.

Treacy, M., & Collins, R. (1999). Hospital nurses' perceptions of health promotion. In M. Treacy, & A. Hyde (Eds.), *Nursing Research Design and Practice.* Dublin: University College Dublin Press.

Tully, A. (2004). Stress, sources of stress and ways of coping among psychiatric nursing students. *Journal of Psychiatric and Mental Health Nursing, 11*, 43–47.

Tyrrell, M. P. (1997). Assessment of acute pain: A study of student nurses' knowledge and attitudes. *Nursing Review, 16*(1), 10–13.

Wells, J. S. G., & McElwee, C. N. (2000). "I don't want to be a psychiatric nurse": An exploration of factors inhibiting recruitment to psychiatric nursing in Ireland. *Journal of Psychiatric and Mental Health Nursing, 7*, 79–87.

Wilkin, K., & Slevin, E. (2004). The meaning of caring to nurses: An investigation into the nature of caring work in an intensive care unit. *Journal of Clinical Nursing, 13*, 50–59.

Wright, S., Courtney, U., & Crowther, D. (2002) A quantitative and qualitative pilot study of the perceived benefits of autogenic training for a group of people with cancer. *European Journal of Cancer Care, 11*, 122–130.

Wright, S., Courtney, U., Donnelly, C., Kenny, T., & Lavin, C. (2002). Clients' perceptions of the benefits of reflexology on their quality of life. *Complementary Therapies in Nursing and Midwifery, 8*, 769–776.

Index

Contents of Previous
10 Volumes

VOLUME 20: Research on Geriatrics

Joyce Fitzpatrick, Series Editor; Patricia Archbold and Barbara Stewart, Volume Editors